LONG LIFE STRATEGY

Ronald M. Caplan, MD

www.rmcpublishingllc.com

Long Life Strategy

Paperback ISBN: 978-1-7350093-0-8
EPUB ISBN: 978-1-7350093-3-9

Interior design by booknook.biz

CONTENTS

PREFACE

THE CENTRAL MESSAGE OF THE BOOK

It is rapidly becoming possible, at the level of the human cell, to prolong life, or possibly even to reverse aging.

The message is a leap beyond the usual strategies for living healthfully, although nutrition, exercise, and disease prevention are covered in detail as well.

Immortality of the living human cell is within our grasp. Genes in the cell control cell aging. There are genes that cause cell death: they are known as self-destruct genes. These genes can be turned off.

Beyond that, various inherited genes predispose each of us to certain life threatening diseases. Genetic manipulation is being developed to negate the effects of these predisposing genes. Some diseases are already being treated this way.

Genes exist in the chromosomes each of us inherits. The end of each chromosome is called a telomere, which is made up of DNA. The telomere prevents mutations (abnormal recombinations of the chromosomes) from happening.

The telomere is maintained and repaired by an enzyme called telomerase. If telomerase is activated, a cell may be induced to become immortal.

If telomerase is inhibited, cells die. This has great implications in cancer treatment: cancer cells multiply in a bizarre fashion indefinitely. Cancer cells eventually take over the host body and kill it. Specifically making the cancer cell die, without damaging the person, is the goal of all cancer treatment.

Every organ and tissue in the human body is made up of specialized cells. Specialized cells arise from the stem cells found in the early developing baby (the embryo) in the uterus. It is now possible to grow new specialized organ and muscle cells from stem cells.

Stem cells are present in the amniotic fluid, which is the liquid surrounding and bathing the developing baby in the uterus. These stem cells from the amniotic fluid can be removed without harm to the baby, and have been shown to be capable of developing into specialized cells.

When a baby is born, a blood sample can be saved and stored indefinitely from the umbilical cord that attached the fetus to the afterbirth, or placenta. If this child unfortunately happens to get leukemia in later life, she or he can get a curative stem cell transplant of their very own cells: a perfect cell match. The stem cells will evolve into new, healthy, blood cells, and the affected person is cured.

The entire field of organ transplantation: the replacement of hopelessly diseased organs by healthy ones will be revolutionized by the availability of new organs that will not be rejected by the body of the person needing the transplant.

Recent studies seem to show that actual reversal of aging can be brought about by regeneration of the thymus gland and immunorestoration.

Survival Strategy

It is finally possible to prolong healthful, useful, enjoyable life beyond the biblical threescore and ten: seventy years. In order to achieve this, each of us needs a survival strategy.

Some components of this strategy can be achieved by the individual, while others involve understanding and being active in issues that impact the whole nation and society.

Each of us can logically expect to survive healthfully to an advanced age only within a stable, advanced, educated society in which random and directed violence is guarded against and largely eliminated. General measures of public health, including the presence of a safe and assured water and food supply, and protection from disease agents by vaccination and other means, must be in place. The environment should be free of debilitating levels of noxious agents.

We should not use substances that can irreversibly harm us. The classic example is cigarette smoking: this one habit, once more prevalent in men, marketed to women as somehow 'equalizing' them ("You've come a long way, baby") has taken lung cancer, which currently in the vast majority of cases is caused by the carcinogens in cigarette smoke – from being a minor factor in women's lives, to being the single greatest cause of cancer deaths in women in our society today.

It is necessary to intelligently differentiate between generally accepted maxims (eat three meals a day and 'snacks') easy fixes (many diets and 'diet' drugs), and what really, by good evidence, works to maintain a healthful existence. To achieve this, it is necessary to re-explore and challenge old concepts: who says three meals a day are necessary, or even healthful for many people? Exercise is good, but long term high impact exercise can be harmful, as a lot of aging athletes can attest.

The concept of preventative medicine has often turned out to be pie in the sky, and a convenient way for politicians and insurers trying to scrimp on health care, to divert public attention from the real issues of identifying and properly treating disease. With some great exceptions, such as prenatal care, to protect women from developing complications of pregnancy, the newly attained ability to immunize young people against some subtypes of the human papilloma virus (HPV) that causes cancer of the cervix and penis, and immunization programs against various diseases, there is really no such thing as what is usually thought of as 'preventative' medicine.

Healthful living can delay the onset of some of the most important disease conditions that are prevalent as people get older, including arteriosclerotic heart and cardiovascular disease, and diabetes.

When people think and talk of 'preventative' medicine, what they are really talking about is the very early diagnosis of disease states. It is then possible to eradicate the disease, or bring it under control, while this is still possible and even easy. In other words, what is being 'prevented' is often the complications and gravity of the disease, and consequent extensive treatment, and not the disease itself.

This is even true in the hallmark and most successful of all 'preventative' medicine programs: the development and almost universal deployment in our society of quality prenatal care for the expectant mother. Incipient disease states in both the mother and her developing child can be diagnosed at earlier and earlier times, allowing for proper treatment to be instituted, before permanent damage is caused. Some conditions of pregnancy can actually be prevented from occurring, by proper care (some of the hypertensive disorders of pregnancy).

There is great resistance to the very early diagnosis of disease in our advanced society, because of the costs involved, and because of the potential for harmful intervention in situations where a disease process is not even yet evident by symptoms and signs. These concerns have to be addressed on a disease by disease basis, but as a general principle, intervening in a disease process early is usually beneficial, and costs per person come down as diagnostic techniques are universally applied: the old mass production approach. The classic example is the Papanicolaou smear. There was great resistance to the adoption of this technique when it was first used for the early diagnosis of cancer of the cervix more than half a century ago. It is now considered perfectly acceptable to absorb the cost of regularly testing every sexually active adult woman by the 'Pap' smear: but DNA probe screening (from the same cervical mucus) for the actual sexually transmitted causative virus of cervical cancer (HPV), which is a far more specific and advanced test, is meeting the same objections today that the 'Pap' smear met half a century ago: it costs too much, not necessary for many women, and leads to overtreatment.

A survival strategy implies that, once a disease condition is found, and found early, that we are knowledgeable about treatment options.

Generally speaking the treatment selected should be evidence based. Ideally, medicine today utilizes treatments that are proven to be beneficial. For most diseases evidence based medicine works: it is logical to use the treatment that has been shown to work.

However, by definition, medicine would never advance if no treatment could be utilized unless it already had been proven to work.

There is an explosion of information, new scientific data, and new instrumentation in both diagnosis and treatment, including robotics and beyond, in medicine today. Controlled studies on selected patients are used to find out which methods and modalities work.

It is often a different matter to find out which modalities are clearly superior: often an evolving technology will not show its superiority in an early stage of development.

A classic example is laparoscopy, or minimally invasive surgery, which has become one of the hallmarks of modern surgery. When it was first introduced it was derided as 'peeking through a keyhole', and competent surgeons contended that they could make adequate diagnoses by simple examination, without resorting to surgery, and that optimal treatment involved bigger incisions for an adequate look and access to body organs. As the instrumentation became increasingly superior, and as surgeons became increasingly adept, laparoscopy became the preferred way to approach many conditions, to the point where the old issues were no longer even debated. In fact, laparoscopy has spread way beyond gynecology, and is a preferred method for many procedures in other surgical fields.

Your Personal Survival Strategy

If a person wants a successful survival strategy, she or he would, where possible, avoid and protect against communicable diseases, whether spread through the food chain, water supply, droplet infection (respiratory diseases), or sexual transmission (for example Human Immunodeficiency Virus: HIV; Human Papilloma Virus: HPV).

The individual would know their genetic background and susceptibility to various inherited states (for example, the presence or absence of BRCA genes for breast and ovarian cancer). The person would be vigilant and be checked for the early onset of such diseases. The person would tend to be not too thin, not obese, and have an adequate intake of known nutrients, including protein and calcium.

Regular exercise with avoidance of excessive high impact workouts would be maintained. Substance abuse, the use of illicit drugs, smoking, and excessive alcohol intake would all be avoided. Each individual would drive carefully and within the speed limit, wearing a seat belt. A pregnant woman would seek competent prenatal care early and regularly and would deliver where evidence shows she would be most safe, and where her baby would have the best chance not only for survival, but for survival in optimal mental and physical condition.

When a disease state inevitably enters one's life (hopefully in much later life), the individual would quickly seek expert help, become knowledgeable about possible alternative treatment regimens, and in most cases go with evidence-based treatment, but not close one's eyes to scientifically valid emerging techniques that might be applicable.

Each person would remember to always keep an inquiring mind and an active body. If an individual does all these things, and their parents were long lived, one just might be the first person to reach, with intact faculties, that theoretical age: one hundred and thirty five, which is not quite double the classical threescore and ten.

The Eventful Journey to Healthful Advanced Age: Hurdles to get by

There are significant life events - hurdles - that must be overcome on the way to an advanced healthy age.

Genetic Makeup

It is possible to know your genetic susceptibility to various important disease states, and to be vigilant throughout life for early signs of appearance of these diseases.

It is even becoming possible to actually alter the genetic makeup, so that disease states can be avoided all together.

Being Born

The passage through the birth canal was, in times past, likened to a 'perilous journey'. Even in our enlightened obstetric age, the intrauterine environment of the developing fetus, and the labor and delivery process, are significant factors leading to the birth of a baby in optimal physical and mental condition.

Childhood Diseases

Many of the scourges of times past, such as poliomyelitis and other communicable diseases, have now been eliminated by the widespread use of appropriate vaccinations, and careful attention to public health. However, there are still significant communicable diseases present in the world, such as tuberculosis. New communicable diseases actually arise: for example SARS (Severe Acute Respiratory Syndrome) and the COVID19 pandemic (Corona Viral Disease 2019).

Accidents

Teenagers and young (and even older) adults often put themselves in harm's way, without adequate protection. Depression and suicide are often neglected pitfalls for young people: the signs should be looked for, and treatment instituted.

Sexually Transmitted Diseases

The most significant of the sexually transmitted diseases today, from the viewpoint of difficulty in treatment and the shortening of lifespan, is AIDS – Acquired Immunodeficiency Syndrome – which opens the individual to a panoply of life threatening infections.

Pregnancy

Although in our modern society, maternal and fetal mortality have been vastly reduced, and most mothers-to-be are at low risk for obstetric complications, debilitating disease, injury, and even death in childbirth still occur. Women who delay childbearing are in a higher risk category for complications of pregnancy, both to themselves and their growing fetuses.

Diseases of Aging

As one gets older, there is an increasing tendency to developing arteriosclerotic heart and vascular disease, hypertension, stroke, diabetes, arthritis and other illnesses that tend to be chronic, and that can be life threatening. Cancer becomes more prevalent. A healthful life style and attention to genetic makeup, along with early diagnosis and treatment are all important in the management of such conditions.

It is now possible to turn previously fatal diseases into manageable, chronic states.

Age Seventy

Statistically, if a person arrives at age 70 mentally and physically fit, relatively unscathed by the passage of time and life events, she or he has a substantial further life expectancy. That seventy year old should have multiple opportunities and goals, and can expect to remain active and fit.

Age One Hundred

There are substantial numbers of people, women more than men, in our society now reaching that age. It is no longer considered to be an almost unattainable milestone. Theoretically, a person might be able to live to approximately the age of one hundred and thirty five, although that age has not yet been attained.

(Next: See Immortality: The Sequel)

References

1. https://www.ncbi.nlm.nih.gov/pubmed/31496122
2. cdc.gov/coronavirus/2019-ncov/downloads/community-mitigation-strategy.pdf
3. Bibliography & Supplemental Bibliography: See www.rcaplanmd.com

CHAPTER 1
LIVING LONGER

The Take-Home Message

To live long and healthfully

As a community we must provide:

- Universal education
- Public health, and attention to mental health issues
- Security for the individual and the society

As individuals we must:

- Avoid high risk behaviors, including illegal drug, tobacco and alcohol use
- Limit diet to a healthful level, preventing obesity
- Exercise moderately
- Get adequate sleep
- Educate ourselves to understand what is available to us medically, and ensure that we get what we need early enough in the disease process
- Understand what 'prevention' really means

The science of medicine must:

- Continue its rapid advance to understand disease at the genetic and molecular level
- Ensure the quality of medical care
- Ensure that treatments offered are based on solid evidence
- Learn to detect those individuals who are prone to various physical and mental disease states, and to intercept disease at an earlier time
- Continue to develop specific treatments that are tailored to arresting each disease process, with a minimum of side effects
- Inform people of the various valid options available for the treatment of their particular condition

We are living in an age of rapidly advancing technology. We are undergoing a revolution in communication and information availability. The human genome is known, disease is understood at a metabolic level, and drugs are created to target the mechanisms of disease.

Imaging can be done to just about the cellular level, and computerization makes diagnoses much more exact. Fiberoptics, laser technology, precise miniaturized instrumentation, and robotics create treatment potential that could only have been dreamed of a generation ago.

All these factors complement one another so that in our industrialized, computerized and linked world people not only have the ability to live much longer than the biblical three score and ten years but start to live healthfully into ages previously thought of possible only for the biblical patriarchs and matriarchs.

It takes educated people to achieve this potential, so attention must be given to the quality of our schools. Attention has to be given to public health. Economic strength in our society is needed if we are to continue to raise the healthy life expectancy of every person.

We must address deficiencies in the educational system, which correlate with poor lifestyle and health habits, pockets of poverty, social breakdown, violent crime, and terrorism.

Overeating, and eating the wrong foods, along with inadequate physical activity, leading to obesity is a major problem in our society. By the year 2000, this had become the second leading actual cause of death in the United States and was threatening to overtake tobacco use as the number one actual cause of death. Alcohol came in third.

Other important countervailing forces are at work. Attention must be given to mental health issues, including depression and suicide. Mental health issues are one factor leading to homelessness, and a factor in many cases of gun violence,

Political rationing of healthcare, especially high technology diagnostic and treatment methods and new drug therapies interferes with the ability to get the finest treatment to those who need it. These are false economies, as the application of these new technologies results in their lower cost per treatment, and ultimately results in a healthier population.

Away from computerized, industrial societies, there are many more problems that impact on the ability to survive healthfully to great age. In the underdeveloped world, these include malnutrition, infectious diseases, air and water pollution, and illiteracy.

Pollution of the environment is present in the industrialized world as well. Products of manufacturing processes get into the water supply, and into the air. "Greenhouse gases" are formed, that include carbon dioxide, sulfur dioxide, and carbon monoxide. Our own mobility, by automobile, and the mobility of goods and services, by truck, plane, ship, and rail, are largely responsible for such emissions. The escape of hydrofluocarbons into our atmosphere is a problem. Nuclear waste products from weaponry and power plants remain dangerous for thousand of years. These are great issues which we have yet to master.

In the United States, a male born in 2019 can expect to live to the age of seventy-six (eighty in Canada) and a female can expect to live to eighty-one (eighty-four in Canada). A woman, on average, can expect to live four or five years longer than a man. While the U.S. numbers are not as good as they are in some smaller population countries with better literacy, less poverty and fewer public health issues, they were still advancing up until approximately 2016, when they started to decline. Some prominent causes of this alarming trend are rampant obesity, drug abuse and suicide.

Some believe that societies in which people live longer have better medical care. There is no better medical care on earth today than exists in the United States of America. The United States, however, is a large, heterogeneous society in which the application of public health measures is not yet uniform. Educational deficiencies in many places and pockets of illiteracy work against our ability to stamp out various infectious diseases. Poverty and malnutrition are still with us. These conditions are on the decline, but still exist. Drug abuse, alcohol abuse, smoking, and crime, especially gun crime, still take their toll. Far too many Americans still get maimed and killed on the highways and byways of this land.

If we are to reach the goals envisioned in this book for our entire population, all of these complex issues will continue to have to be addressed.

UNITED STATES: FEMALE POPULATION 2010

Number of women 65-69 years of age	6,582,716
Number of women 70-74 years of age	5,034,194
Number of women 75-79 years of age	4,135,407
Number of women 80-84 years of age	3,448,953
Number of women 85-89 years of age	2,346,592
Number of women 90-94 years of age	1,023,979
Number of women 95-99 years of age	288,981
Number of women 100 years and over	44,202

*US Census Bureau, 2010

UNITED STATES: MALE POPULATION 2010

Number of men 65-69 years of age	5,852,547
Number of men 70-74 years of age	4,243,972
Number of men 75-79 years of	3,182,388
Number of men 80-84 years of age	2,294,374
Number of men 85-89 years of age	1,273,867
Number of men 90-94 years of age	424,387
Number of men 95-99 years of age	82,263
Number of men 100 years and over	9,162

*US Census Bureau, 2010

It is important when using numbers or statistics to understand how and when those numbers were derived, how accurate they are, and what they mean. For instance, by the 2000 United States census, men are stated to have a life span of 74.24 years, and women are stated to have a life expectancy of 79.9 years. Those numbers were projected to change in the 2025 census, so that men would have a life expectancy of 78.4 years, and women would have a life expectancy 83.7 years. One of the keys to these numbers is that the life expectancy is calculated from birth. When a baby is born, if it is a male, it can be expected on average to live 76 years, and if it is a female it can be expected on average to live 81 years. Various societies, and even states within the United States, define a live birth differently.

In our society, a fetus that is born even significantly preterm, or premature, is defined as alive from the time of birth and figures into the overall life expectancy figures. Other societies do not enter a fetus into their statistics as living unless it has attained twenty-eight weeks of intrauterine life prior to birth, or has lived for at least seventy-two hours, or even up to one year, after birth. Obviously, such definitions not only impact upon how intensively a society tries to save its preterm infants, but also impacts upon the life expectancy figures. Infants that are born markedly preterm have a greater chance of not surviving the immediate hours, days, and weeks of early life. The inclusion of significantly preterm babies in our statistics alters the life expectancy figures. A country that excludes such infants in its calculations will come up with significantly higher life expectancy figures, both for men and for women.

Everybody has a life expectancy. All of us are survivors. A woman who has survived as a fetus in the womb, entry into the world via the labor and delivery process, the vulnerabilities of infancy and childhood including childhood diseases, the temptations and risk taking along with the questionable judgments of adolescence, the bearing of children during her own reproductive years, the societal pressures of conflict and even war, nutritional problems including malnutrition, epidemics, endemic disease states in the population such as tuberculosis, the so called degenerative diseases, and arrives at the age of eighty in relatively good health with no life threatening conditions present, has a significant life expectancy. She can expect to live not only the biblically prescribed three score and ten years, but significantly beyond her attained age of eighty. There are well over a million women living today in the United States over ninety years of age, and the numbers of people living beyond one hundred years of age is significantly growing and expected to grow even more.

Women live significantly longer than men in our society. Some of the reasons for this phenomenon are well known, and others are not. The greatest single barrier to the longevity of women historically has been childbearing. The advent of modern prenatal care during pregnancy, coupled with great advances in obstetrical care during the labor and delivery process, and good postpartum care, have almost entirely taken away the real fear of maternal death during childbirth in modern industrialized society. Morbidity, or sickness, related to pregnancy, or exacerbated during a pregnancy, still has a role in the longevity of women. Women still lose their lives during pregnancy and childbirth. In our society today, such deaths tend to be limited to women who are at high risk because of various severe medical conditions. Even a vast majority of those cases today can be handled in tertiary care medical centers and brought through labor and delivery unscathed.

Some of the disparity in the life expectancy between men and women can be explained by higher risk behavior for men, especially young men, in our society. Men still are disproportionately on the front lines of the armed forces, where they are potentially in harm's way. There is the violence that has been prevalent, notably among young men, especially in our urban areas. Hopefully, there are signs that this violence has been abating. There are vehicular accidents, which are a major factor in the loss of life among young people. Suicide and drug overdose are significant risk factors for our youth.

Men in our society have disproportionately tended to take on jobs and occupations that are physically hazardous, including such things as mining, construction, and working with hazardous materials. The stress of the workplace has often been cited as a factor in reducing life expectancy. It will be interesting and instructive to see if the dramatic entry of women into all occupations including the armed forces changes the long term survival figures. Of course, it cannot be forgotten that war now affects civilian populations, so that the armed forces are not the only ones at risk in armed conflict.

Whether women have a genetic superiority to men in longevity is unknown. It is true that men generally have increased muscle mass and increased bone mass, which may affect cardiac load. Men are more prone to life threatening disease states such as heart attacks at an earlier age than women are, although cardiovascular disease and heart attack are a prominent threat to women as well. Neither sex should neglect regular evaluations of the heart and cardiovascular system. Some degree of the risk of heart disease has been attributed to life style and eating habits. A diet that is high in saturated fat can be a factor. Obesity is certainly a factor in limiting life expectancy.

Smoking is definitely an important contributing factor to the incidence and severity of cardiovascular disease in our society. In the United States in the year 2000, tobacco was the leading actual cause of death. Traditionally, men in our society smoked much more than women. This trend has been reversed, as smoking has become commonplace among women in our society. Women are paying the price with a marked increase in disease states such as lung cancer.

There is some question as to whether women have a hormonal advantage. At one point, in some studies, men were even given small doses of female sex hormone, estrogen, in order to determine whether this would protect them against heart disease. In fact, these men were not protected from heart disease. Hormonal regulation and balance within the body is complex. For example, various types of androgens, which are male sex hormone, are also present in females, but generally in much lower amounts. There is to date no evidence that the hormonal differences between men and women lead to differences in life expectancy.

However, it is probable that hormonal signals from the brain, both in men and women, do cause youthfulness to persist.

Middle Age

The term middle age, as it is commonly used, is a euphemism. We speak about certain things and think about certain things in ways that make us more comfortable. Strictly speaking, if the average life expectancy of a woman in the United States is eighty years of age, then middle age would be forty. No one in the United States at age forty nowadays considers themselves middle aged. More often, you will hear fifty and sixty- year olds speaking about themselves and thinking about themselves as middle aged. Happily, the reality is beginning to catch up with the wish. We are living longer and staying healthy and fit longer. However, there are countertrends in our society that work against this, notably the tendency to overeat and obesity.

The American Association of Retired Persons (AARP) accepts membership from anyone aged fifty and over. Social Security normally kicks in at age sixty-two or over, depending on whether the person is still employed. Medicare defines an eligible senior as anybody sixty-five years of age and over.

Euphemistically, we refer to that part of life after attaining the age of say, sixty-five years, as the "Golden Years". If you look at the statistics, these years can be anything but golden. Many people tend to be on fixed incomes that were adequate when they started out but lose their buying power as inflation takes its toll. Various chronic disease states are prevalent in older people. These can impact on quality of life, and increase the expense required for medical care and medications. There can be expensive lifestyle changes, including the need for personnel and laborsaving devices required for personal care. Families, once close-knit in our society, tend to become far flung, with limited access to the ones we love: children and grandchildren. We may lose friends, or even a beloved spouse.

Lifestyles

We may look back longingly at the idealized extended family where several generations of family members lived happily together under one roof. Unfortunately, today in our society we are often lucky if the nuclear family - parents and children - stick together. This alteration in family living, patterns and lifestyle occurred for various complex reasons. With relative wealth and mobility, Americans, who treasure their independence, ventured out on their own to new and exciting places, as they attained adulthood. They started their own families, often far from their roots.

Inheritance issues concerning the ownership of farms and businesses left many children with the need to look for their own opportunities far from their parents.

The great migration westward to the Pacific Coast has now slowed, but adventurous souls are still making their way to new places, including the States near the Rocky Mountains, and to the western Canadian provinces. The southern United States has been a focal point of migration for years. It is possible in years to come that the push will be northward.

A large part of the migration to the southern United States has been by older people whose children have grown to adulthood and left home. Yearning for sunnier climes, these seniors have changed the demographics and population density of the State of Florida and other areas. Happily, there has been a migration of younger people and families to such states as well, offsetting the imbalance.

The downside to all of this is that many of us have lost immediate access to one of the primary pillars of support for each other - our close family members. There are, however, increasing signs that a lot of us are beginning to rethink this process.

With fewer great lands left to open up and explore, the realization that the grass is not always greener elsewhere, and with the increasing ability in this computer and information age to work where you are, some young adults are opting to stay where they are, and more older adults are rethinking the wisdom of moving far from children, grandchildren, friends, and the doctors and hospitals who treat them in times of illness.

In fact, many older people are opting to stay in the homes where they raised their families. This can become an expensive option, especially if the need arises to bring in additional people to care for not only the people, but for the property as well. Some of these expenses are reimbursable by insurance if they are medically necessary, and various agencies, such as visiting nurse services, do exist to help with medical problems at home.

If the home is large enough, and zoning laws permit, it is not uncommon to find parents and married children with there own offspring all under one roof. Some families find that these traditional relationships and living patterns can work well.

In the main, both parents work in today's society. The ability to have babysitting by the most trustworthy people to be found – grand-parents - is a real advantage. The grandparents are usually happy to be of help and to be with their grandchildren. The grandchildren know they are loved and secure, and have wisdom and kindness imparted to them on a daily basis. If grandparents live independently nearby, within easy commuting distance, the advantages of proximity remain, including mutual security.

Warehousing people, and lumping all older people together in one category, are outmoded concepts. There are huge numbers of older people today who are healthy, happy, and productively working at either formal jobs, or involved in a myriad of tasks and activities ranging from childcare to consulting, from travel to sports.

The ideal is to live independently of strangers, and happily most older people can do this, especially if they have family support in their later years, as well as appropriate medical care and household help as needed. Of course, this can be expensive, and at some point, assisted living does become necessary for some, for medical, social, and economic reasons.

CHAPTER 2
AGING: IT CAN BE DELAYED… AND REVERSED?

The Take-Home Message

- Immortality does exist for body cells.
    - Stem cells evolve into the specialized cells that make up all the cells of the human body
- Genetic makeup is important in determining how long we live.
    - Genetic manipulation to change the odds is possible
- We are each genetically unique
- Environment, including the life of the fetus in the womb, is important in determining longevity and health
    - Environment can be changed to our benefit
- We can scan the body to a precise level, identifying possible disease very early
- Targeted drugs now do exist that go directly to receptors on affected cells, blocking disease at a microscopic level, anywhere in the body that the disease is present
- It is possible to grow new, healthy tissue

People have been searching for immortality since history was first recorded, and probably before that. Legends, myths, and stories in various cultures refer to the immortality of the gods, and the loss of immortality. The Bible speaks of the patriarchs as living to ages measured in hundreds of years. Early explorers came to America, looking for the Fountain of Youth.

It is only very recently that scientists have come to realize that the concept of the immortal living cell is not only possible, but true.

The very first reaction I got from a professional reading a draft of this book was "He's got to be kidding". I am not kidding. Immortality is not just a hope or a religious belief or a futile dream. For the cells which make up every part of our bodies, immortality is an achievable state. There is a cautionary note: watch what you wish for.

Cell death, which is a normal occurrence, is caused by genes. These genes are known as "self-destruct" genes. It is possible to turn off these genes, so that the cell does not die.

Each of us inherits chromosomes from our parents. Genes exist in the chromosomes. The end of each chromosome is called a telomere. The telomere prevents abnormal changes, called mutations, from happening.

The telomere is maintained and repaired by telomerase. By activating telomerase, it is possible to make the human cell immortal. On the other hand, if telomerase is inhibited, the cell dies. That is the double-edged sword. The hallmark of cancer is bizarre, out of control cells that live too long. In order for the human body to function properly, it is important that abnormal and malfunctioning cells be removed. Keeping cells alive that normally would die could have major consequences.

On the other hand, making specific cells die could be very helpful. Cancerous cells multiply and keep on multiplying. The cancerous cells eventually take over the body and kill it. The ability to specifically make cancer cells die without damaging the body should be the goal of all cancer treatment.

The ability to alter the lifespan of the cell could radically change life and health.

What we will be able to expect from our doctors will be changed. In fact, these changes are already taking place and represent a revolution in medicine.

When I first became a medical doctor, there were no imaging techniques beyond x-ray. There was very little in the way of prenatal diagnosis, beyond our ability to diagnose by palpating, or feeling, the fetus within the mother. Our diagnostic senses and skills were highly tuned, but we were limited. Minimally invasive surgery was not yet developed. The very first cancer marker was just being developed for use with patients, by Dr. Phil Gold and his colleagues. The cause of cervical cancer was still unknown. Mapping the human genome was in the realm of science fiction.

What a physician does when she or he sees a patient for a checkup is an evaluation of whether or not the patient has a disease or diseases, and the extent to which those diseases have progressed. As well, the physician evaluates what the future may hold for the patient in developing new disease states. The physician recognizes what is normal, and what is abnormal. The physician is then in a position to inform the patient that she or he is healthy, or conversely what disease is present, what the prognosis is, and the options available for getting the best possible results with treatment.

When a disease state is diagnosed, the physician basically has three options. One is to simply watch the condition to ensure that it does not progress, and to counsel the patient on steps that could be taken, such as a modified proper diet and other lifestyle modifications, that would help the condition.

Advanced imaging techniques and minimally invasive surgery allow the physician to watch conditions that not too long ago would not have been diagnosed in time for relatively simple treatment, or that would have required full scale major surgery for diagnosis.

The second option is the treatment of the condition with drugs or medications. The third option is corrective surgery.

For approximately 50 years, antibiotics that kill germs or bacteria have increasingly become available. Bacterial infection, although still a danger, does not pose the life threatening risk to the same extent that it did in ages past.

Antiviral drugs are available to treat dangerous viral infections, although there are still many viral diseases that cannot be effectively treated or treated at the level which we would wish.

Vaccines, of course, have long been available for certain classic viral illnesses. A vaccine triggers the human body's own immunity to a specific virus: when that virus does enter the body it is killed before it can do harm.

Classically, surgery was used to remove abnormal growths or tumors, or to cut out diseased organs.

In trauma cases, surgery was used to close off bleeding blood vessels and to remove damaged organs and limbs.

Although these categories of surgery are still needed, modern surgery focuses on the repair of organs and reconnection of even tiny blood vessels, with the use of microscopes, video cameras, and precision often tiny, tools. Many surgeons have mastered minimally invasive techniques and robotic surgery: the surgeon works at a console, directing instruments placed in the patient.

Physicians and surgeons are now nearing the point where they will be able to introduce new cartilage into damaged joints, regrow bone, induce damaged heart muscle to repair itself, and give people with damaged vital organs, such as the kidneys and the liver, the ability to grow new replacement cells.

Based on what we know today, and the treatments for disease now available, it is possible for people in our society to live much longer, possibly even to the theoretical age of approximately one hundred and thirty-seven years.

This may seem fanciful, but as new understanding and the ability to manipulate the workings of the human cell increase, even that age may be surpassed.

In order for people to be able to live meaningfully to great age, there will have to be availability of replacement parts for worn out joints and the ability to grow healthy new tissue to shore up failing organs.

It was not too long ago that the four minute mile was thought to be an impossible goal. Some suggested that in order to achieve it, athletes would have to use oxygen tanks. Nowadays, world class athletes break this barrier routinely.

The first two men who climbed 'unconquerable' Mount Everest were hailed as heroes. Now, successful climbs of Mount Everest are mentioned in the press in the context of delays and difficulties encountered because of the numbers of climbers.

Goals that are thought to be impossible, and obstacles that are labeled unconquerable, are often attained and overcome.

In medicine, we are now progressing beyond the point of making people "feel better about themselves", and "looking their best", to actually being able to offer people longer, more productive lives.

Countervailing forces in society, notably among them rampant obesity, drug abuse and suicide,
have to be addressed.

It is possible to decrease the incidence of the serious diseases that traditionally occur as we age – including heart disease, stroke, and cancer. When these diseases do occur, it is often possible to manage them as chronic conditions for long periods of time.

A healthy, active, fit, person, free of disease, will obviously feel better about herself/ himself, and will tend to "look their best".

The Genetic Blueprint

The human genome has been likened to the blueprint of a human being, heretofore known only to God. It is really the sequence of massive numbers of genes which determine human characteristics and behavior. The recent mapping of the human genome has great implications for the understanding of the natural aging process and its variation from person to person.

DNA makes up the chromosomes that carry the genes. There are 46 chromosomes in each body cell. However, the egg, or ovum, which is the human female sex cell, in its ready to mate state only carries 23 chromosomes, one from each pair of the woman's chromosomes. Similarly the human sperm, which is the male sex cell, carries 23 chromosomes, one from each pair of the man's chromosomes.

When egg and sperm unite, a unique new individual is formed who carries 46 chromosomes, half of which are derived from the mother, and half of which are derived from the father. The mother has two X chromosomes, so that one of her X chromosomes is in each egg. A man carries an X chromosome and a Y chromosome, so that each of his individual sperm carries either an X or a Y chromosome. If a Y carrying sperm successfully unites with the egg, an XY individual results, and the embryo is male. If an X bearing sperm unites with the egg, which always is X bearing, then the resulting child is XX, and therefore female. The ancient male rulers who discarded wives because they could not produce sons were grossly misinformed: the Y chromosome comes from the father.

Our genetic makeup, of course, is only the beginning, and the new baby lives in our environment. The environment can influence health, well-being, and long life, starting with the environment in the womb before the baby is born. Good nutrition and adequate oxygenation are necessary within the womb. Once the baby is born, environmental influences only become more complex.

The search for prolonged life drove some of the early explorers to American shores. Specifically, they were searching for the fabled Fountain of Youth. Ironically, these early explorers brought with them communicable diseases to which the native people of the Americas were highly susceptible. They also brought sexually transmitted diseases for which there was little effective treatment at that time. Consequently, populations of native Americans were ravaged. While the early explorers did not raise their own life expectancy, they managed unwittingly to lower drastically the life expectancy of the people who were already here.

Over the centuries however, because of the vast natural resources and the protection of the North American continent from foreign wars, as well as the unique freedom of the political system, as well as a sometimes enlightened immigration policy, and with the abolition of the ultimate repression in the form of slavery, Americans are finally achieving a life expectancy that surpasses that of the three score and ten years alluded to in the Bible.

Allowing people to enter our shores in the short run can lower the average life expectancy, because of their often low socioeconomic status. However, infectious disease in that population of legal immigrants can now be ruled out and, in fact, that newly arrived population is often better screened than people already living here. There are, however, loopholes in the screening process. Tuberculosis is a problem in much of the world, and unfortunately, many strains of tuberculosis are now drug resistant, so that the condition must be treated rigorously and long term. One of several sources of drug resistant tuberculosis strains is the former Soviet Union. Immigrants from Russia, as well as immigrants from all other countries, are required to supply chest X-rays to prove they are pulmonary tuberculosis free. However, they are allowed to bring their own X-ray films, rather than be screened under strict American supervision. It is easy enough to buy 'clean' chest X-rays from another individual, and have the prospective immigrant's name applied to the film. There is now drug resistant tuberculosis in the United States.

In the longer term, immigrants have built this continent by their innovation, motivation, and hard work, directly and indirectly leading to better living conditions and a longer life span for all of us. We are all, after all, immigrants a few generations removed.

In this modern world, it is practically impossible to prevent serious disease from arriving on our shores. A recent example of this is the emergence, and arrival into the United States, of the corona virus, which can be spread from person to person and can be fatal. One of the major industries in North America today is tourism. As well, the United States is one of the world's most important destinations for business travelers, as well as for politicians and diplomats. There are approximately forty-nine million visits a year to the United States, and, of course, few of these visitors have been screened for tuberculosis. The government is now taking steps to get advance passenger lists from foreign air carriers. Such lists are helpful in preventing terrorism, including bioterrorism, but probably do not have an impact on disease prevention. Within the close confines of an aircraft, passengers seated near an infected person, or even at a distance depending on the air circulation system, are in danger of getting infected themselves even prior to their arrival into the United States. Older Americans, who love to explore and travel, do put themselves at some risk.

Travel to a country with less rigorous public health measures than are in effect in the United States and Canada creates the risk of returning with a wide range of diseases. Tropical medicine experts are kept busy by returning travelers. Travelers should check with a doctor or hospital prior to leaving North America for a foreign destination to ensure that proper inoculations are done and should carry appropriate medication with them. It is sensible to have the name of a qualified medical professional at the destination, if possible.

If a serious medical condition suddenly occurs or worsens overseas, the care received will be at the level available at the destination. The sick person might not be able to quickly return home. This can be a major problem on a cruise, days out from any major port. The cruise line should be asked about the level of competence and country of origin of medical personnel on board, and the level of facilities available to deal with medical emergencies.

Strategies for Prolonging Life

Each of us carries our parents' genetic material. If parents are long lived, and other members of the family tend to be long lived, there is a good chance for an individual to be long lived. In order to achieve this expected long life however, harmful environmental influences have to be avoided.

On the other hand, if family members including parents tended to die young, there is no need to despair. More often then not, this would have been due to harmful environmental influences. For example, people in our society tended to die in their forties to fifties from heart attacks. Behavior modification, including not smoking, eating properly, and exercising properly, has eliminated much of that risk. Cholesterol (LDL: low density lipoprotein) lowering medications are in wide use. Regular medical checkups and the use of advanced technologic and diagnostic tools now allow doctors to identify the population at risk for heart attack. Advanced minimally invasive and open surgical techniques are used to correct partial blockages of the vital coronary arteries, although rigorous attention to the absolute indications for such procedures is necessary. It is now quite common to meet people of a certain age who have had coronary bypass procedures and who are leading perfectly normal lives. Not too long ago this would have been impossible.

Ironically, our ability to treat diseases can result in a shortened lifespan for following generations. Juvenile diabetes and congenital heart disease are examples of diseases that we can now thankfully treat, allowing people with these conditions to live healthfully into their reproductive years. Any gene they carry that predisposes to the condition can then be passed to their children.

Gene Therapy:

However, genetic manipulation is now becoming possible. Individuals with genes predisposing them to life threatening disease will be able to undergo procedures to nullify the effects of those genes. Certain disease processes can already be treated in this way, including Fabry's disease, an enzyme deficiency.

Preimplantation Genetic Diagnosis (PGD):

When the first "test tube baby" was born, more than thirty-five years ago, it was thought to be a miracle, and many ethical considerations were raised, along with a long list of doubts.

I learned a valuable lesson in the 1970's when I edited Advances in Obstetrics and Gynecology, a textbook for specialists. Attempts were being made at in vitro fertilization, the fertilization of a human egg by sperm in the laboratory. The plan was to develop one of these eggs, implanted in its mother's womb, to full development: a baby.

I spoke with some noted scientists working in the area. I heard that it couldn't be done with the available knowledge and technology, and that the attempts being made smacked of pseudoscience.

Shortly afterwards, the first successful baby born by this technique was announced in England. An entire new era had begun in reproductive medicine.

I now know that even the most brilliant and ethical scientist can have a natural bias against work that is not their own. The mindset is "I didn't think of it, so it can't be done". Unless their thoughts at the time are recorded, they soon forget that they ever minimized the work.

Once it was apparent that a new field of medicine and hope for countless couples had been created, former critics tended to join in and use their talents to make rapid advances in the science.

Looking back, the concept was quite simple, and the baby had nothing to do with a test tube. In a case when a woman's egg and a man's sperm cannot naturally get together, classically where the fallopian tube is blocked, but in many other situations as well, the woman's egg is extracted from her ovary before she ovulates. The egg is then incubated (warmed) in a laboratory along with the man's sperm. One of the sperm naturally penetrates into the egg, fertilizing it. The fertilized egg is then placed back into the woman's uterus, where it naturally implants and grows.

The science of assisted reproduction has now grown way beyond those beginnings. It is now possible, under a microscope, to place a single sperm directly into the egg, fertilizing it.

As the egg in the ovary matures, the genetic material it carries is reduced. Only one chromosome from each pair of the woman's chromosomes is present in the ready to mate egg. The rest of the chromosomes, the other one of each pair, is separated off into a small microscopic structure called a polar body. The polar body contains the half of the woman's genetic material that is left behind and will not be inherited by her baby. It is possible to look at the chromosomes contained in this cast off polar body. If the mother has a detectable gene defect on one chromosome and this defect is on a chromosome in the polar body, then the egg itself, which will become the baby, did not get that gene and the baby will not be affected.

It is possible to select an egg from the mother that does not carry her own defective gene, and to use that egg for fertilization. The fertilization of that particular egg is then accomplished by micromanipulation, inserting her mate's sperm directly into the healthy egg. This technique is called ICSI (Intracytoplasmic Sperm Injection).

In an ongoing pregnancy, it is possible to carry out genetic diagnosis relatively early by sampling (biopsy) of the placenta.

Small amounts of fetal DNA that are present in the pregnant woman's circulation can be analyzed, to see if there is fetal aneuploidy (abnormal number of chromosomes).

Maintaining Long Life:

We must, as individuals and as a society, eliminate those forces that shorten the lives of so many of us. Highways, vehicles, and drivers must be made to perform more safely. Accident prevention in the home is important. The home should be equipped with smoke and carbon monoxide detectors. Public buildings should be protected with such things as sprinkler systems, fire rated doors, and wide stairwells for escape.

We should keep the Four Horsemen of the Apocalypse in mind. We are not yet at the stage where we have eliminated war and strife, without compromising our own safety and liberty. Many of our people died in this way in the twentieth century, and continue to die, in this twenty-first century, in spite of our great advances in other fields.

Attention must be paid in each community to seemingly mundane things like the water supply and levels of sanitation. The complex infrastructure of our society, including water reservoirs, pipelines, sewage treatment plants, and power plants must be maintained and upgraded. The general level of education must be high enough so that people understand what must be done to keep us all safe and disease free, including how to limit the spread of sexually transmitted and other communicable disease.

We must strive to eliminate gun crime from our society. The level of violent crime in our society is simply unacceptable. In some places, older people, who are often slower and weaker, are considered prey at the time of their lives when they should be honored and respected.

Mental health issues should be addressed, so that the level of suicide is decreased. Unfortunately, there is a significant incidence of suicide among older people. There are much better ways, including medication, available today to deal with depression, hardship, and the rigors of life.

We are all of us survivors. We have outlived the potential for childhood infectious disease, now largely obviated in our society by various vaccines and public health measures. Most sexually transmitted diseases are now curable or at least manageable. Even acquired immunodeficiency syndrome (AIDS) has become more manageable in recent years. A person in a long term monogamous relationship is in little danger of getting that. Even health care workers on the front lines of the disease, provided proper precautions are taken, can be protected.

The person who is older and healthy has made it past the danger point of getting many hereditary diseases, although there is still a risk for such things as adult onset diabetes, heart disease, cardiovascular disease, and cancer.

A person who does not smoke and did not work in a hazardous environment, is much less likely to get a disease caused by carcinogens in the environment. However, a sun worshiper does have an increased risk of skin cancer.

We are all at risk for degenerative diseases such as arthritis. A person who is older and not experiencing much difficulty with such a condition probably will get by without significant damage. Imperfectly understood disease conditions of the central nervous system, including Alzheimer's Disease, which are a risk in later years, fortunately will not affect the majority of us earlier on.

All in all, it is beginning to look like the age of seventy is an important milestone. A person who can get by seventy in relatively good health is well on the way to longevity.

There are more people in our society living healthfully over a hundred years of age with sharp minds and a good quality of life than ever before in our history. With what we know today, it might even be possible for people to live to be a hundred and thirty-seven years of age. We do not know of anybody who has made it that far yet, but we are hopeful. Beyond that is the stuff of science fiction.

The Genome:

We each have our own genome, differing in subtle ways from that of everyone else, except those of us who are identical twins. Identical twins are true clones of each other: they have exactly the same genome. The genome is a person's complete DNA sequence.

The sequencing of the human genome was actually performed on a relatively small group of people. In the case of the sequencing done by the Public Consortium, no single individual was analyzed. That DNA analysis was carried out on different individuals for various parts of the genome.

The Human Cell:

In every cell in the human body, the center or nucleus contains 46 chromosomes arranged in 23 pairs. Chromosomes themselves can be seen with an ordinary microscope. The chains of DNA (Deoxyribonucleic

Acid) which make up these chromosomes, are not so easily seen. At this point, we are down to a molecular level. The DNA strands are arranged in a twisting double helix manner, something like a tight spiral staircase, or ladder. This ladder shape actually has little steps or rungs. Each step or rung of the ladder holds only two of four separate nucleic acid bases. They are arranged in pairs on each rung of the ladder of DNA. These are called base pairs. The four nucleic acids involved, are adenine (A), cytosine (C), guanine (G), and thymine (T). They code the sequences of the amino acids that, in turn, make up the proteins that are the building blocks of our bodies.

The human genome project, which involved vast ingenuity, much money, and enormous computer capability by both the public Human Genome Project, headed by Francis Collins, and a private company called Celera Genomics, which was headed by J. Craig Venter, have placed approximately three billion of these bits in their proper order on the chromosome.

The sequence looks like an unending series of the letters A, C, G, and T.

Bioengineering:

We are still nowhere near the point where we can build a human being from a plan of four nucleic acids or bases. However, the understanding of aging, disease, and specifically designed drugs to combat disease, not to mention the ability to deal with defective genes that cause disease, is rapidly becoming within our power. For years now, scientists have been capable of rearranging DNA molecules, manufacturing recombinant DNA. This is the basis of bioengineering.

There are approximately twenty to twenty-five thousand genes in each of us that are essential for the formation of proteins. A gene is a section on a DNA molecule. The function of most genes is still unknown. A major challenge and opportunity for scientists in the years ahead will be to increase our understanding of how the human body functions. Genes carry the code for the manufacture of the proteins that make up our bodies. The various tasks that need to be carried out as part of the life process are carried out by these proteins. Proteins are the building blocks of our cells. They facilitate the chemical reactions of life by serving as organic catalysts, or enzymes.

The end of each chromosome is called a telomere. The telomere, which is itself a DNA sequence, gives stability to the end of the chromosome. Abnormal recombinations of the chromosomes are therefore prevented. Telomerase is necessary for the maintenance and repair of the telomere. Telomerase does this by helping in the transfer of genetic code information between nucleic acids.

Telomerase appears to have an essential role in the immortality of cells. If telomerase is inhibited, the telomere can be shortened, and the cell can die.

If telomerase is activated, the cell may become immortal. This, of course, has almost unbelievable implications in the possible control of the aging process of cells, which make up every organ and tissue in our bodies. The discovery of the Fountain of Youth again beckons.

On the other hand, if telomerase is suppressed, cells die. This has great implications in cancer treatment, as a hallmark of cancer cells is their ability to multiply in a bizarre fashion indefinitely. If a cancer cell can be made to die, without damaging the human host, then a great leap will have been made in cancer treatment. It goes without saying that ridding ourselves of the threat of cancer will increase our life expectancy substantially.

There is, however, another way to look at cancer. Cancer cells are effectively deteriorated cells that look like they are growing old. In that case, a treatment for cancer may actually involve activating telomerase, helping the cell to stay young and not to deteriorate into a malignant type.

It is almost impossible to overestimate the significance of the decoding of the human genome. From one side, we are beginning to understand the makeup of the human being at a molecular level. From the diagnostic side, we are approaching the molecular level in diagnostic capability with such tools as the PET scan (positive emission tomography), which can identify sites in the human body of increased metabolic activity, which can mean that cancer cells are present. Magnetic resonance imaging (MRI) can already show the structure of the human body at an anatomic level, identifying small disease sites and their structure. Computerized axial tomography (the CAT scan) does much the same thing by a different technique.

Designer Drugs:

We are rapidly entering an era of designer drugs. These drugs can be specifically targeted to patients based on their genetic profile, in much the same way as the television market has been fragmented into niche markets that cater to your individual taste. The History Channel is most usually watched by people who have been around awhile. It is not MTV.

The coming designer drugs will specifically target problem cells in the human body based on the individual's genetic makeup. They will be much more effective and less toxic than many presently available drugs. There will be unanticipated side effects and complications that will have to be evaluated and taken into account.

Nanotechnology:

It might even become possible to deliver medications to body cells by the use of microscopic nanomachines, measuring only billionths of a meter in size, powered by biomolecular motors using ATP for energy formation. ATP is key in the metabolism of glucose (sugar). This is the exciting new field of nanotechnology. Such machines may have tiny propellers, or may use cilia, the microscopic hair like projections of altered bacteria, for getting around.

Thoughtful people have always asked, 'Are we interfering with the natural order of things?' The first person to pick up a stone or a stick and ward off a predator was interfering with the natural order of things. That person was making a statement: he or she refused to be prey, or lunch. Penicillin was first discovered by Fleming, and other antibiotic therapies quickly followed, allowing us to be able to destroy the bacteria that had caused epidemics of disease for untold centuries, killing us. That was interference with the natural order of things.

Advances in public health, prenatal care and proper obstetrical care for pregnant women, that largely eradicated death in childbirth for both mother and child, brought us to the massive worldwide population explosion that now confronts us. Again, we interfered with the natural order of things.

Vaccines became available to eradicate viral diseases. Now we are in an era where antiviral drugs are available. We can attack disease on a submicroscopic level. Viruses are particles that cannot even be seen under a microscope, but require visualization by electron microscopes, or more recently genetic fingerprinting by DNA probes. These techniques are now clinically available, to the great benefit of modern medicine and the people it serves. It is certainly an interference in the natural order of things. We can now battle our submicroscopic enemies.

If specific areas of our genetic material are defective, we are now rapidly approaching the point where the damage can be repaired, with the potential of almost unlimited benefit to humankind. No longer will we have to treat cancer with traditional shotgun chemotherapy that drives the healthy cells of the patient almost to the brink of death in the theory that the faster growing and uncontrolled cells of the cancer will perish first. The new treatments will be aimed specifically at the disease process if its source is a defective gene or genes, sparing the person from damage while the disease is eradicated or controlled.

We have learned to control our bigger natural enemies with relatively primitive techniques. We live longer and are confronted by much smaller unseen enemies that we are learning to control by sophisticated and elegant means. This will mean that more of us will be living much longer.

Questions will have to be answered on how this impacts on the very makeup of our populations. Concepts like mandatory retirement age in the early sixties will fall by the wayside. A person will stay productive and healthy much longer. We will have to examine how vast numbers of us will coexist with our grandchildren and great grandchildren. Fortunately, these issues evolve over time, and science and technology, and hopefully society, progress in all other areas as well. Ultimately, larger answers will be found.

We are on an unending exciting search. Europeans in the middle of the last millennium, intent on shortening their trade routes, instead discovered what they called a 'New World' which in fact were the American continents. The world in its entirety is now the center of our existence.

We are just beginning to realize that the whole solar system with its vast trove of resources and secrets is becoming available to us in the attainable future. Just the search for these secrets has already yielded a vast dividend in expanded technology, much of which has been applied to the medical sciences. Beyond that, there are countless unknown other worlds, but that is for another time.

Proteomics:

Another step in learning how we are built and function is the study of proteomics, the analysis of the proteins that are made by the genome. The proteins, formed of amino acids in sequences, themselves are molecules with specific functions. Some repel and kill invading organisms. Other protein molecules are capable of repairing tissue, or actually building it. However, just having the blueprint does not mean we are yet capable of erecting or building a human body, or making it function.

Regenerative Medicine:

The promise of regenerative medicine is just that: it is becoming possible to regrow new organs and tissues from stem cells that are present within each of us.

We are at a stage where we are beginning to have available bioengineered tissue derived from related donors, which can be grafted on to an individual. The first uses are in burn victims who need new living grafted skin, and people with eye damage in the cornea who require new tissue. The future possible applications are many and exciting.

Because of its structure, each protein has a distinctive and very complex shape. Various molecules can fit into the little nooks of the protein. Targeted drugs work by binding on to these receptor sites on the cell to prevent unwanted molecules in the body from locking into these sites. Drugs specifically targeted to the abnormal cells of a tumor can carry small doses of lethal substances which can then kill the cell. Nanotechnology is advancing. Microscopic drops are being developed that can select out dangerous bacteria and kill them.

Even a beginning knowledge of the genome and of the proteins it designs will yield increasing and vast benefits to medical science, allowing us to be healthier and to live longer, productively.

Erythropoietin, which stimulates the formation of red blood cells, is produced by recombinant DNA technology. The human erythropoietin gene is put into mammalian cells, essentially yielding copies of erythropoietin. The resulting drug is Epoetin Alfa (Epogen, Procrit). Aranesp (Darbepoetin) works similarly. These drugs stimulate the formation of erythrocytes, or red blood cells in anemic people. There is the downside risk of thrombotic events, including myocardial infarction (heart attack) and blood clots. These proteins, because they stimulate blood cell formation, cannot be used in people who have myeloid leukemia, which is a cancer of the blood cells.

White blood cell production can similarly be stimulated. Neupogen (Filgrastim) encourages white blood cell production. Serious side effects, including rupture of the spleen, are possible.

Drugs may become available that can stimulate the growth of bone, nerve, and brain cells.

Drug Risks:

Drugs and medications of any type should only be taken under the direction of a qualified physician, who understands the possible benefits and risks in light of your individual situation.

Every drug has possible downside risks and complications, even old standbys like aspirin.

This is especially true in pregnancy, or when pregnancy is even contemplated, or possible. Many drugs should not be used during pregnancy because of harmful effects to the fetus or the mother. In many other cases, possible risks of the drug must be carefully weighed, in consultation with a qualified physician, against benefits that might be achieved in treating a specific disease or condition.

Stem Cells:

There are now various ways to create new cells to replace damaged ones. The entire human body, of course, is made up of cells that have differentiated into specialized types to perform various functions. For instance, there are oxygen carrying red blood cells, infection fighting white blood cells, white blood cells that are the basis of the immune system, nerve cells, muscle cells, and so on. Each individual cell has a center, or nucleus, that contains genetic material within the chromosomes.

New cells are formed in the marrow of bones including the sternum (breastbone), and part of the pelvic bone structure (the iliac bones). These not yet specialized, parent cells are called stem cells. It has now become possible to induce bone marrow cells to become neurons, or nerve cells. The fact that these new nerve cells can probably be obtained from the bone marrow of the exact person who needs the replacement nerve cells has the potential of getting rid of the major problem of transplanting replacement organs. That problem is host versus graft rejection. In the transplantation of organs today, commonly the transplantation of kidneys, hearts, and even liver and lungs, as well as less common procedures, such as the transplant of limbs (arms and legs), the body recognizes the transplanted organ as foreign, and treats the transplant as it would any foreign substance. It tries to reject and kill it. Therefore, people who need transplanted organs must receive tissue that is closely matched to their own and must be treated with drugs to suppress the immune system. This opens the person getting the transplant up to a whole host of infections. Rejection of the transplanted organ or tissue is still possible.

The ability to create new cells of the specific type needed by a particular individual from their own bone marrow cells gets rid of this rejection problem.

Embryonic stem cells are immortal and renew themselves. The embryo is the early developing baby in the uterus. The cells are called stem cells because they are as yet undifferentiated cells capable of becoming the different specialized cells that make up the human body, including nerve cells, muscle cells, blood cells and organ cells.

When a baby is born, its umbilical cord is cut. Within that umbilical cord are immature stem cells from which it is possible to create new blood cells. It is now possible to save and freeze these umbilical cord cells for future use. This technique can revolutionize the treatment of leukemia. At present, a person with leukemia who needs stem cell replacement must find a perfectly matched bone marrow donor. This can be an almost impossible task. If the parents at the time of a birth have the cells from the umbilical cord saved and frozen, and their offspring did develop leukemia, she or he could get bone marrow replaced with stem cells derived from their very own umbilical cord. This would be a perfect match. Some parents are now having umbilical cord stem cells saved, for the future benefit of their children.

Stem cell transplants are used in replacing the cancerous blood cells of leukemia patients with healthy donor stem cells that then create a new line of healthy blood cells. The use of stem cell transplants has now gone beyond this well recognized use. For instance, promising results with stem cell transplantation has been seen in people with kidney cancer.

Angiogenesis:

Stem cells from bone marrow are probably involved in angiogenesis, the creation of the blood vessels that can bring nourishment to malignant tumors. Other stem cells from bone marrow evolve into red and white blood cells. VEGF (Vascular Endothelial Growth Factor) includes six types of protein made by tumors that cause stem cells to leave the bone marrow and go to the tumor. Antibodies can be made that block VEGF receptors. An antibody is being tested that interferes with the VEGF protein itself.

Stem Cells and Cloning: The Promise and The Threat:

All the cells that make up all the tissues and organs of the human body arise from stem cells. The primary female sex organ, the ovary, is totipotential. It is capable of producing any type of specialized cell found in the human body. The ovum (egg) of the female, when mated with the male spermatozoon forms a distinctive new cell, the zygote. The zygote, as it divides and multiplies, rapidly differentiates into distinctive and specialized cells that form the organs and all the working parts of the new individual.

By the end of the second month, all major features of the developing embryo are recognizable, and all the main organ systems have been laid down.

Everybody ultimately dies of organ failure. Eventually, an organ necessary for life ceases to function. Medicine has advanced to the point where failure in a single organ can be overcome. Today people often live until there is multisystem organ failure. The kidneys, heart, liver and lungs are all vital organs. The brain is the ultimate vital organ. The body can live independently without upper brain function, but of course unknowingly, in a coma.

Organ Transplant:

The ability to transplant healthy organs to replace severely damaged, diseased vital organs was a major breakthrough in medicine. Pioneering cases were sometimes done by transferring the healthy organ from an identical twin. An identical twin is a true clone, whose tissues are an exact genetic duplicate of those in her twin sister. The already fertilized egg split into two, and two genetically identical individuals grew into embryos.

Transplanting organs from one identical twin to another, although surgically challenging, presented no immunologic problem. There was no danger of the individual receiving the organ recognizing the transplant as a foreign substance, setting off a rejection process. However, limiting transplantation to identical twins in which only one member of the pair had a seriously diseased organ, made the procedure a medical curiosity because the vast majority of people could not be helped.

Methods, including tissue typing, and the use of immunologic suppressing drugs, were developed, and are now widely used so that people with severely damaged organs now often have the option of receiving a healthy donor organ by transplantation. Women with transplanted kidneys now can essentially lead normal lives, and in fact, often have babies of their own. I was privileged years ago to successfully deliver the first baby ever born to a woman who had undergone a kidney transplant from an organ donor who had donated the kidney upon death.

Organs for transplant are most often obtained from newly deceased persons who have donated organs, and who are on support of their vital functions until the organs are removed. Otherwise, the organ is donated by a friend, relative, or other sympathetic person who is willing to undergo major surgery, and lose all or part of a vital organ, such as a kidney.

The lists of people awaiting suitably matched donor organs is long. The potential recipients are seriously ill, and often succumb before a suitable donor organ can be supplied.

Even when the donor organ is available, significant surgery to introduce it and a lifetime of immunosuppression is necessary to maintain it unharmed by attack in the body of its new host. In spite of all efforts, rejection of the organ may take place, and the long awaited transplant may fail.

The shortage of organs available for transplant can be solved by the use of stem cells. A stem cell is an undifferentiated cell that has the potential to become a specialized cell with a specific function, such as a blood cell or a muscle cell. Stem cells can be induced to evolve and specialize into the specific type of cell needed: nerve cells (neurons), heart muscle (myocyte) cells, and so on.

Introduction of healthy new cells might be enough: surgical transplantation of an entire organ could become unnecessary.

Furthermore, rejection of these healthy new cells would not occur if the stem cells from which they evolved came from the intended recipient.

This can be achieved by using stem cells already present in the individual, such as bone marrow stem cells ordinarily destined to become circulating blood cells. These cells can be induced to become nerve cells (neurons). Stem cells present in the heart do evolve into heart muscle (myocytes). Other body cells can be induced to differentiate into muscle cells, presenting another avenue of approach.

The most obvious, and controversial, way to obtain stem cells genetically identical to an individual is from a clone. Sheep and other animals have been cloned. Most recently, and inevitably, human embryos have been cloned. The technique involves the removal of the genetic material from the nucleus of a fertilized egg cell and replacing it with the genetic material from a mature cell of the adult to be cloned. It is possible to introduce the cloned egg into the uterus of a female who will carry the fetus to term. A new individual results, if the cloning is successful, that is an exact genetic copy of the donor. However, the cloned egg used to create stem cell lines has never been brought to that step.

Human cloning is ethically challenging, at the very least, and the use of that clone for organ harvesting would be morally repugnant. As usual, the science fiction writers were way ahead of the scientists (often they are the scientists): "The Boys from Brazil" quickly comes to mind. Not only do we have the ability to genetically replicate the worst among us, but we can weaken the genetic biodiversity which strengthens us as a species. The epic, unspeakable horror of the previous twentieth century, in which pseudoscience combined with fascist politics to promote a 'master race' coupled with the conscious policy of destroying 'inferior' races, has made us all look askance at genetic dabbling.

However, it is not necessary to go to such extremes in order to realize the vast potential benefits of stem cell research.

Federally funded stem cell research in the United States is currently limited to the use of already existing stem cell lines. The creation of new stem cell lines from human embryos is currently prohibited. Canadian guidelines are somewhat more liberal. Inevitably, research will be done in countries where the legislation is least restrictive. Major funding in biologic research worldwide does emanate from the United States, and therefore American opinion and guidelines do carry much weight.

A large supply of unused frozen embryos, created for in vitro fertilization (IVF), exists. Many of these embryos are destined never to fulfill their potential to grow into babies, and to be eventually destroyed. Such embryos have been used to create the existing embryonic stem cell lines.

Creating a specific cloned embryo of an adult woman who needs a transplant, and then using the stem cells of that embryo to differentiate into the specific tissue she needs, destroying the embryo in the process, instantly brings up moral and ethical considerations. In a society where abortion on demand was long fought for and eventually achieved, the choices might appear obvious.

It is possible to derive stem cells from an embryo without destroying it. For example, in order to detect whether an embryo is genetically normal, before implanting it into the mother's womb, it is possible to remove a cell from the cell mass of the dividing fertilized egg and examine its chromosomes microscopically. The embryo does go on, in spite of the removed cell, to develop normally. However, if this was a cloned embryo, a human baby that was a cloned copy of an existing adult would be born.

In a less controversial way, it is possible to induce an unfertilized egg to divide, so that stem cells can be derived. It is not possible currently for a human egg that is unfertilized to progress to a live human being. Therefore, it cannot really be argued that the destruction of this dividing egg represents the elimination of a possible person.

In an exciting development, scientists at Wake Forest have shown that stem cells present in the amniotic fluid which surrounds the developing fetus in the mother's uterus can be removed and induced to grow into specialized cells. There is no harm to the developing baby. As a matter of fact when a woman is in labor and her "water breaks", it is this amniotic fluid which is naturally and painlessly released.

Such advances change the whole tone of the moral and ethical dialogue.

Can Aging be Reversed?

Human trials have recently been conducted administering recombinant human growth hormone (rhGH) to people to reverse immunosenescence.

Immunosenescence is age associated immune change with a reduction in peripheral blood naïve cells and an increase of memory cells, along with the inflammatory changes that accompany aging.

Recombinant DNA technology involves rearranging DNA molecules. A recombinant DNA molecule is constructed from segments obtained from different DNA molecules.

Growth hormone (Somatotropin) is a substance secreted mainly by the pituitary gland at the base of the brain and carried by the bloodstream to other organs which it affects (end organs).

Growth hormone can influence growth and regeneration of the thymus gland., a lymphoid gland of the immune system located in the neck that produces T-cells (T-lymphocytes), which are immunologically competent white blood cells responsible for cell-mediated immunity.

The human trials showed protective immunologic changes, improved risk for some age-related diseases, and some decrease in epigenetic age, which is different than one's chronologic age.

Epigenetics is the study of the regulation of genes. As we age, our DNA increasingly undergoes a process called methylation. The amount of methylation in DNA can be assessed, giving a picture of one's age. Each five year increase in DNA methylation age has been said to be associated with an eight to fifteen percent increase in mortality. However, the association between DNA methylation age and age-related disease and longevity is inconclusive at this point.

It is true that growth hormone, as its names suggests, is a driver of childhood growth. Growth hormone does help maintain body tissues and organs throughout life. As we age, the amount of growth hormone produced declines. At this point, human growth hormone (HGH) treatment is only advised for adults with a true deficiency because of a particular medical condition.

There are significant risks to HGH treatment, including insulin resistance and diabetes, and breast tumor growth.

References

1. www.S3.amazonaws.com/cdn.smfm.org/publications/224/download-491f0e6962960848d2097447abS7a024.pdf ACOG Practice Bulletin Number 163, May 2016
2. www.ncbi.nlm.nih.gov/pubmed/26287791
3. www.ghr.nlm.nih.gov/primer/testing/nipt
4. https://www.ncbi.nlm.nih.gov/pmc/articles/PMC4966880/
5. https://www.ncbi.nlm.nih.gov/pmc/articles/PMC6826138/
6. https://www.sciencedirect.com/topics/neuroscience/epigenome
7. https://epi.grants.cancer.gov/epigen.html
8. https://clinicalepigeneticsjournal.biomedcentral.com/articles/10.1186/s13148-019-0656-7

9. https://www.peprotech.com/en/recombinant-human-growth-hormone
10. https://www.mayoclinic.org/healthy-lifestyle/healthy-aging/in-depth/growth-hormone/art-20045735
11. https://www.cdc.gov/coronavirus/2019-ncov/index.html?CDC_AA_refVal=https%3A%2F%2Fwww.cdc.gov%2F-coronavirus%2Fnovel-coronavirus-2019.html
12. Bibliography & Supplemental Bibliography: See www.rcaplanmd.com

CHAPTER 3

DISEASES OF AGING AND THEIR PREVENTION

The Take-Home Message

- Stop smoking
- Eat healthfully
- Women, men and their physicians must pay attention to the prevention of, and early detection of, heart and cardiovascular disease
- Methods for the early detection of breast and ovarian cancer do exist – but better methods are needed

The diseases that we confront as we enter a more mature age group fall into several broad categories. Some of these are specific to women because of their unique physiologic makeup and anatomy. Others are common in both men and women, but the incidence may vary between the sexes for various reasons that may or may not have something to do with basic physiology and the interplay of lifestyle and environment. A particular public awareness of the given disease condition, with the attendant political activism, and private and public money spent on it, does not necessarily have a lot to do with how pervasive the disease is in the society, and how damaging it is. For example, lung cancer has become one of the leading causes of cancer deaths, not to mention illness, in women. Although attention is lately being paid to the root cause of this condition, namely smoking, and to its early diagnosis and eradication, these efforts to date have been relatively modest compared to the huge publicity and resource allocation that has been deservedly given to breast cancer in women.

As more and more diseases are better understood, and are able to either be prevented, cured, or at least controlled, we are confronted with new diseases and challenges in our older years. People have traditionally thought that if they could only get past the life threatening conditions that were most prominent at a given time in history, they would enter on a bright new future. This is only partly true. We have now reached the stage of confronting a host of so-called degenerative disease processes that tended not to be a problem for most of our ancestors, simply because they did not live long enough for those diseases to become a factor.

The most pressing problem historically for the human race was malnutrition. Getting enough to eat and maintaining a diet that contained all the essential nutrients, was a constant challenge for our ancestors in most places on earth. Unfortunately, it is still a major problem today. Malnutrition is still, unfortunately, present in our world in this new millennium, and natural disasters such as floods and crop failures exacerbate the problem. In our own society, pockets of poverty still exist and our nutrition is still suboptimal. Permanent damage to the individual can result. A striking proportion of our population, most notably women and girls, have eating disorders such as bulemia, which is self-induced vomiting, and anorexia, which results in a failure to eat sufficiently to maintain health and body weight. Overeating and obesity are rife in our society, and if malnutrition is properly defined it means just that: bad nutrition. Poor eating habits encourage the early onset of various disease processes commonly thought of as occurring in an older population, including heart disease, arteriosclerosis, hypertension, diabetes, and even cancer.

The prevention, early diagnosis, and aggressive treatment of heart disease in women has had far too little attention paid to it, and right up to the present time insurance companies tend to balk at paying for it. Sophisticated diagnostic modalities are necessary to make the early diagnosis that necessarily precedes early and effective treatment.

The early diagnosis of that silent killer, ovarian cancer, has so far eluded us. Part of the reason is that the diagnostic tests currently available, such as the blood tests CA 125 and CA 19-9, which are cancer markers, are nonspecific. That means that a positive test does not necessarily mean that cancer is present, and a negative test does not mean that the cancer is not present. Ultrasonography to look at the ovaries is an excellent way to pick up early enlargement of these structures. However, there is still much discussion in the gynecologic community as to the specific meaning of subtle changes in the ovaries picked up on routine ultrasonography. The insurance companies have seized upon this very often as a reason not to pay for routine ultrasonographic screening of the ovaries in more senior women, which at this time is probably the best means available for picking up early tumors when they are still removable with a high possible cure rate. As it now stands, the vast majority of ovarian cancers are not discovered until they are in so-called stage III, when the disease has already spread, the treatment options severe, and the long term outlook less than optimistic. The same is true of lung cancer, where only recently programs have gotten underway to pick up lung cancer at a very early totally resectable stage by fast computerized axial tomography (CAT scan). Many of those screening programs that do exist tend to start the screening at too late an age, when many tumors have already progressed. As usual, the insurance companies are generally averse to picking up the cost.

It is interesting that companies that call themselves euphemistically "Health Maintenance Organizations" (HMO's) tend to balk at any new advance that can lead to the early detection and successful treatment of diseases that threaten peoples' lives. They conveniently label any new test or treatment they do not wish to pay for as 'experimental' or unproven. They are adept at limiting access to new drug therapies.

Introducing single payer nationalized health care by the government, without any provision for the continuation of private medical care, could be a regressive step. It has been shown in other major societies, most notably in Britain, and more recently in Canada, that total governmental control of a single payer system can result in a significant layer of bureaucracy for managing the system. Control can become cumbersome and costly. Failure to maintain sufficient facilities notably in the areas of emergency care and high technology diagnostics and treatment can result. Criminalization of health care professionals for alleged overutilization gets written into law as a method of cost control. Rationing of health care results. Stifling of innovation is accompanied by papers in the scientific medical literature citing cost effectiveness, which is often spurious

The 'Canadian Model', often touted in the American media, owed much of its early success to the high level of medical expertise available in Canada prior to the onset of government controlled single payer medicine. Canadian society is smaller and more homogeneous than its United States counterpart, so that a government controlled single payer system had a better chance of working. As the system took up a huge part of the government budget, de facto rationing of resources resulted. Long waits have inevitably resulted, limiting access to the most modern medical modalities. As a result, for-profit medical facilities have sprung up on the United States side of the long US-Canadian border, where more affluent Canadians can now go to obtain state of the art medical care from practitioners who are often their former Canadian doctors who have emigrated to the United States. Thus, the idealistic and well intentioned refusal to allow even the slightest hint of a "two-tier" medical system, where citizens who desired it and could afford it had quick access to quality care actually resulted in an even less egalitarian system, where the wealthier and most mobile citizens simply went across the border. A strong movement has arisen in Western Canada to mitigate these unforeseen effects, and to finally allow private ambulatory surgical centers to have a role in Canadian medicine.

If the United States ever puts such a single government payer plan into place, Americans will have no such safety valve of available care just across the border that patients can use. Considering that a huge proportion of medical advance and technology currently emanates from the United States, a bureaucratic stifling of that effort and innovation could be expected as well, to the detriment of all us, and indeed to the whole world.

It is estimated that 3.65 trillion dollars was spent in the United States on medical care in 2019. Twenty cents of each of those dollars are paid to doctors who, in turn, often have their own offices and facilities to maintain, and for clinical care. Creating a government single payer system would potentially make medical care the single largest item in the U.S. budget. Other societies have seen these costs become responsible for massive per capita deficits, and even a decline in the value of their currency. This can result in a weakened economy, with even less ability to meet the health needs of the people. Decision making becomes slow and cumbersome, with taxing authorities unwilling to make the necessary expenditures to keep rapidly evolving technology available to the public.

On the other hand, millions of Americans presently have no health insurance at all, and this basic problem in our society must be addressed. Various solutions have been proposed, which can be implemented without destroying a diverse medical system with practically unlimited choices for each patient that is presently at the forefront of technology and treatment and is presently nimble enough to be capable of rapid evolution of new therapies.

At present, universal health care coverage incorporating varying amounts of flexibility is proceeding in the United States on a state by state basis, with California being a notable recent proponent.

The continuing answer to the early diagnosis and conquest of the diseases that ravage us is far more likely to come from the free and diverse private sector, with governmental support and supervision only where necessary.

The popularization of advanced technology, as the computer industry and information industry have shown, quickly leads to moderate prices for incredible technologic breakthroughs that are within the reach of every person. The same can be true of medical tests and treatments that are now exotic and expensive. As the hardware and the software are streamlined and available to the mass market, the prices will inevitably and quickly come down. The economic benefit in the medium term will be stupendous. The longer productive lives of older people will bring continuing contributions to society. We will be less reliant on heroic and often fatal treatments that are far more expensive than any sophisticated diagnostic technique or early interventional procedure.

CHAPTER 4
HEART DISEASE AND HYPERTENSION

The Take-Home Message

Heart Disease

- Coronary artery disease is a significant concern
  - It can be prevented, helped, or delayed in onset
  - It can be effectively treated
  - Prophylaxis against heart attack is easily available for most people who need it
  - Better early diagnosis is available
- Congestive heart failure can be effectively treated
- Heart transplantation is no longer experimental
- Heart muscle actually undergoes repair, and new heart muscle can be grown

High blood pressure (hypertension)

- Is increasingly common as one ages
- It can be prevented, helped, and delayed in onset

High cholesterol (hypercholesterolemia)

- Is associated with obesity
- Genetic factors are involved
- It can be prevented, mitigated, and treated effectively

Stroke

- There are two different mechanisms: hemorrhage, or blood clot
- Early identification of people at risk, and specific treatment for them, is possible in some cases
- Prompt treatment is of vital importance

Aneurysm

- Weakening, and bulging, of a blood vessel wall
- Early diagnosis and treatment is important

Heart Disease

There are of course, many different types of heart disease. The type of heart disease most of us are concerned about as we get older is coronary artery disease. The coronary arteries are the branching arteries that supply blood and oxygen to the muscle of the heart itself. Arteriosclerotic plaques form in the walls of the coronary vessels and bulge into the channel, narrowing it and eventually blocking the channel (lumen) completely. There is inflammation in the wall of the blood vessel. Myeloperoxidase is an enzyme that helps convert LDL (low density lipoprotein) into a form that leads to cholesterol deposition. The heart muscle being supplied by the affected artery is deprived of oxygen, becomes ischemic and can die. This is a classic heart attack, manifested by severe pain, and is a life threatening situation. If the victim of the attack survives, a scar remains in the area of the affected muscle interfering with the normal conduction of electrical impulses across the heart. This can lead to abnormal heart rhythms.

Fortunately, it has now been shown that the heart does actually undergo repair. Heart muscle cells (cardiac myocytes) do divide after myocardial infarction, replacing the damaged heart muscle (myocardium). Stem (primitive) cells are present in the heart which can evolve into heart muscle (myocytes). As well, new blood vessel growth does occur in the damaged heart.

Risk factors for coronary artery disease can be found even in children and young adults. A high level of LDL formerly known as "bad" cholesterol is one of these factors. Cholesterol metabolism is a complicated affair. Too much LDL is definitely not good. On the other hand, HDL cholesterol, formerly simplistically known as "good" cholesterol, is not always "good". If LDL is high, no matter what the HDL level is, it is important to get the LDL level down.

There are, in fact, people in Italy with low HDL-C (high density lipoprotein cholesterol) who have little in the way of atherosclerosis and seem to live long. These people are born with a variant apolipoprotein A -1 (Apo A –I Milano). This substance is now in an experimental drug that has been shown to make atherosclerosis in the coronary arteries of the heart significantly regress.

Cigarette smoking is a risk factor for the development of atherosclerosis in the coronary arteries that supply the heart, as well as large arteries in the body. With smoking, there is a risk of myocardial infarction and stroke.

Young adults, who are not fit, and often obese, have a higher risk of getting cardiovascular disease. Fortunately, improving fitness can modify that risk.

Other well known risk factors for coronary heart disease are obesity, and chronic disease conditions such as diabetes and high blood pressure (hypertension). There is some suggestion that sleep deprivation, or, conversely, too much sleep (greater than nine hours each night) may somewhat increase the risk of heart attack.

Angina Pectoris:

Coronary arteries can go into spasm even in the absence of arteriosclerosis, leading to a lack of proper oxygenation of the heart muscle.

Nitroglycerin has classically been used to alleviate the chest pain on physical exertion known as Angina Pectoris. Nitro-Dur is a skin (transdermal) patch. The drug acts on the smooth muscle of the vascular system, opening (dilating) blood vessels, reducing the load on the heart, and increasing the blood flow to the heart itself. However, delivered transdermally, the nitroglycerin will not stop a heart attack (myocardial infarction). The use of nitroglycerin in an actual heart attack has not been established. The potential drop in blood pressure with use of this drug should be monitored.

Ranexa (Ranolazine) possibly acts by causing the heart to use glucose instead of fatty acids for energy. The glucose gives more energy with the same amount of oxygen. Changes in the electrocardiogram with severe consequences can occur with this medication, so its use tends to be limited to cases in which other anti-anginal drugs don't work.

Beta blockers, which take up the receptor sites that control blood pressure, are used in angina as well. Blood pressure and heart rate are reduced, so that the heart does less work. Like all other drugs, the administration of this class of drugs has to be carefully controlled by a physician, especially in view of the fact that it is the heart muscle itself, as well as adequate blood circulation , that is at risk. In pregnancy, there is risk to the fetus, as well as to the newborn at birth. As with all drugs and medications in pregnancy, it is important that a qualified physician, who can weigh the possible risks and benefits of taking the drug, is consulted.

In acute coronary syndrome, chest pain occurs at rest, along with changes in the electrocardiogram and echocardiography. Perfusion studies, in which a radioactive isotope is injected to study flow through the heart muscle (myocardium) show alteration. The syndrome can rise to the level of an acute heart attack, or myocardial infarction, which means that heart muscle actually dies. Then biochemical tests of cardiac function, such as serum creatine kinase, become abnormal.

The risk of heart attack (MI, myocardial infarction), stroke, and death can be reduced in people with acute coronary syndrome by taking aspirin daily, possibly along with Plavix (clopidogrel),. Clopidogrel prevents platelets from sticking together: so-called platelet aggregation. Platelets are small fragment-like structures that are present in the blood stream that are necessary for blood coagulation (clotting). Of course, bleeding problems can occur in people taking these types of medications.

Statins, such as Lipitor (atorvastatin), which lower lipid levels and are generally used where cholesterol levels are abnormally high, may be used by physicians in acute coronary syndrome to reduce the recurrence of ischemic events, in which the heart muscle is oxygen deprived. This class of drugs cannot be used in pregnancy, as they inhibit the biosynthesis of cholesterol, which is essential for fetal development.

Arteriosclerotic coronary artery disease, affecting the arteries that supply the heart muscle, can be prevented to a large extent, and its onset delayed. A regular program of aerobic exercise, coupled with a sensible diet is necessary. One of the single most important factors in the causation of this disease is smoking. A person who already smokes cannot undo what has been done but can certainly quit to prevent the ongoing insult. Ideally, the smoking habit should be stopped before it starts. This is a message that should be conveyed to children and grandchildren.

Taking baby aspirin daily has become a widely prescribed measure for preventing permanent heart damage and heart attack. Older people who regularly take aspirin seem to be at a lower risk for death than people who do not take aspirin. It is important to consult with a physician as the anticoagulant properties of the aspirin can lead to serious side effects, such as severe bleeding or hemorrhage from the gastrointestinal tract.

Much attention has been given in the past to personality types and to the repercussions of having a certain personality type on the susceptibility of getting various diseases including coronary artery disease and ulcers of the duodenum. The duodenum is the part of the small intestine closest to the stomach outlet. It has now have been shown that the ulcers were in the main caused by a germ called H.Pylori, and that personality type has nothing to do with it. People were actually placed into programs such as psychotherapy and biofeedback, when all the time all they needed was a couple of weeks of antibiotic therapy. We have now in our collective memory conveniently forgotten about our former misinformed approach to ulcer disease.

On the heart disease issue, things are more complex. No infectious agent has yet been identified that has anything to do with arteriosclerotic heart disease. There were studies that showed that high powered executives did have a higher risk of arteriosclerotic heart disease. However, when someone thought of selecting out the actual bosses or owners from the rest of the executive pool, it was found that the people who actually had the ultimate power and control tended to live longer.

Historically, most of the studies on arteriosclerotic heart disease and its treatments were done on men. There was a relative lack of information on how best to treat women with arteriosclerotic heart disease. Considering that older women have a significant chance of getting arteriosclerotic heart disease and considering that this disease process carries a significant death rate, it was important to develop knowledge concerning women and their propensity for this condition. It is lately being learned that giving supplemental estrogen to women does not decrease the risk of getting arteriosclerotic heart disease and in fact makes the risk of getting heart and cardiovascular disease greater.

There is a familial and genetic propensity to getting arteriosclerotic cardiovascular disease. The promise of genetic manipulation in the future to control that risk is a very exciting possibility. For example, a drug to lower levels of an enzyme (organic catalyst) Lp-PLA2 (Lipoprotein-Associated Phospholipase A2) that is associated with a high risk of coronary artery disease, is being tested.

We have not yet achieved good screening programs to identify people who are at greater risk for arteriosclerotic heart disease. Stories of people who have had perfectly normal electrocardiograms, and within twenty-four hours have had severe heart attacks, are well known and true. The thallium stress test is a far better way of identifying those individuals who are at risk of the disease. The possibility of getting such a test should be discussed with a doctor. More recently, the advent of high speed computerized axial tomography (CAT scan) to image the coronary arteries in the heart and to actually see the arteriosclerotic plaques in the arteries, has become available. Unfortunately, many insurance companies refuse to accept this procedure as a standard screening procedure for arteriosclerotic heart disease although the procedure has already been shown to be life saving for some people. If someone is willing to pay for the test, and is within reach of a medical center, they should be able to arrange for it. A problem with this test is that all the data required to show who needs repair of the coronary arteries is not yet developed. Obviously, as more and more people are screened by the technique, the data base will become fully developed.

Very small implantable cardiac monitors are now in use that continuously transmit data to a bedside console that in turn transmits data to the cardiac unit in a hospital.

Heart Failure:

Congestive heart failure is another form of heart disease that affects many older individuals. The heart in failure is not sufficiently strong to properly circulate the blood, with consequent fluid accumulation in dependent areas such as the legs and feet, and in the lung bases. In acute heart failure, the lungs fill with fluid. This is an emergency situation known as pulmonary edema.

The classical and still predominant treatment for chronic heart failure is the use of drugs derived from digitalis, to strengthen heart muscle contraction.

Natrecor (nesiritide) is a genetically engineered protein that works in properly selected cases of heart failure by reducing lung fluid and reducing blood pressure . An increase in deaths can occur with this drug, so patient selection needs to be careful.

Heart Transplant:

If the heart muscle has undergone widespread damage, or has widespread disease within it, such as cardiomyopathy, heart transplantation has become the state of the art answer. This is no longer an experimental procedure. The surgical techniques for heart transplantation, as well as for kidney and even lung transplantation, are now well worked out and available at major tertiary care medical centers throughout North America. The major problems of the body rejecting transplanted tissue because it is a foreign substance that is not genetically identical to the body's own tissue, remain. However, great advances have been made both in preoperative tissue matching and in the formulation of drugs that damp down the rejection process.

Growing New Heart Muscle:

It is now possible to grow new heart muscle from other body cells. Those other cells are induced to differentiate into muscle cells. The new heart muscle is genetically identical to all the body's other cells, and therefore will not be rejected. Furthermore, the new heart muscle can be genetically altered to prevent cell death: we are approaching the immortal cell, and possibly the immortal heart.

Gene Therapy:

A virus carrying genes that improve the ability of the heart to pump blood can experimentally be injected into the coronary arteries supplying the heart. It may become possible to place various types of stem cells into the heart muscle that then will evolve into new heart muscle cells (myocytes). As well, growth factors placed into the heart muscle might improve blood flow to the heart.

Gene therapy shows promise in forming a natural living cell lining for arterial grafts and damaged arteries.

The Artificial Heart and Medical Cardiac Support:

Research on smaller and more efficient mechanical artificial hearts continues. There are also mechanical devices that assist the efficient pumping of the failing heart (Mechanical Cardiac Support).

Surgical procedures that remodel the heart can be done on the failing heart so that only well performing parts of the heart are effectively pumping blood.

Once the diagnosis of arteriosclerotic coronary artery disease is made, the physician can discuss the steps that must be taken to retard the progression of the disease and to actively correct the problem.

This will depend on a number of factors, including other health problems that may exist, and the severity of the condition at the time of diagnosis. Behavior modification with particular attention to diet and exercise should be addressed. Various medications may need to be used. If high blood pressure (hypertension) is present as well, various antihypertensive medications may be suggested. If cholesterol is out of the acceptable range, as it often is, a cholesterol lowering medication should be used. In fact, it has now been shown that the regular use of Lipitor (atorvastatin) can be useful in the prevention of heart attack.

Hypertension

The cause of most cases of high blood pressure (hypertension) is still unknown. There may be complex hereditary factors at play. Obesity predisposes to hypertension. One of the more striking known causes of high blood pressure is kidney disease (renal disease). Diabetes can be associated with kidney complications and with high blood pressure.

Probably, more than half of all postmenopausal women eventually have to deal with hypertension, as the tendency to get high blood pressure increases with each passing decade. It is important for the doctor to rule out the known causes of high blood pressure before a diagnosis of essential (primary) hypertension is made. The word "essential" is simply a way of saying that the cause is unknown. If the cause can be determined, the treatment obviously is aimed specifically at the known problem. It used to be thought that only the bottom number of the blood pressure was significant for the diagnosis of hypertension (diastolic blood pressure). However, the top number (systolic blood pressure) is important as well.

Hypertension that is left untreated can result in permanent damage. The greatest concern is the possibility of having a stroke, which is a cerebrovascular accident. Heart disease affecting the coronary arteries which nourish the heart is seen with high blood pressure.

Outlying blood vessels in other parts of the body can be affected as well (peripheral vascular disease). The kidneys and the eyes may be damaged by hypertension.

Hypertension is divided into four stages, with Stage I being the mildest. Stage IV hypertension carries the risk of imminent danger and severe consequences, including cerebrovascular accidents, or stroke.

In mild cases, lifestyle changes can be beneficial in reducing the blood pressure. Smoking should be eliminated. A healthful diet, including fruits and vegetables, should be followed, with gradual weight reduction, especially for obese individuals, to an appropriate weight level. A sedentary lifestyle should be changed. Sensible aerobic exercise should be gradually undertaken under the supervision of appropriate medical professionals who are aware of the individual medical condition.

Diuretics:

Diuretics are drugs that increase the output of urine by working at the level of the kidney tubules. The tubules basically make up the kidney and secrete and reabsorb substances. Diuretics remove excess fluid from the body. Thiazides, such as Hydrodiuril (hydrochlorthiazide) are a class of diuretics. When using such drugs, it is important that the potassium level in the blood is carefully checked on a regular basis, and that potassium is properly replaced. This may be accomplished by eating potassium rich foods, such as bananas. Sometimes, potassium intake must be supplemented by pills.

Of course, the use of diuretics, potassium, and all other drugs or supplements must be carefully monitored by a physician. For example, the use of one class of antihypertensive drugs, ACE inhibitors, may actually raise the potassium level. As potassium levels that are too high or too low may both be dangerous, it is important for the physician to monitor the situation. Self medication can be a dangerous thing.

Monoclonal Antibody:

Repatha (evolocumab) given by injection is a human monoclonal immunoglobulin G2 (IgG2) that binds to PCSK9 (human proprotein convertase subtilisin kexin 9), inhibiting it from binding to the LDL (low density lipoprotein) receptor. This increases the number of LDL receptors available to clear LDL from the blood. Consequently, LDL cholesterol levels are lowered.

Beta Blockers:

A class of drugs called beta blockers are widely used to control high blood pressure. Inderal (propanolol hydrochloride) is such a drug. The drug goes to and fills up the receptor sites in the autonomic nervous system, which controls blood pressure, so that receptor stimulants cannot attach there. All human cells have specially shaped sites where specific substances will normally attach, like a key in a lock. Beta blockers probably act at the level of vasomotor centers in the brain, at the level of the kidneys to inhibit release of a substance called Renin, and at the level of the heart to reduce cardiac output (work).

Again, physicians weigh benefits against possible risks and known contraindications before prescribing these drugs. In pregnancy, there are risks to the fetus and the newborn .

Ace Inhibitors:

Depending on the individual case, the class of drugs known as ACE inhibitors, such as Vasotec (enalapril) Prinivil (lisinopril), Mavik (trandolapril), and Altace (ramipril) may be prescribed. Such drugs should not be used by pregnant women, because of the risk of harm and death to the developing fetus. As a matter of fact, no drug or medication should be taken by any woman who might be, or might become, pregnant, without checking with her doctor first.

ACE refers to the angiotensin-converting enzyme, which is inhibited by these drugs. They work to lower blood pressure by stopping the formation of a substance called angiotensin II, which constricts (tightens) blood vessels, partially shutting them off.

Like all prescription drugs, ACE inhibitors should be carefully used only on the direction of skilled physicians who are aware of possible side effects. For example, in people of a specific genotype who have had reopening and stenting of the coronary arteries, treatment with ACE inhibitors may make the coronary arteries more prone to closing again (Restenosis).

Angiotensin Receptor Blockers:

Other drugs, called A.R.B.'s, block the angiotensin receptor, so that angiotensin cannot attach there. Diovan (valsartan) is an angiotensin II antagonist that blocks the binding of angiotensin II to the AT1 receptor in tissues including vascular smooth muscle. Another such drug is Cozaar (losartan). These drugs carry the same warning of severe harm to a developing fetus and should not be used in pregnancy.

ACE inhibitors and ARB's can prevent heart attacks and strokes. These drugs can be useful in preventing or delaying the appearance of diabetes. They seem to have some positive effect on retaining skeletal muscle mass as people age. ACE inhibitors are better than calcium antagonists in preventing coronary artery disease and heart failure.

Calcium Channel Blockers:

A class of antihypertensive drugs that had been widely used, calcium channel blockers, actually increase cardiovascular risk, including the risk of angina and heart attack.

It is important to look at the big picture. Antihypertensive medications are not the whole answer to high blood pressure. High cholesterol must be lowered. The tendency to be overweight should be corrected.

Daily aspirin should be considered to prevent the tendency to blood clots. Good kidney function must be maintained.

Hypercholesterolemia

It is not merely the total high cholesterol levels in the blood that increase the risk of plaque formation in the arteries resulting in arteriosclerotic disease, with an increased chance of getting heart attack and stroke. Substances called low density lipoproteins (LDL) are elevated in this condition. That is why LDL was formerly known as 'bad' cholesterol. High density lipoproteins (HDL), formerly known as 'good' cholesterol, tend to be at lower than normal levels with arteriosclerosic disease. However, a high level of HDL is not always a good thing. The optimal balance of these lipoproteins should be maintained, but it is most important to bring down high levels of LDL, no matter what the HDL level. Genetic predisposition does play a role in the levels of these lipoproteins.

A major public health problem associated with arteriosclerotic disease in America today is obesity. Smoking is another factor that increases the propensity to heart disease and stroke. The natural way to decrease the tendency to heart disease and stroke is to maintain a healthy diet and to keep to a regular pattern of aerobic exercise. The American diet generally tends to include far too much saturated fat. Hydrogenated oils, found in margarine and snack foods tend to be a major culprit. Fast food chains classically fry with these substances, although attempts have been made recently to cut down on this practice. Unfortunately, as children many of us are conditioned to eat foods high in saturated fat and salt, which we then think of as tasting good our whole lives.

It is important that mature adults regularly have the cholesterol level checked, including levels of HDL and LDL. The doctor will advise necessary dietary modification. However, it is difficult for most people to modify eating habits that have been established over a lifetime, and often difficult to maintain an ideal weight.

People who eat more fish have a lower risk of coronary heart disease. Fish oil supplements containing Omega-3 fatty acids can be beneficial as well, as Omega-3 fatty acids probably give the fish its protective effect.

Fortunately, there are drugs available that can reduce very low density lipoprotein concentration (VLDL), and encourage the LDL receptor. Increased uptake of LDL-C (low density lipoprotein cholesterol) and decreased production of this substance results. The amount of LDL circulating in the blood is reduced in consequence. At the same time concentrations of HDL-C (high density lipoprotein cholesterol) are increased. Higher concentrations of HDL seem sometimes to be protective against heart attack and stroke. However, the situation is more complicated than this. White people often have a mutation in a gene called the cholesteryl ester transfer protein gene. People with this gene mutation have an increased risk of cardiovascular disease when their HDL is high.

Statins:

The drugs that reduce low density lipoprotein and encourage the LDL receptor are known as statins. This group of drugs includes Lipitor (atorvastatin), Zocor (simvastatin) and Mevacor (lovastatin).

Statins reduce the inflammation of atherosclerosis. The coronary arteries that supply the heart muscle are therefore less likely to get blocked. Lipitor has now been shown to be capable of stopping the progress of atherosclerosis.

The natural pathways of cholesterol biosynthesis are very important to fetal development. Statins should not be used during pregnancy

Beyond the statins, research is continuing on drugs that can lower LDL-C levels and levels of triglicerides in other ways.

Cholesterol Inhibitors:

Zetia (ezetimibe) inhibits the intestine from absorbing cholesterol. LDL and triglycerides are lowered, along with apolipoprotein B (Apo B) which is a major protein in LDL.

Vytorin is a combination of Zetia and Zocor.

Bile Acid Sequestrants:

WelChol (colesevelam) is an example of this class of drugs that bind bile acids in the intestine, so that they are excreted. This in turn triggers increased conversion of cholesterol to bile acids in the liver. LDL cholesterol (LDL-C) gets used in this process and is cleared from the blood, lowering LDL levels.

There is an increased need for vitamins and nutrients in pregnancy. The effect of WelChol on the absorption of vitamins in the pregnant woman is not known.

Angiography:

If one or more coronary arteries is significantly clogged, it may become necessary to undergo a procedure to correct this. Microinvasive techniques now exist. These are performed either by an interventional radiologist or by a cardiologist specifically trained to do these procedures. These techniques involve threading small devices through the blood vessels and into the clogged arteries to reopen the channels. Angiography is a technique used to place dye into the coronary arteries, which are the blood vessels of the heart. Narrowing or blocking of these arteries can then be seen radiologically. A stent, which is a mesh made of stainless steel, can then be placed under direct Xray visualization into the narrowed blood vessel. The stent may be coated with a drug that discourages regrowth of cells in the artery wall. A balloon inside the stent is then inflated, opening the mesh of the stent into place around the inside of the vessel wall to keep the blood vessel open. The balloon is then removed. There are specific indications that should be followed for stent placement.

This technique, called PCI (percutaneous coronary intervention) is a heart saving, often life saving procedure that should often be used when a coronary artery is blocked in a classic acute heart attack. MI (myocardial infarction) refers to the impending death of heart muscle (myocardium) when the blood vessel nourishing it with oxygen blocks off. A plaque of arteriosclerosis in the blood vessel wall ruptures, sending its contents into the channel of the vessel. Platelets stick to the artery's wall and a blood clot (thrombus) fills the vessel, blocking it.

Bypass procedures performed by cardiac surgeons quite routinely now use blood vessels taken from other parts of the body to effectively go around the blocked channels and create open paths for oxygen carrying blood to get to and nourish the heart muscle.

It is now possible to use the vein accompanying each coronary artery to bypass the compromised artery, by opening into the vein, changing the direction of its blood flow.

Robotic Surgery:

Coronary artery bypass procedures can now be done by robotic minimally invasive surgery. The use of robotic arms, by the surgeon seated at a console, visualizing the organ being operated on in three dimensions on a screen is being used in a wide variety of procedures. Robotics allow the surgeon to make fine, tremor-free movements with small articulated (jointed) instruments.

The big advantage of robotic surgery is "motion scaling". The surgeon at the console makes large hand movements, which the computer translates into tiny precise microscopic movements at the tips of the instruments placed within the patient.

Laser beams can be used to create new channels in heart muscle, improving the blood flow to the heart. (Transmyocardial Laser Revascularization; TMR).

Advanced drugs are now available to help prevent blood clotting during some interventional procedures. For example, ReoPro (abciximab)is a monoclonal antibody that stops blood platelets from getting together, or aggregating, thus preventing blood clots and oxygen deprivation to the heart.

In cases of gradually advancing arteriosclerotic coronary artery disease, the body itself will build new channels, called collateral circulation, to the heart muscle. This happens after a heart attack as well. The first heart attack in a relatively young individual can be a particularly dangerous situation, because collateral circulation has not had the opportunity to form. Therefore, the area of potential death of heart muscle can be much larger.

When a heart attack does occur, it is necessary that supporting intervention is quick and sure. Many people now take cardiac life support classes. If they are confronted with an emergency situation, they can be of immediate assistance until professional help arrives by ambulance. Modern intensive care and cardiac care units are equipped to take care of these emergencies. Monitoring is instituted, and appropriate support is given so that vital signs are maintained. Specific drugs that prevent and dissolve blood clots in the vessels may be administered. More and more, angiography is quickly done to see the blocked artery, and PCI is performed to open it. Pretreatment may be done with lower dose Retavase (reteplase) which dissolves the clot. Retavase. is a form of Tissue Plasminogen Activator (TPA) produced by recombinant DNA technology.

TNKase (tenecteplase) is available for use in cases of acute myocardial infarction (heart attack). It is produced by recombinant DNA technology. It, as well, is a form of TPA.

Plavix (clopidogrel) can decrease actual heart attack and stroke in cases of acute chest pain. It is used to prevent blood clotting after angioplasty. The drug prevents platelets, a blood clotting component, from aggregating.

As protection or prophylaxis against such an event, a baby aspirin a day is often prescribed by doctors. This regimen should only be undertaken on the advice of a physician, as the aspirin does interfere with the blood clotting mechanism, and there may be other conditions present which would be adversely affected by this treatment. A woman in the menopausal age group, having a bleeding problem, should discuss this issue with a qualified gynecologist.

Of course, it is wise to seek the advice of a qualified physician before taking any drug or medication that interferes with the normal blood clotting mechanism. This is especially true if pregnancy is contemplated.

Stroke

It is important to differentiate between two different types of stroke. There can be actual hemorrhage into the brain tissue, or a blood clot can occur in one of the vessels of the brain, leading to the death of the brain tissue nourished by that vessel. In either case, the symptoms may be similar, causing the loss of various functions depending upon which area of the brain is affected. These may include paralysis and a loss of speech. Immediate emergency care is of course required. The treatment will be dependent upon the mechanism. A hemorrhage cannot be treated in the same way as a blood clot.

Unfortunately, replacing estrogen and progesterone (Hormone Replacement Therapy, HRT) in postmenopausal women increases the risk of getting a stroke.

Elevated levels of homocysteine, an amino acid building block of protein, seem to be related to the risk of stroke. Elevated levels of homocysteine seem to be related to heart attack risk, as well.

Taking Vitamins B6 (pyridoxine), B10 (folic acid) and B12 (cobalamin), lowers homocysteine levels, causes plaque in the carotid blood vessels in the neck to regress, and restores the function of the lining of vessels. There is a genetic propensity to elevated homocysteine levels. Homocysteine levels do, however, go up in stroke patients, so that the elevated levels may be an effect of the stroke, rather than a cause.

The goal in treatment of a stroke, once it has occurred, is to prevent, as much as possible, the death of brain cells that have been deprived of oxygen. That is why early diagnosis and treatment are so important.

The prompt use of TPA (tissue plasminogen activator) in a stroke caused by blood clot can be of vital importance. TPA dissolves blood clots by converting a protein, plasminogen into plasmin. This substance cannot, of course, be used in strokes caused by bleeding into the brain, as the problem would be made worse.

It is possible to deliver thrombolytic (clot-dissolving) agents directly into the clot in the artery, with visualization of the clot by angiography.

A promising approach in stroke patients in whom brain cells have already died is to transplant new brain cells. One approach is to use stem cells taken from bone marrow, and convert them into neurons, which are nerve cells. Such cells could be important not only in treating stroke victims, but also people with brain and spinal cord injury, and people with Parkinson's disease.

There is a well known condition called Transient Ischemic Arteriospasm (TIA). The name is quite descriptive. Blood vessels in the brain constrict, partially closing down, causing a transient and temporary loss of function to the specific area of the brain served by those vessels. This can result in temporary loss of speech, vision, or paralysis. The neurologist will perform appropriate examinations and imaging studies, and then treat the condition, usually with medication. Again, it is important to rule out any significant underlying cause and to make sure that the diagnosis is accurate. The possibility of having an aneurysm or tumor must be ruled out.

It is important to identify people with significant disease in the major blood vessels supplying the brain, the carotid arteries, so that the narrowing caused by arteriosclerosis can be corrected surgically, preventing a stroke. The classic, reliable, surgical procedure utilized to achieve this is carotid endarterectomy. Carotid endarterectomy is a technique in which the arterial lumen (opening) through which the blood flows, is widened. Carotid angioplasty may be done, placing a balloon in the artery and inflating it, to increase the size of the opening, which is then held open by a stent. A stent is a structural support placed within a blood vessel that holds the vessel open.

Aneurysm

An aneurysm is a weakening in a wall of a blood vessel, so that it bulges out. The threat is that the weakened, bulging area can burst, causing a hemorrhage. Brain hemorrhage can occur in this way.

Another relatively common site of aneurysm is in the aorta. The aorta is the main blood vessel that carries blood from the heart to the other arteries in the body. An aortic aneurysm may be thoracic, in which case it occurs in the chest behind the lungs, or abdominal, where the aorta overlies the spine behind the abdominal organs. Smoking increases the risk of getting an aneurysm in the abdomen.

Modern cardiologists and radiologists have the diagnostic capability of discovering these aneurysms before they can do damage, and neurologists and radiologists have the same capability for the diagnosis of aneurysms in the brain. Depending on the location of the aneurysm, it can then usually be operated on by a neurosurgeon if it is in the brain, or a cardiovascular surgeon if it is in the thoracic (chest) or abdominal areas. In the brain, clips may be applied to the affected blood vessel so that it no longer carries blood. Some aneurysms, notably at the base of brain, are congenital. In other words, the person is born with the problem, which often does not become evident until there is leakage of blood into the brain and symptoms occur. Very precise radiosurgery techniques have now been devised to specifically deal with such problems.

In the abdominal and thoracic areas, the weakened area of blood vessel is removed and replaced with a synthetic implant, which then carries the blood in a normal fashion. Minimally invasive techniques are being used in some cases. Laparoscopy, and robotic surgical techniques may be employed.

It is even now possible to "patch" a weakened bulge in the abdominal aorta, the main artery from the heart. The patch, which is really a stent graft that opens within the aorta, is inserted closed into the blood vessel from the inside, through a major artery in the groin area: the iliac artery. This technique may lower the risk of the procedure.

This technique may also be used in the diseased iliac artery itself. The iliac arteries are the major vessels supplying the legs and the pelvis.

Peripheral Artery Occlusive Disease:

It is not only the large, "important" arteries in the body that are affected by arteriosclerosis. Smaller arteries serving the limbs, down to the fingers and toes, can become narrowed and blocked.

Regular physical activity is one good way to help prevent this problem. It is important not to smoke. Surprisingly, people who drink one half to one alcoholic drink per day seem to have a lower risk of this problem.

People with arteriosclerotic disease in the legs tend to have arteriosclerosis throughout the body, and are at risk for heart attacks. It is important to diagnose this often unrecognized problem and to start treatment.

A simple test is the ABI (low ankle-brachial index). This is a calculation made from the measurement of the pulses in the feet by Doppler ultrasound evaluation of the blood flow.

People with narrowing or blockage (occlusion) of arteries in the leg are treated with cholesterol lowering drugs. Aspirin may be recommended to prevent blood clotting (thrombosis). Plavix (Clopidogrel) prevents blood platelets from coming together (aggregating), preventing blood clotting.

It sometimes becomes necessary with this condition to do bypass surgery. Vein grafts, usually taken from the affected person, are used to get around blocked areas. Angioplasty and stents can be used, depending on the specific blood vessels involved.

Varicose Veins (Venous Stasis):

The valves in the veins of the legs can be damaged, and blood that should be returning to the heart remains in the veins. This is called venous stasis. The veins bulge out, resulting in the well- known, and much disliked, bluish varicose veins.

The problem can now often be treated endoscopically, interrupting the affected veins. It is possible in some cases to actually correct an incompetent vein valve.

The classical treatment of varicose veins was known as vein stripping, actually removing the damaged vein. Such veins can now be treated with radiofrequency or laser.

Thromboembolism:

People with poor venous circulation in the legs are at some risk of developing blood clots (thrombosis). When bits of clot break off, they travel in the blood stream to the heart, and then possibly to the lungs. A blood clot in the lung is called a pulmonary embolus (PE). This is an acute, life-threatening emergency. It is now known that long airline flights, with prolonged sitting, can increase the risk for blood clots in the legs and pulmonary embolism. Elastic compression stockings can be helpful. Drugs that lessen the chances of blood clotting may be needed.

Pulmonary embolism can now be diagnosed quickly by spiral CT (cat scan).

References

1. https://www.ncbi.nlm.nih.gov/pmcarticles/PMC6361748/
2. www.repathahcp.com/
3. Bibliography & Supplemental Bibliography: See www.rcaplanmd.com

CHAPTER 5
CANCER

The Take-Home Message

- Early diagnosis and treatment is vital: act decisively
- Very specific DNA cancer markers for early detection of cancer are becoming available
- Know the characteristics of a person's individual tumor cell, to see if targeted therapy is available
- Immunotherapy to treat cancer is a reality
- Specific drugs do exist that can go directly to the cancer cell
- Keep the tumor tissue removed at surgery for further testing
- Stay away from carcinogens that cause cancer
- Test for gene mutations that cause susceptibility to cancer
- There are drugs available that can protect against breast cancer
- Cancer can be converted from a killer to a chronic disease condition
- Anticancer vaccines now exist

Beyond heart and cardiovascular disease, the biggest danger confronted by older people is cancer.

When my mother founded the Cancer Research Society in Canada more than seventy years ago, in 1945, she was motivated by her own mother's untimely early death from breast cancer.

She was interested in finding the 'cause' and 'cure' for cancer by encouraging funding in the United States and Canada for institutions and research scientists. Her dream is not yet fulfilled, but we have come a long way in understanding the mechanisms involved in various cancers, and even the cause of some cancers.

Cancer is a multitude of disease conditions with various causes and many manifestations that have a common characteristic. Cell growth becomes bizarre and out of control. The disease process can spread to various parts of the body. When vital organs are affected, so that they no longer can function properly, death can quickly follow.

The common pathway in cancer is the disruption of cell genetics, so that the genes responsible for orderly cell death at the end of the normal life span of the cell do not operate. Normally in the body, new cells are formed by an orderly process of cell division. These cells mature, age, and eventually die, to be replaced by new cells that are constantly being regenerated in an orderly fashion. This is one of the major reasons why the decoding of the human genome is so important. If the genes at fault in a cancer can be determined, then they can be dealt with so that the cancer cells will not be immortal. At the same time, genes will be able to be identified that govern the aging process in an individual, so that normal cell lines will be able to be kept normally growing and regenerating, thus greatly prolonging life expectancy. Obviously, there is much research work to be done in this area.

Genes that cause a predisposition to various types of cancer have already been identified. Notably, the HER- 2 gene which can be present in women, leads to an increased risk of breast cancer. That is not to say that all women with the HER-2 gene will definitely get breast cancer. However, there is a drug, Herceptin (trastuzumab), which is effective against breast cancer in women who carry the HER-2 gene. This is an exciting example of the new generation of specific designer drugs that are aimed at populations who have a specific disease process. There will be a virtual explosion of such effective targeted treatments of various diseases in the future.

It is not now as important to know the site at which a cancer originally arose, as to know the cellular and receptor status of the tumor cells in each affected individual. In other words, the tumor itself is tested for specific cellular characteristics. Herceptin, a monoclonal antibody created by recombinant DNA technology, binds to the human epidermal growth factor receptor HER- 2 , inhibiting proliferation of the tumor cells that overexpress HER-2. It is now becoming evident that Herceptin can be used as well in women with lung cancer who express the HER - 2 gene.

Like all drugs, Herceptin must be used with care by competent physicians. One of the notable complications can be cardiac (heart) dysfunction. In pregnancy, consultation with qualified physicians is required to weigh the possible benefits against risks to both mother and her growing fetus.

Monoclonal antibodies go directly to receptor sites on the cancer cell surface, blocking the cell from dividing. The next generation of drugs will include monoclonal antibodies that not only bind to the cancer cell, but also carry a substance that will destroy it. In other words the drug will not simply retard the progress of the cancer, it will destroy it: the word 'cure' may begin to have real meaning in certain types of cancer.

Lung Cancer

There is nothing so helpless as a physician who prides herself or himself as being a healer, watching a beloved one die of a devastating disease. I was in that position. My wife, at too young an age, with incredible determination and bravery, coped with lung cancer, and treatments including multiple major surgeries, radiation, and chemotherapy that left her incapacitated and outwardly changed, but never took away her inner beauty, grace, or compassion. She finally succumbed after seven years.

We do know characteristics that predispose people to various types of cancer. The most glaring example of this is lung cancer. This disease, which has become a predominant killer of women as well as men, is almost totally preventable. It has only recently been publicized that lung cancer is as great, or a greater, threat to women than even breast cancer, or cancers of the female reproductive organs. A root cause in a vast majority of cases is smoking. There is recent evidence that smoking by women may be even more dangerous than smoking by men.

It is easier to never start smoking than to stop after the addictive effects have taken hold. However, societal pressures and peer pressure do impact heavily on teenagers and preteens. Cigarette advertising, although now targeted away from children in America, is still prevalent. The desire to be "cool", adult, and socially accepted can outweigh counterpressure from physicians, family, and ostracism by public facilities and restaurants. The desire to curb appetite and hunger, and to remain thin, often unreasonably thin, is a significant factor in young women and girls. I am often struck by the numbers of young women on 'break' standing outside office buildings, smoking.

Once smoking has started, of course, cumulative lung damage occurs. It is still better to stop, even after many years of smoking, to prevent the continuous insult to sensitive tissue and the exposure to carcinogens.

Various patches containing nicotine, such as Nicoderm are effective in many cases to help stop smoking. Smokers can gradually wean themselves from the oral gratification of the habit, without having to undergo sudden nicotine withdrawal. There are, of course, possible side effects to the use of these patches, including increased heart rate and blood pressure.

It is well known that smoking in pregnancy is harmful to the developing fetus, as well as to the course of the pregnancy, and to the mother herself. It is better whenever possible to use behavior modification measures rather than to resort to the use of Nicoderm or Zyban during a pregnancy. A knowledgeable physician should be consulted before using these, or any other drugs in pregnancy.

Zyban (bupropion) has been advocated for smoking cessation. This medication is essentially the antidepressant Wellbutrin. There is an increased risk of suicidality in adolescents with Major Depressive Disorders who take this, or some other antidepressant drugs. Bulemic and anorexic people should not take this drug, because of a heightened chance of seizures.

Tobacco smoke carries carcinogens that get into the breathing passages of the lungs, called bronchi. The smoke also travels into the actual air sacs themselves, which are called alveoli. The use of filtered cigarettes does not help. Smoke particles are simply smaller and therefore can get further into the lung tissue. Various terms describe the site of the lung cancer, the virulence of the cancer cells, and the stage to which it has progressed.

Bronchogenic carcinoma means that the cancer has developed primarily in the breathing passageways leading from the air sacs towards to the trachea, or windpipe. The usual cell type of lung cancer is called non-small cell cancer (NSCLC). A minority of lung cancers are small cell lung cancers.

Cancer Stage:

The stage of the cancer refers to how contained the cancer is or how far it has spread, when it is first diagnosed. A Stage One tumor is confined to its area of initial growth and has not spread to nearby lymph nodes or to distant organs. Any cancer is capable of breaking through the boundaries of the initial tumor and invading local organs and tissues or getting into the lymphatic system which is a drainage system in the body leading into connected lymph nodes. These are small nodules that are designed to fight infection. Here the tumor cells multiply and divide, enlarging the lymph nodes. As well, cancer cells spread through the blood stream to distant organs.

Common sites for the spread of lung cancer, and many other cancers, include liver, brain, and bone. The heightened metabolic activity of these very active cancer implants, called metastases, can be picked up by sophisticated diagnostic tests such as PET scan (positron emission tomography). Bone metastases can be picked up by bone scan. Small metastases, often in lymph nodes, can be picked up by CAT scan (computerized axial tomography) or MRI (magnetic resonance imaging).

Tumors are deemed to be resectable or nonresectable. A resectable tumor is one that can be completely removed at surgery. In lung cancer, if it is detected early, which is still unfortunately in the minority of cases, the first line of treatment today is to remove the tumor. In modern centers, this is usually preceded by mediastinoscopy. Using very small incisions, the thoracic surgeon places a fiberoptic scope directly into the mediastinum, which is the area surrounding the heart, major blood vessels, and trachea (windpipe). The surgeon can get a good idea of the stage of the disease before doing full scale surgery and can better plan for that surgery.

Early Diagnosis of Lung Cancer:

Traditionally, chest x-rays were used to scan large groups of people for chest disease when tuberculosis was widespread in our society. However, these screening programs were stopped. Nowadays, we have 'fast' spiral CT scans that pick up even tiny early lung tumors, when they are still Stage I with an excellent survival rate. The spiral CT scan can even determine the size of atherosclerotic plaques in the heart blood supply (coronary arteries) that usually cause no symptoms until a coronary artery is effectively blocked and heart muscle dies – a heart attack. There is much discussion concerning how the widespread use of 'fast' spiral CT scans will greatly increase the cost of medical care, and even lead to 'unnecessary' procedures including surgery to remove small lung masses that turn out to be benign, and excessive numbers of procedures to open coronary arteries. Of course, HMO's tend not to pay for spiral CT scans in people without symptoms, on the basis that the test is not 'indicated', and, of course, costly.

HMO's also tend to create Rating Lists of physicians who participate in their plans. Often, physicians whose cost of treating patients is lower get a higher approval rating than other physicians. This practice has triggered governmental investigation of some HMO's .

Still, many sophisticated people are going for this fast, painless, non-invasive, and informative test. The whole point is to discover major disease early, before symptoms are present. How to make use of the information you obtain should, of course, be discussed with a qualified consultant, such as a lung specialist (pulmonary medicine), a lung (thoracic) surgeon, or a cardiologist if heart disease is discovered.

Tumor Grade:

Depending on the Stage and Grade of lung cancer, the surgical treatment is often followed up with radiation. Chemotherapy might be added on an individualized basis. The Grade of the tumor refers to how bizarre the cells have become. Grade I cells do not look much different from normal cells. Higher grade cells bear little resemblance to any normal tissue and show evidence of very active cell division in their chromosomes which are present in the nucleus (center) of each cell. Obviously, the worse the Grade, and the higher the Stage, the less chance the person has of long term survival.

Many exciting treatments, however, are becoming available for people with lung cancer and other cancers. Radiation, even though it is now carefully applied with the aid of computer programs, inevitably damages normal tissue along with cancer cells. Traditional chemotherapy, unfortunately, does the same thing.

Immunotherapy to Treat Cancer:

From modest beginnings, immunotherapy has now advanced to the point that there are suggested possible treatments for various Stages and Grades of malignant tumors, alphabetically from A: acute lymphoblastic leukemia to V: vulvar cancer.

There are basically five types of immunotherapy:

Immune checkpoint inhibitors:

Checkpoints are a part of the immune system that prevent immune responses from being overly strong and destroying healthy body cells. Inhibition of checkpoints allows the body's own immune cells to respond more aggressively to cancer. Checkpoints include the PD-1 protein present on T-cells.

T-cell transfer therapy (adoptive cell therapy):

Heightens the ability of the body's own T-lymphocytes to act against a cancer. Immune cells are taken from the tumor, enhanced, multiplied outside the body, then reinserted into the affected person intravenously.

Monoclonal antibodies:

It is now possible to identify specific receptor sites in tumor tissue that can be attacked by antibodies. These so-called monoclonal antibodies are directed to specific sites on the cancer cell surface.

"Monoclonal" refers to the fact that the antibody protein is derived from one clone of cells, all of which are identical. Such drugs are now under very active development, and many are now available. The drug will not cause damage to any cell that does not have the specific receptor that is being attacked in the cancer cell.

Unfortunately, even these drugs are not totally specific, because normal cells in the human body often share the same receptor being targeted in the tumor cell. However, the side effects tend to be minimal in relation to the life saving effect of the monoclonal antibody.

One such drug specifically attacks tumor cells bearing endothelial growth factor (EGF) receptor. The drug binds to the receptor on the cell surface, blocking the cell from dividing. Obviously, this drug, Erbitux (cetuximab) a recombinant monoclonal antibody, works only on those cancers that contain that specific receptor. There are, however, significant numbers of tumors that do have that specific receptor. Promising results have been reported in tumors of the head and neck, and in colon cancer, although no data shows increased survival in the colon cancer cases. Studies were undertaken for lung cancer, and pancreatic cancer. Complications included infusion reactions and cardiopulmonary arrest.

As Erbitux is an inhibitor of the EGF Receptor which is operative in prenatal development, it can be harmful to a developing pregnancy.

Ironically, when Erbitux was first made experimentally, no major drug company was found that would bring it through the rigorous FDA approval process and to market.

A smaller venture company, called Imclone, did back the drug, then called C 225, and tried for years to take it through the approval process. Experienced oncologists did note that the drug did slow down tumors, with minimal side effects. However, the FDA found Imclone's application to be deficient, and rejected it. The price of Imclone shares plummeted, and the Chief Executive Officer, Sam Waksal, went to jail.

A major drug company, Bristol- Myers Squibb, in the meantime, had effectively taken control of the Erbitux trial, and the FDA finally approved the drug. As a final irony, the price of Imclone shares went up again.

My own wife, after all else failed, was placed on Erbitux on a compassionate use basis, when it was proven that her lung cancer cells had EGF receptors. Her disease remained stable for a few years, then broke through again. A final course of Iressa (gefitinib) could not contain it.

As cancer treatment progresses, targeted treatments will be used much earlier, so that cancer patients will be spared the debilitating, often permanent side effects of radiation, chemotherapy, and radical surgery.

The FDA walks a fine line. There is always this or that claim of a miracle drug that cures cancer, often promoted by charlatans who prey on the most vulnerable and suggestible: people who are dying of cancer and are desperate.

Even the most well intentioned scientists can put great effort into possible anti-cancer treatments that at first seen promising, but in the end turn out to be useless or worse.

It is essential that controlled scientific studies statistically prove that a drug has real beneficial effect before it is released for use.

On the other hand, all bureaucracies seem to place an inordinate amount of faith in 'paperwork' – or nowadays computer communications – that properly fit into the prescribed forms. There is an almost prohibitive cost, as well as a long passage of time, needed to satisfy the requirements of the FDA.

Iressa (gefitinib) may be taken orally. Although it is not a monoclonal antibody, it does block intracellular events secondary to EGF receptor activation. Although Iressa can cause reduction in the size of tumors in people with advanced lung cancer, it has not been shown to significantly increase their life expectancy. Interstitial lung disease, including pneumonia, can be a complication. The drug can cause fetal harm if used in pregnancy.

Tarceva (erlotinib) inhibits the EGF Receptor. Tarceva may work against lung, ovarian, and head and neck tumors. The use of this drug in pregnancy should be avoided.

These drugs have been approved by the FDA for use in specific patients with non-small cell lung cancer who do not respond to chemotherapy. Tarceva has been shown to prolong survival in non-small cell lung cancer patients. Interstitial lung disease, including pneumonia, and an increased incidence of heart attack can be complications.

Checkpoint Inhibitors that are used in advanced non-small-cell lung cancer (NSCLC) are Tecentriq (atezolizumab), Imfinzi (durvalumab), Opdivo (nivolumab) and Keytruda (pembrolizumab).

Sending monoclonal antibodies to receptor sites in cancer cells is something like sending a soldier into battle unarmed, to place his or her body in the way of an invasion. It makes sense to give the soldier a weapon to kill the invader.

Monoclonal antibodies can be attached to a radioactive isotope. When the antibody attaches to the tumor cell, the radioactivity then specifically kills that abnormal cell. This is the targeted 'hunt and kill' approach that has been sought after for years.

One such drug is Zevalin (ibritumomab tiuxetan) which may be used to treat certain cases of non-Hodgkin's lymphoma in conjunction with Rituxan. One form of Zevalin uses the radioisotope Indium -111, and the other form uses Yttrium-90. Both forms of Zevalin are given during the treatment regime .Severe side effects , including effects on essential components of blood, do occur. If Zevalin is used, a woman should avoid becoming pregnant, as her fetus could be harmed.

Major side effects, including fatal infusion reactions, can occur with the use of Zevalin in conjunction with Rituxan (rituximab). Rituxan is a genetically engineered monoclonal antibody that targets the surface of B lymphocytes, a form of white blood cell.

Malignant B lymphocytes are present in cases of B-cell non-Hodgkin's lymphoma. Rituxan use in pregnancy can result in immunosuppression in the child. The risks in pregnancy must be carefully weighed by qualified physicians against any possible benefit.

Bexxar (tositumomab) is another radioactive monoclonal antibody that can be used in certain refractory cases of non-Hodgkin's lymphoma. The radioactive component is Iodine I-131. Severe side effects, notably impacting essential components of blood, occur with this drug as well .It should not be used in pregnancy : it can harm the fetal thyroid gland.

Generators of alpha particles that are the size of molecules, delivered by monoclonal antibodies into cancer cells are called targeted atomic nanogenerators.

Treatment Vaccines:

Cancer cells contain tumor-associated antigens that are not found at all, or only found at low levels, in normal cells. Vaccines made from a person's own tumor cells are then given back to the affected person, leading to an enhanced immune response against the tumor itself.

Dendritic cell (a type of immune cell) vaccines are made from the dendritic cells of the individual cancer patient.

Alternatively, a vaccine can be made from tumor associated antigens found on cancer cells of various people who have a specific type of cancer. This type of vaccine could theoretically cause an immune response in anyone with a cancer producing that antigen. This is an experimental technique.

Immune System Modulators:

These agents stimulate the immune system so that it more efficiently attacks tumors and responds to viruses. Intron A (Interferon Alfa-2B) produced by recombinant DNA technique is one such drug. It may be used in certain cases of leukemia, lymphoma, melanoma, AIDS-related Kaposi's sarcoma and genital warts. However, side effects of the use of this and similar drugs can be fatal.

Proleukin (Aldesleukin) is produced by recombinant DNA technology. It is a form of Interleulkin-2 which activates cellular immunity and inhibits tumor growth. It can be used in certain cases of renal (kidney) cell cancer, Severe side effects may be fatal.

Antisense Technology:

Genes that are active in cancer formation may be turned off by the introduction of actual pieces of the genetic code. This is called "anti-sense" technology.

PTK's (protein-tyrosine kinase) regulate signaling in the cell. When PTK signaling is disrupted by genetic alteration and mutation, malignant transformation of the cell can result.

Gleevec (imatinib mesylate) is a drug that binds receptors in chronic myelogenous leukemia. It is a tyrosine kinase inhibitor. It blocks the 'abl' signaling protein, which causes overactive cell division in this disease. The drug inhibits the activity of a growth factor receptor called the 'c - kit' receptor, and therefore also works against gastrointestinal stromal tumor, which is a rare form of stomach cancer. Side effects of Gleevec include toxicity to liver and blood cells. Gleevec should be avoided in pregnancy, as it is hazardous to the fetus.

Gene Therapy:

Gene therapy is an exciting approach. Cancer cells multiply by unrelenting cell division, so that there is unrestrained growth of the tumor mass. Often, there is a mutation of a gene called p 53 in tumor cells. Normally, the p 53 gene elaborates the p 53 protein, which prevents abnormal cells from dividing. Even in cancer cells where this gene has not mutated, the p 53 protein is inactivated in other ways.

The p 53 protein may have a role in the aging process. Too much p 53 protein may result in premature aging. A balance has to be maintained: you do not want to have too little p 53, nor too much. The p53 protein stops cell division and triggers cell death, as well as repairing damaged DNA. These functions are important in ridding the body of potentially cancerous cells. At the same time, these same functions can hasten the aging process.

A promising treatment that can be used involves inserting p 53 into an adenovirus from which the contents have been removed. The adenovirus is the virus that causes the common cold. The altered adenovirus with the p 53 is then administered. The p 53 then prevents the abnormal cancer cells from dividing. This treatment has shown promise in causing regression of lung, head and neck, and possibly ovarian tumors.

It may become possible to use altered viruses themselves to attack cancer cells. For example, an adenovirus with a damaged gene called Onyx-015 will grow only in cancer cells.

The FHIT gene (fragile histidine triad gene) resides at a site on the chromosome that is fragile and susceptible to carcinogens in the environment, including the carcinogens in cigarette smoke. Loss of this gene results in FHIT- negative cancer cells. This phenomenon can be present in lung, stomach (gastric), and kidney (renal) cancer, as well as other cancers. FHIT is introduced into cancer cells by using an adenovirus. FHIT protein is then made, suppressing tumor function and causing cancer cell death.

Breast Cancer

In spite of recent advances, breast cancer still remains a devastating disease to women. Factors that increase the chance of getting breast cancer include a high fat diet and a tendency to obesity. There is specific genetic propensity to the disease in people who carry the HER-2 gene. Taking female sex hormones increases the possibility of getting breast cancer. Women who take hormonal replacement therapy in the postmenopausal years should be aware of this risk. There are no easy answers with any drug, hormone, or medication. There are always risks and benefits.

Alcohol consumption is associated with increased breast cancer risk. Women who consume alcohol tend to have increased estrogen and androgen levels, but other mechanisms may also be involved, including associated dietary habits.

The Gail Model Risk Assessment Tool is a computerized program that is available to doctors to help assess individual risk for breast cancer. It takes into account race, age, age at first menstrual period, and the mother's age at which her first child was born, if indeed the woman did have children. An important factor incorporated into this program is whether a so-called first degree relative, that is, a mother, sister, or daughter, has breast cancer. It also takes into account previous breast biopsies that may have been done, and whether these biopsies had atypical hyperplasia, a type of abnormal growth pattern. The estimated risk, as a percentage, in the next five years, and the risk of breast cancer up to age ninety, is then calculated. The woman and her doctor can then use this information to help guide future management, including the possible use of medication to help stave off the disease.

It is now possible for women, by taking a blood test, to find out whether they have mutations in BRCA genes. BRCA is short for breast cancer. BRCA 1 and BRCA 2 are cancer susceptibility genes. Mutations in these genes can cause a heightened susceptibility to breast and ovarian cancer.

BRCA 1 in its normal state may actually be a tumor suppressor gene. BRCA 2 in its normal state may work in a similar manner. Significant mutations in these genes are most common in women of Ashkenazi Jewish descent. Testing for these mutations gives more specific risk information than can be obtained from computer risk models. Many insurers will now pay for this type of testing.

It is becoming evident that certain genotypes may be at greater risk for breast cancer. Transforming growth factor B (TGF-B) inhibits mammary (breast) cell lines. A change in the receptor for TGF-B can lead to a greater risk of breast cancer in white women aged 65 years and older.

It has been shown that SERM's (specific estrogen receptor modulators) are somewhat protective against the formation of breast cancer. Many women in the postmenopausal years use these newer drugs instead of traditional hormonal replacement therapy with estrogen or progesterone. However, Soltamox (tamoxifen) which is a SERM, tends to increase the incidence of uterine (endometrial) cancer, as well as the risk of sarcoma of the uterus - a rarer, more virulent tumor. Therefore, the state of the lining of the uterus has to be carefully monitored by a gynecologist.

Side effects include an increased incidence of stroke and pulmonary embolism. Pregnancy should be avoided, as tamoxifen can cause fetal harm.

Evista (raloxifene)is a SERM that has not been shown to increase the incidence of endometrial cancer (cancer of the lining of the uterus). There is a risk of deep vein thrombosis and pulmonary embolism. Its use in pregnancy should be avoided due to the possibility of fetal harm.

In the postmenopausal women, much of her naturally circulating estrogen is derived from the adrenal glands that sit atop the kidneys.

These endocrine glands make androgens, notably androstenedione and testosterone. A class of enzyme called aromatase encourages the conversion of androstenedione to estrone, a form of estrogen. Aromatase inhibitors are now used to prevent this conversion, and therefore lower the levels of circulating estrogen. These drugs have now been shown to lower the recurrence of cancer in breast cancer patients. In other words, they can be used in prevention of recurrent cancer. Femara (letrozole) and Arimidex (anastrozole) are two currently available drugs of this class. They are not hormones. Use of these drugs can result in decreased bone mineral density, increasing the chance of bone fracture. Usage of these drugs in pregnancy should be avoided, due to the possibility of fetal harm.

It is thankfully possible to detect most breast cancers at an early stage, when the tumor is still small and confined. Every woman should know how to do breast self examination. Far more early tumors are discovered by women themselves than by their doctors, who only get to examine the woman at arbitrarily spaced intervals.

Breast Self Examination:

A good time to examine yourself is after the menstrual period, if you still menstruating. If you no longer menstruate, you should examine yourself at least once a month. Examination should start standing up in front of a mirror with your arm raised behind the head to see if there are any abnormal looking areas, or areas where the skin seems pulled or dimpled. If there is any nipple discharge, you should immediately see your doctor. Examination then continues, lying flat on a firm surface with your arm behind your head. Using the index and middle fingers of the opposite hand, gently roll the breast tissue under your fingers starting in a circular fashion from the nipple and areola (the pigmented area around the nipple) then making wider and wider circles until your fingers end up in the armpit area (axilla).

It is important to get to the armpit area, because the breast is actually teardrop shaped, and there is breast tissue in the axilla, as well as lymph nodes. Have your doctor show you how to properly do breast self-examination. The first time you examine your breasts, the chances are you will not have a good sense of what you are feeling, but if you do examinations on a regular basis, you will quickly be able to discern if there is any new lump or different feeling. If there is even the slightest question in your mind as to what you are feeling, see your doctor. It is much better to go to the doctor once too often than once too seldom. Fortunately, many lumps or tumors turn out to be benign cysts, fibroadenomas, which are solid, benign tumors, or other benign conditions. However, it is always important to rule out cancer promptly.

Mammography:

Mammography has been widely available for years and is a great standby in the early diagnosis of breast cancer. Your doctor will advise you as to when you should start having mammography on a regular basis. Mammography as a technique is not only dependent upon the imaging equipment used, but also dependent on the expertise of the radiologist who reads the films. Mammography is done with X-rays, and radiation taken into the body is cumulative and forever. However, modern digital mammographic studies use little radiation comparatively, and lifetime doses are calculated so that untoward levels of radiation will not occur.

More often now, mammographic studies are supplemented by the use of ultrasound. This technique gives a different look at the breast tissue using sound waves. Obviously, there is no radiation in this technique, but the technique has not reached a level where it can be used instead of mammography. A number of other diagnostic techniques have been tried over the years, such as thermography which gives a heat map of the breast. Unfortunately, such other techniques have not as yet proven useful in the early diagnosis of breast tumors.

Magnetic resonance imaging (MRI) is now becoming much more important, especially in defining the extent of tumor.

The presence of small amounts of calcium, microcalcifications, in the breast, may require biopsy for diagnosis. Biopsies of this type today may be image-guided. An imaging technique called stereotaxis is used to pinpoint the questionable tissue in three dimension. A vacuum-assisted biopsy is then carried out. This technique is called DVAB (stereotatic-guided directional vacuum-assisted biopsy).

It is now possible to use galactography in women with an abnormal nipple discharge. This technique can pinpoint the source of the discharge. The discharge itself is then sent to the cytology laboratory. Microscopic analysis can then detect abnormal cells, including malignant cells, in the smear.

Even in the absence of abnormal breast discharge, a small (micro) catheter can be inserted through the nipple into the milk ducts in women at high risk for breast cancer. Cells are then washed out and sent to the cytology lab for evaluation. This technique can be used in the early detection of breast cancer.

Early diagnostic techniques have reached the level where in situ cancers can be diagnosed. An in situ carcinoma is a tumor in which cell change has occurred, but the abnormal cells have not penetrated even microscopically outside the boundary of the tumor. In other words, no invasion of surrounding tissue has taken place. Unfortunately however, so-called lobular carcinoma in situ can be located over a widespread area of the breast. Strategies for dealing with this type of in situ cancer include vigilance and watchful waiting to make sure that it does not turn to a more virulent type of tumor. Removal of the affected breast tissue can be undertaken and the breast reconstructed with implants and plastic surgery.

Specific estrogen receptor modulators (SERMS) are being prescribed for selected women who have been diagnosed with breast carcinoma in situ. Treatment should be individualized in consultation with a qualified breast surgeon, mindful of the possible drug risks, including those previously noted in this Chapter.

For more aggressive breast tumors, the first line of treatment usually involves removal of the tumor tissue (lumpectomy) with subsequent radiation if necessary and drug therapy, including drugs such as Soltamox (tamoxifen), and Herceptin (trastuzumab). Femara (letrozole) inhibits the manufacture of estrogen in the body, and is used in therapy of breast cancer in postmenopausal women. Aromasin (exemestane) which blocks the formation of estrogen from androgens, has been shown to improve disease – free survival in postmenopausal women with breast cancer. It can cause fetal harm in pregnancy.

At the time of surgery, lymph node dissection is also often undertaken in the axillary region (armpit), both to make the diagnosis as to the extent to the disease process, and also to try to ensure that there is no further spread to the lymph nodes in the region of the armpit.

In more severe cases, radical mastectomy, in which the entire breast is removed along with the surrounding lymph nodes including those in the axilla may have to be done. Even in these cases, nowadays careful breast reconstruction with the use of implants and tissue flaps is possible.

Targeted immunotherapy drugs used in breast cancer, targeting HER2 receptors on breast cancer cells, are Herceptin (trastuzumab), Perjeta (pertuzumab) and Kadcyla (ado-trastuzumab emtansine)

Tecentriq (atezolizumab) is an immune checkpoint inhibitor that can be used in breast cancer treatment.

As in all cancers, the word cure is rarely used. It is well known that even when there is no ostensible disease process left, that months or years later there can be recurrence of the disease at local or distant sites in the body. Anybody who has had treatment for cancer needs to be followed up by the operative surgeon and an oncologist, who is a specialist adept in cancer therapy, often throughout life. A follow up will include appropriate sophisticated scanning at timed intervals individualized to the specific case.

Making Cancer Manageable:

If the disease recurs, all is by no means lost. Thankfully, we have reached a stage where many cancers never seem to recur after initial effective treatment. If cancers do recur, they can often be effectively treated by further surgery, radiation, chemotherapy, or newer drug therapies such as monoclonal antibodies. Thus, oncologists nowadays, in many of their cancer patients, even if they have not cured the disease, have converted it from a killer into a chronic disease condition. The chronic condition can then be adequately managed over many years in the same way that any chronic disease process can. You see many people walking around today and functioning quite normally, and leading productive lives, who in years past would not have been with us. The ability to turn lethal disease into a manageable chronic process has been one of the great medical advances of recent years.

Cox – 1 and Cox – 2:

It has recently been shown that newer drugs that are effective in arthritis, such as Celebrex (celecoxib) which is a Cox-2 inhibitor that inhibits the Cox-2 enzyme, have an anti-tumor effect. These drugs work in arthritis, and potentially atherosclerosis, by inhibiting inflammation. They do this by inhibiting prostacyclin production. Prostacyclin (PGI 2) causes opening of blood vessels and prevents accumulation on the vessel wall of the platelets that cause blood clots. This is a potential two-edged sword, because reduction of these effects may lead to increased blood clotting events. Aspirin itself is a Cox-1 inhibitor which accounts for its gastrointestinal toxicity. Aspirin has anti - blood clotting as well as pain relieving and anti-inflammatory activity. The side effects of Cox - 2 inhibitors include an increase in untoward cardiovascular events, including heart attack. Celebrex use has been associated with deleterious effects on the fetus in pregnancy. The use of aspirin and similar drugs may lead to bleeding complications.

It is important that the use of any drug, including aspirin, be discussed with and managed by a qualified physician. Whenever there is even a possibility of pregnancy, this becomes even more important.

Cancer of the Uterus

As women get into their more senior years, they are much more prone to develop cancers of the reproductive organs. Cancer can arise in the lining of the uterus, or womb. This lining is called the endometrium, and therefore this cancer is called endometrial carcinoma. There is a precursor condition to endometrial cancer called hyperplasia of the endometrium. Hyperplasia simply means overgrowth. The type of hyperplasia that most commonly is associated with cancer formation is adenomatous hyperplasia, which means glandular. If you think of the lining of the uterus as a lawn, then in hyperplasia the grass is growing too thick and too fast.

Most tumors in the wall of the uterus are fibroids and are benign. However, malignant tumors can arise in the wall of the uterus, and they are called sarcomas. These tumors tend to be particularly virulent, but rare. The use of Soltamox (tamoxifen) to prevent recurrence of breast cancer can, unfortunately, increase the risk of getting sarcoma, as well as the risk of endometrial cancer.

Colon Cancer

Colon cancer is one of the more common malignancies encountered by people of middle age and beyond. Predisposing factors may include a high fat diet and eating grilled food that has a charred surface. There is definitely a genetic predisposition. A genetic mutation predisposes to HNPCC, or hereditary nonpolyposis colon cancer.

Ironically, my own mother, who spent her life searching for a cancer 'cure', was, at an advanced age, diagnosed with colon cancer. She died shortly after having the tumor removed at surgery. Before she died, she was able to speak to my own daughter, who was about to lose her mother from lung cancer, about her own experiences as a young woman coping with the untimely loss of her mother.

Colonoscopy:

The good news is that colon cancer is quite easily detectable at an early stage, and treatable with a high degree of success. The bad news is that the public at large seems to have a general aversion to undergoing colonoscopy. The disease process often starts in polypoid lesions. In other words, bulbous growths arise on the inner lining of the large bowel, or large intestine. These growths are on stalks. A thin, fiberoptic flexible instrument called a colonoscope is gradually advanced through the rectum all the way up to the cecum, which is the place where the small intestine meets the large intestine. A complete examination of the entire large bowel can be easily performed, quite comfortably with mild sedation, by an adept gastroenterologist or bowel surgeon. Commonly growths can be photographed and removed through the scope by cutting the stalk of the polyp, therefore removing the tumor totally. The polyp is then sent to the pathology lab for identification. Sigmoidoscopy, in which only the lower part of the large intestine, namely the rectum and sigmoid colon, are visualized, is no longer thought to be adequate, because some cancers arise higher up in the large intestine. Like any cancer, if the disease is not diagnosed early enough, the cancer will spread, invading the wall of the intestine and then spreading to lymph nodes. Treatment at that stage, is of course, much more complex, often requiring colostomy. The prognosis in more advanced cases is much less favorable, but with intensive treatment, long survival can still often be obtained.

There are now even less invasive procedures available to visualize the large bowel. A tiny catheter can be inserted into the rectum through which air can be sent to inflate the large bowel, and the wall of the colon is then visualized by helical CAT scan technique with three dimensional reconstruction. This is virtual colonoscopy. However, if an abnormal growth is discovered in this way, a resectoscope will still have to be introduced in order to remove the tumor.

The classic treatment of colon cancer is surgical resection of the affected part of the colon.

Now, beyond surgery and chemotherapy, immunotherapy is available.

Targeted monoclonal antibodies that can be used in colon cancer include Avastin (bevacizumab), Erbitux (cetuximab), Vectibix (panitumumab), and Cyramza (ramucirumab).

Opdivo (nivolumab) and Keytruda (pembrolizumab) are checkpoint inhibitors that may be used in colon cancer.

Cancer Markers:

The first available cancer marker by blood test was the CEA antigen. The test, however, is not entirely specific for colon cancer.

It is now possible to obtain DNA from a simple blood sample. Most of the free DNA in the plasma of people with colorectal cancer comes from the actual tumor. This should become a specific test for the detection of colon cancer, and also could be used to tell how well treatment is working. It should be possible to use this exciting technology in detecting and following other cancers as well.

A very basic test for colon cancer consists of checking the stool (feces) sample for traces of blood at the time of a rectal examination.

Anyone who is positive for blood in this test should be checked for the possibility of colon cancer.

The stool sample can be evaluated in a much more sophisticated way for the actual presence of a gene, the APC (adenomatous polyposis coli) gene, in colon cells. If the APC gene has mutated, there is a significant chance that colon cancer may, or already has, developed.

It is now possible, in certain cases of colon cancer, to remove part of the large bowel (colon) with minimally invasive surgery by use of the laparoscope. The laparoscope is a fiberoptic telescope that is inserted through a small incision into the abdomen. The scope is then attached to a television monitor, so that the operating surgeon and assistants can view their surgical manipulation easily.

Prostate Cancer

This cancer that becomes commoner in men as they age is discussed in the next Chapter: The Reproductive Organs.

Bibliograhy:

Bibliography and Supplemental Bibliography www.rcaplanmd.com

https://www.cancer.gov/about-cancer/treatment/types/immunotherapy

https://www.cancer.gov/about-cancer/treatment/types/immunotherapy/cancer-treatment-vaccines

https://www.cancer.gov/about-cancer/treatment/types/immunotherapy/immune-system-modulators

https://www.cancer.gov/about-cancer/treatment/types/immunotherapy/checkpoint-inhibitors

https://www.cancer.gov/about-cancer/treatment/types/immunotherapy/t-cell-transfer-therapy

https://www.cancer.gov/about-cancer/treatment/types/immunotherapy/monoclonal-antibodies

https://www.cancerresearch.org/immunotherapy/cancer-types/colorectal-cancer

https://www..breastcancer.org/treatment/immunotherapy

https://www.cancer.org/cancer/lung-cancer/treating-non-small-cell/immunotherapy.html

https://www.webmd.com/lung-cancer/lung-cancer-immunotherapy-right-for-me

https://www.cancerresearch.org/immunotherapy/cancer-types/ovarian-cancer

https://www.cancer.gov/about-cancer/treatment/types/immunotherapy/checkpoint-inhibitors

CHAPTER 6
THE REPRODUCTIVE ORGANS

The Take-Home Message

- Early diagnosis and decisive treatment is the key
- A sexually transmitted virus, HPV (human papilloma virus) is responsible for most cervical cancer, precancer and penile cancer. It is easily detected by DNA probe, often before there is significant cell change seen on a "Pap" (Papanicolaou) smear.
- A vaccine that prevents HPV infection is available
- DNA probes are highly precise
- The Pap smear was one of the great early advances in true "preventative" medicine: cervical disease was detected microscopically before it turned to cancer, or at an early stage of cancer. Women could be and were effectively cured by definitive treatment. However, Pap smears have both false positive and false negative results.
- Never take abnormal bleeding for granted; it must be evaluated.
- Bleeding after the menopause (postmenopausal bleeding) must be evaluated.

- Menopause means the menses have stopped. Irregular or abnormal bleeding around the time of the menopause is not a normal symptom of the menopause.
- Ovarian tumors may occur at any age, although they are commoner in older women.
- Minimally invasive surgical techniques have proven to be a great advance in the diagnosis and treatment of disease of the reproductive organs.
- The diagnosis of prostate cancer by PSA testing is still controversial.
- Sexual function and satisfaction can persist in later life

Great advances have been made in the early diagnosis and treatment of tumors of the reproductive tract.

The outer part of the female reproductive tract is the vulva. The vulva consists of the outer lips, the labia majora; the inner lips, the labia minora; the opening of the passage from the urinary bladder to the outside, the urethra (the opening itself is called the urethral meatus). On either side are tiny openings of the ducts of the Bartholin's glands, and near the urethral opening are other small glands, called Skene's glands. Above the urethral opening, within the folds of the labia minora, is the clitoris, the sensitive, erectile organ which has an important role in female sexual response.

The bottom of the vaginal opening, towards the rectum, is called the fourchette. The area between the bottom of the vagina and the top of the rectal opening is called the perineum.

Just inside the vaginal entrance or vestibule, is the hymeneal ring, the vestiges of the hymen. Even in the virgin the hymen, an intact ring, has a central opening through which the menstrual flow exits.

Further up, the vagina and rectum are closer together anatomically. There is gradually less bulk to the perineal body, which is triangular in shape, so that the vagina and rectum are separated by a relatively thin rectovaginal septum.

The opening, or os, of the cervix, which is the passageway leading into the uterus (womb), protrudes into the top, or vault of the vagina. The cervical os is normally closed. Mucus does secrete from glands in the cervix though the os. The vagina, of course, has secretions as well, as do the Bartholin's and Skene's glands. The vagina is naturally lubricated by these secretions. The outer vulva does contain sebaceous glands as well.

The uterus itself is contained within the pelvic cavity, which is the lower part of the abdominal cavity. As the pregnant uterus enlarges, it enters into the abdominal cavity beyond three months (twelve weeks) of pregnancy, and the trained physician can then palpate (feel) it on abdominal examination. Of course, on pelvic examination, the gynecologist can ascertain important characteristics of even the normal uterus. The trained gynecologist can usually describe the size, shape, position and consistency of the uterus, as well as its mobility. A normal uterus is not rigidly fixed in its position but can be gently moved.

The lowermost area in the pelvic cavity behind the uterus and in front of the rectum is called the "cul de sac". This is an important area where disease conditions, classically endometriosis and infections, can cause adhesion formation. Adhesions are fibrous and connective tissue bands that hold organs together, limiting mobility and causing obstruction. Enlarging tumors of the uterus or ovaries can be found in the cul de sac. A complete pelvic examination by a gynecologist assessing the health of the pelvic organs includes a rectal examination, so that the cul de sac can be evaluated.

The fallopian tubes enter into each side of the uterus near its top, or uterine fundus. The primary female sex organs, the ovaries, are attached to the sidewall of the pelvis on each side by a ligament that contains their blood supply, and on the other side by another ligament to the uterus itself. The ends of each fallopian tube has moving, fingerlike projections, that rest very close to the ovary. These are the 'pickup' mechanism of the egg (ovum) released during ovulation by the ovary. The egg is then wafted down the tube. The fallopian tube is a dynamic, fine, living structure, with muscular contractions of its wall. Inside it has cells that secrete fluids, and tiny microscopic, hairlike projections called cilia on cells that help move the egg, on a precise schedule, to its meeting with sperm that swim up the reproductive tract from the vagina, through the cervix, into the uterus, and finally into the fallopian tube, where fertilization occurs.

The fertilized egg then continues to move through the fallopian tube towards the uterus.

The fertilized egg reaches the inner lining of the uterus when it has developed to the point when it is ready to implant into the mother's uterine wall.

If the structure and function of the fallopian tube is damaged or destroyed, even though the tube is still open, the vital timing mechanism can be lost, and the egg is still in the fallopian tube when it is ready to implant. Tubal pregnancy results. The thin tube wall cannot sustain the pregnancy, and eventually the tube wall will rupture, with hemorrhage (severe bleeding) into the abdominal cavity.

Tumors (Abnormal Growths)

Tumors can, and do, arise at every level of a woman's reproductive tract.

Any ovarian tumor in a woman during the pre-menopausal and menopausal years should be looked at with great suspicion. There are many types of ovarian tumors, both cystic (fluid filled) and solid.

There is great confusion about this. Most cysts are benign, but on the other hand, many ovarian cancers have a cystic, or liquid component. It is vital to diagnose and treat ovarian cancer at the earliest possible stage, because once it has spread to the stage where most ovarian cancers unfortunately are still diagnosed, treatments become particularly severe and the outlook can become very serious.

Tumors of the fallopian tube, which is the tube leading from uterus towards the ovary, are rare, but do occur.

The Cervix

Cancer of the cervix (mouth of the womb), often starts in sexually active women at a younger age. It is now known that a majority of cervical carcinoma is caused by HPV (Human Papilloma Virus) and its many subtypes. In other words, it is a sexually transmitted disease. However, there is often a long time, measured in years, between the infection and the appearance of a full blown cervical carcinoma. Thus, it is essential for every woman to continue to have screening with gynecologic examination, Papanicolaou smear, and when necessary screening with DNA probes for Human Papilloma Virus into her senior years.

George Papanicolaou was a research scientist who was acquainted with my mother through her work in funding and encouraging cancer research.

When Papanicolaou first described his pioneering work in the early diagnosis of cervical cancer by looking microscopically at smears taken from the cervix, he was a long way from getting the 'Pap' test accepted as a mass screening tool for the early detection of cancer of the cervix.

Dr. Ernest Ayre, an entrepreneur, started the National Cancer Cytology Center in New York and Florida. He was one of the key people instrumental in popularizing the use of the 'Pap' smear as a clinical tool. After his death, his wife, Ann, continued his work. For some years, I served on the Medical Advisory Board of the National Cancer Cytology Center.

It soon became apparent that cervical cancer, detected early, did not require radical surgery, and that there truly was a high cure rate – still a difficult thing to say in most cancers.

Huge bias had to be overcome. Just multiplying the number of sexually active women in the United States and Canada by the average cost of a 'Pap' smear made the cost of addressing the problem seem insurmountable. A whole infrastructure of laboratories, trained technicians and pathologists was needed. Of course, if you subtract from this cost the pure saving in not having to radically treat women in danger of dying from advanced cervix cancer, not to mention the time lost from productive work by women affected by the disease, the numbers looked better. As well, as systems were put into place to efficiently mass screen the population, the relative cost of the test came down dramatically. The saving of women's lives and preserving women's health: priceless. (But only to a society that values each human life above all).

Unfortunately, any time a new diagnostic technique comes up, no matter how self-evident its value, the same 'cost' argument is brought up.

The other big argument against any new diagnostic test is that early diagnosis will lead to needless, often dangerous treatment to large numbers of women. As well, the 'yield' from the test is looked at, to see how much money and time is invested in order to find each of those women who do have the problem. These are legitimate concerns, but they are politicized.

It is important that any woman who feels no symptoms but has been told that she has an abnormal test, have a serious discussion with an appropriate expert, in this case a gynecologist, to know what her options and risks are. If she is not satisfied or still has questions, a second opinion from another qualified expert should be obtained. A wealth of information is available today, notably on the Internet. It is important, however, to know what level of expertise is behind each web site, or book or magazine. Even a so-called 'peer review' medical journal cannot address itself to your particular individual situation.

At about the same time that the 'Pap' smear was being popularized in North America, European physicians were experimenting with directly looking at the cervix under magnification, with an instrument called a colposcope.

As a medical engineer once told me, there are competing technologies available to tackle just about any problem. It is often almost arbitrary what method is picked for general use.

It took many years until gynecologists came to realize that the 'Pap' smear and colposcopy were complementary. Women with abnormal 'Pap' smears should have the cervix looked at by a trained gynecologist using the colposcope, to see the most abnormal appearing areas, which are then biopsied for diagnosis.

All the while, even in the early days, it was evident that cervical cancer had something to do with sexual intercourse. Nuns were virtually free of the disease. Specialized populations were similarly spared. For example, it was known that in Ireland, then a poor, largely observant Roman Catholic country with a dowry system, there was a lower incidence of cervix cancer. It took a long time for a poor family to acquire the dowry. Consequently marriage, and often first intercourse, did not occur until a woman was in her thirties.

This all seems antiquated today, but it did give clues as to where to search for the cause of this serious disease that was killing women.

The scientific breakthrough of DNA probes capable of not only detecting viruses but of typing them has totally changed the situation.

We now know that the vast majority of cervical cancers are caused by the sexually spread Human Papilloma Virus (HPV). A benign condition known as CIN (cervical intraepithelial neoplasia) caused by HPV can, and often does, progress to cervical cancer.

HPV also causes cancer of the penis in men.

Those of us who early on tested our patients for HPV with DNA probes – a quick and painless test that just takes some mucus from the cervix – were ironically faced with all the same criticisms, economic and otherwise, that were initially faced by doctors using the revolutionary 'Pap' smear all those years ago. Having first being exposed on an almost daily basis to these arguments that were frustrating my mother's work before I was even teenaged, I was bemused by 'having deja vu all over again', to quote Yogi Berra.

Now, many leading gynecologists are leaning towards thinking that DNA probes for HPV virus should be the new gold standard in mass testing for the early diagnosis of cervix cancer and precancerous conditions, and that the 'Pap' smear, that has saved so many women's lives and health, will be phased out.

Papanicolaou did make one of the great contributions to preventative medicine in women when he created the Papanicolaou smear test. Even though this classic test, which was first described almost one hundred years ago, is low tech by today's standards, it still remains a most valuable screening tool for pre-malignant and malignant conditions of the uterine cervix, or mouth of the womb. This test has the advantage of being painless, relatively fast, and relatively cheap. As well, it can be done by a host of medical professionals. Like many tests, the Papanicolaou smear can have false negative and false positive results. That is, if disease is present, the Papanicolaou smear does not necessarily detect it, and if disease is absent the Papanicolaou smear may be positive. If however, it is properly used simply as a screening test, it will identify a population of women at risk for cervix disease who can then be more exactly diagnosed and appropriately treated by more sophisticated means.

There is regrettably, however, a common misuse of the test. It is not appropriate, when the test is abnormal, to wait and then repeat the test at a later date. The reason for the abnormality should be determined. If it is determined by more sophisticated means that no abnormalities exist, then of course no treatment is necessary. Follow up testing where there has been an abnormal Papanicolaou smear involves the use of the colposcope. The gynecologist looks at the magnified cervix and sees if there is abnormal cell structure. The gynecologist can then take small biopsies of the abnormal areas of the cervix. This is done as an office procedure, with the patient awake and often lightly sedated. Discomfort tends to be minor. The biopsies are then sent to the pathology lab for diagnosis. As well, the gynecologist takes tissue from the canal of the cervix to ensure that there is no disease there.

The advent some years ago of DNA probes for Human Papilloma Virus have become an essential part of the diagnosis in disease of the cervix. The test itself is quick and painless, taking a small amount of secretion from the cervix. It is then sent to a lab for DNA analysis. The virus is subtyped to see if one of those types is present that is more likely to cause cervical cancer. Other types are commonly associated with sexually transmitted venereal warts.

Treatment can be undertaken to get rid of the virus long before cancer develops. Some of these HPV infections may regress spontaneously, much like other viral infections in the body that are essentially killed by the body's immune system. However, this should not be taken for granted. If patient and doctor decide on watchful waiting, retesting should be carried out before the disease condition can become widespread and dangerous. Unfortunately, the types of HPV likely to cause cancer are less likely to regress.

Once a cancer of the cervix is present, it tends to invade locally, blocking vital organs such as the ureters which are the passages from the kidneys to the urinary bladder. Cervical cancer has been, in the past, a significant killer of women, many of whom are tragically quite young. The classic treatment is surgery, which can be radical, depending on the extent of disease and its spread. Radiation is also used, as well as chemotherapy where indicated. The immune checkpoint inhibitor Keytruda (pembrolizumab), which targets the PD-1 protein on T-cells, may be used in advanced cervical cancer.

Premalignant cell change in the cervix, which is called CIN (cervical intraepithelial neoplasia), usually can be treated quite simply by removing the tissue in the place where the virus likes to live in the cervix. This area of the cervix is called the transformation zone, where under normal circumstances there is cell activity, as the outside lining of the cervix grows into the canal of the cervix as a woman gradually gets older (metaplasia). This tissue can be removed quite simply by loop excision. An electric current heats a fine wire loop so that it can cut through tissue. This however, has the disadvantage of obscuring the margins of the removed tissue with a cautery burn, so that the pathologist cannot be sure that all the affected tissue has been removed. Therefore, depending on the individual case, it may be elected to excise the tissue surgically without the use of the loop. This is called a cone biopsy of the cervix. Cervical tissue that has undergone some cell change and is benign can often be eradicated by simple techniques such as laser beam excision, guided by magnification with the colposcope, or by cryosurgery, which is a relatively simple freezing technique.

There is now a vaccine against types of the HPV virus, and much hope is being held out that eventually cancer of the cervix will be a rare condition, of historical interest only.

Gardasil 9 is a Human Papillomavirus Recombinant Vaccine. The vaccine protects against the 16 and 18 subtypes of the HPV virus that cause 70% of cervical carcinoma and precursors of cervical cancer. The vaccine also protects against the 6 and 11 subtypes that cause genital warts, as well as cell changes in the cervix. In addition, it protects against HPV types 31, 33, 45, 52 and 58 that cause ten to twenty percent of cervical cancer. It is recommended for use beginning with children aged as early as nine, and up to twenty-six years of age for previously unvaccinated adults who have not already been exposed to, and developed antibodies to, the HPV virus. Gardasil is not recommended to be used during pregnancy.

There seems to be some level of apprehension in the society presently that the administration of the vaccine to children will somehow lead to earlier sexual contact and promiscuity. There may also be misgivings about long term effects. Unfortunately, the HPV virus is currently widespread in the population, with significant consequences to women, including cancer. Education about the benefits along with familiarity with the vaccine should serve to ensure that people get protected by the vaccine before they are exposed to the virus. After all, most of the same parents having misgivings at present ensured that they protected their children at an early age by immunization against various other dangerous diseases. Boys as well as girls should be vaccinated to protect against penile cancer and genital warts, and to break the chain of sexual transmission of dangerous subtypes of HPV virus.

Abnormal Bleeding

Common sense tells us that diagnosis comes before treatment. This allows the physician to properly attack and treat the cause of any problem. Unfortunately, women in the age group of the menopause are also in the age group most at risk for various disease conditions, including endometrial cancer. The early symptom and hallmark of endometrial cancer is abnormal bleeding from the vagina, especially bleeding that occurs after the menopause, even if it is just a little spotting or staining. A woman who has not yet reached the menopause is abnormally bleeding if her periods are too long or too heavy or if she is passing blood clots. Spotting, staining, or bleeding in between the periods is similarly abnormal. With any such symptoms, a woman should see her gynecologist. Appropriate investigations, tests and examinations should be done to find the cause of the bleeding. It is not enough simply to do a cursory pelvic examination and to state that the periods can be regulated by a birth control pill. Birth control pills are for birth control. Prior to giving this or any other treatment, the determination must be made as to whether or not disease is present. By ultrasonography, the actual thickness of the lining of the womb (endometrium) can be measured. Bulging or asymmetry in the inner cavity of the uterus can sometimes be seen. Any accumulation of fluid or blood in this endometrial cavity can also be seen. Ovarian size can be determined as can uterine size, and the characteristics of these organs can be determined. If abnormal cells are being shed from the uterine lining they may turn up on the Papanicolaou smear, although this test is really designed to get cells from the cervix or from the canal of the cervix only. If there is any doubt, actual endometrial tissue must be examined under a microscope, by a pathologist.

Endometrial biopsy is a minimally invasive office procedure. A small, flexible, soft hollow instrument is placed in the endometrial cavity and tissue obtained, usually by suction. Assuming that the entire womb lining has one pattern, which is often not the case, then the tissue obtained by this technique will be representative of the entire womb lining and give the doctor sufficient information upon which to base treatment. If the situation is more complex, as it often is, more sophisticated techniques, such as videohysteroscopy should be used. A fiberoptic telescope is placed through the partially opened cervix into the uterine cavity. A small television camera is then hooked to a color television monitor so that the entire uterine cavity can be seen, magnified. Abnormal areas can be biopsied.

Alternatively, sonohysterography can be carried out. Fluid is injected into the uterus and sonography is used to observe the lining of the uterus. The drawback to this technique is that no actual sample of uterine lining is taken for diagnosis.

Abnormal menstrual bleeding in women prior to the menopause is being treated in some European centers by the use of a device inserted into the uterus that continuously releases a progesterone - like substance (levonorgestrel). This system is currently used in the United States for contraception only. Progesterone is often used in North America orally or by injection to achieve the same purpose. Prolonged use of progesterone can lead to a decrease in bone mineral density.

Unremitting bleeding in a woman who has not yet reached the menopause, and who has been proven by actual biopsy of the endometrial lining to have a benign problem, may be treated by ablation (removal), or destruction of this endometrial lining. Of course, she must know that she cannot have any more pregnancies following such a procedure. Removal of the lining by cautery under hysteroscopic guidance with a small instrument called a "rollerball" is an accepted way of doing this. The lining may be destroyed by heat (bipolar desiccation) or by inserting a heated solution through a balloon inserted into the uterus (hydrothermal ablation). The lining may be frozen by a technique called cryoablation. All these techniques may result in difficulty in the diagnosis of a subsequent endometrial cancer, as the hallmark symptom of early endometrial cancer, abnormal bleeding, may not be present. These procedures may not be curative in a significant percentage of cases, and hysterectomy (surgical removal of the uterus) may eventually become necessary.

Cancer of the Uterus

As in any cancer, the early diagnosis of endometrial cancer, which is commonly referred to as uterine cancer, is important. If a diagnosis of a precancerous condition – hyperplasia - is made, the only treatment necessary might be hormonal treatment with progesterone. It is well known that unopposed, unabated estrogen stimulation of the uterus can cause endometrial cancer.

In Stage One endometrial cancer, total hysterectomy, that is removal of the uterus complete with the cervix, can be curative. However, radiation is often needed in these cases as well. In order to be certain of the staging, it is often advisable to do lymph node removal at the time of surgery. Removal of the uterus with surrounding tissue and lymph nodes is referred to as a radical hysterectomy. The increasing sophistication of magnetic resonance imaging (MRI) may make such extension of the surgery unnecessary, if it shows that no other tissues or lymph nodes are involved. It is important to discuss any proposed surgical approach at length with the gynecologic surgeon, or gynecologic oncologist.

Immunotherapy may be utilized in advanced endometrial cancer. For example, the checkpoint inhibitor Keytruda (pembrolizumab) may be used in certain advanced endometrial cancers. The checkpoint inhibitor Opdivo (nivolumab) has been utilized as well. The monoclonal antibody Avastin (bevacizumab), a VEGF inhibitor, has been used alone (monotherapy) or in conjunction with chemotherapy. These are just some of the approaches being tried, with some success.

Sarcoma of the uterus is thankfully much rarer, as it is a particularly virulent disease process. There are several types of this disease that arise in the muscle and the connective tissue of the uterus. Any uterine growth that has been diagnosed as a benign fibroid but is rapidly increasing in size should be regarded with suspicion. Definitive treatment is removal by total abdominal hysterectomy at an early stage. Lymph node dissection is also usually advised, and radiation is utilized as well. One of the reasons that sarcomas of the uterus are such virulent tumors is that they may represent only one end of the spectrum. If women undergo hysterectomy for ostensibly benign disease, which is usually fibroid formation, the uterus is sent for examination to the pathologist. Where there are many fibroids in the uterus, the pathologist will often microscopically only examine representative fibroids, or those which look particularly suspicious to the naked eye. It is quite possible that small fibroids with sarcomatous change are removed that are never identified. A patient is then pronounced cured, and in fact usually is.

Fortunately, many sarcomas initially present as polypoid growths in the cavity of the uterus leading to abnormal bleeding patterns. Again, it is vital not to ascribe any abnormal bleeding in a woman in the pre-menopausal or menopausal years as being part of normal menopause. The menopause means that the periods get lighter, shorter, and further apart and either eventually or suddenly stop altogether and forever. Other change in the bleeding pattern should be regarded with suspicion. Polyps, which are most usually benign, very often present with bleeding or spotting in between the periods. Although they do not cause an enlargement of the uterus that can be felt on ordinary gynecologic examination, they can often be seen by ultrasonographic visualization. This noninvasive, simple test is widely available, and should be used when necessary. A small endocervical polyp that is protruding through the opening of the cervix can easily and quickly be removed, usually as an office procedure. If there is a larger polyp in the uterine cavity, it is more ideally treated in an outpatient surgical facility, where proper visualization can be done by means of a videohysteroscope, the base of the polyp seen, and the polyp removed. On the off-chance that there is sarcomatous change in the polyp, it is still usually necessary to do surgery including hysterectomy and lymph node dissection and possibly follow-up radiation. The chance of long term survival without recurrence in a woman whose disease has been found in this way is greatly enhanced. In such women, very little remaining disease is usually found in the uterus when it is examined in the pathology lab.

Ovarian Tumors

The large group of diseases known as cancer of the ovary are still dangerous. Genetic predisposition does play a role, but outside of that the cause remains largely unknown. The ovary is by its nature a totipotential organ. In other words, any tissue or organ in the human body can be made out of ovarian tissue. This of course makes sense, because each new human life starts as an ovum, or egg, which is then fertilized by a sperm. Ovarian tumors, both benign and malignant, can have the traits of many tissues within the human body. In cancer, the growth has gone awry and has a bizarre appearance with abnormal forms. Ovarian tumors can arise in women at any age, regrettably even little girls, but are most common in women beyond the menopause. Users of a contraceptive pills may have a somewhat lowered incidence of ovarian cancer.

For now, our best hope dealing with ovarian cancer is early diagnosis. Unfortunately, we have not as yet attained even this step. Ovarian tumors, in at least fifty percent of cases, are silent, with no symptoms at all until they have already spread. The only symptoms when they do occur, can include menstrual periods that are too frequent because of the disturbance in the hormonal output of the ovary. Symptoms can also include discomfort in the pelvic region, and later, swelling and protrusion of the abdomen, as an enlarging tumor presses on other pelvic contents and gradually grows into the abdominal cavity. There are tumor markers available which can be checked by a simple blood test. These markers are known as CA 125, and CA 19-9. These tests are not specific, in that people with ovarian cancer, especially the early ovarian cancer which the gynecologist is trying to detect, may test negative, while people with various benign conditions, such as endometriosis may test positive.

A blood test now exists that can profile proteins by identifying them and their patterns. The proteomic pattern that distinguishes ovarian cancer can be identified by computer analysis. This new bioinformatics tool seems to be quite precise in correctly identifying even early cases of ovarian cancer. The computer is actually trained to identify whether a blood sample contains the protein pattern for ovarian cancer by first using training samples from patients with ovarian cancer, and samples from unaffected women. This technique is a significant advance over simply testing the blood for one substance that may be a cancer marker.

Pelvic examination even by the most qualified gynecologist, is notoriously unreliable in picking up early ovarian tumors. The normal ovary on average measures approximately three by two by one centimeters, or a little over one inch in its greatest measurement. Prior to ultrasonography, the common wisdom was not to remove an ovarian tumor until it was estimated by an examining gynecologist to be at least five centimeters in diameter, which is approximately two inches. Even a tumor of that size can be missed on ordinary pelvic examination, even by the most experienced gynecologist. The situation is made more complex by the fact that a woman in the reproductive years builds up follicles in the ovary every month, one of which becomes dominant and eventually releases the egg. Follicles are fluid filled structures surrounding eggs, and of course they are perfectly normal. After the egg is released the follicle regresses and the ovary goes back to its normal size. The gynecologist must be prepared not only to be able to feel the enlarged ovary but to diagnose whether the enlargement is a temporary, normal process, or an abnormal growth. The best way to do this at present is by means of ultrasonography. Most ultrasonography is done with the ultrasound probe placed on the woman's abdomen, and this tends to be accurate for measurements of the uterus. It is essential, in order to accurately measure the ovaries and to get as much information as possible about any enlargement, to use a transvaginal ultrasound probe. This involves a qualified technician or the doctor placing an ultrasound probe directly into the vagina so that the ovaries can be closely imaged. This complements the pelvic study with the abdominally placed probe. The test is usually painless.

Ultrasonography has become increasingly sophisticated. Real time ultrasonography allows the sonographer to see the image of the ovary as the test is being done. Color flow Doppler technology shows the actual pulsing of blood through the ovarian vessels. The characteristics of this flow become suspicious when a malignant tumor is present.

Three dimensional ultrasonography now is available, so that the characteristics of an ovarian cyst can be looked at in greater detail, and the actual volume of fluid within the cyst accurately calculated.

Physicians now speak of four dimensional ultrasonography, referring to a three dimensional image seen "as it happens", time being the fourth dimension.

Magnetic resonance imaging and computerized axial tomography can also be used to image the ovaries. When an ovarian tumor has been discovered, CAT scan and MRI are useful in determining whether lymph nodes have become enlarged and whether other organs in the body such as the liver have been affected.

Routine ultrasonographic screening of large populations is not yet economic. As well, there is not yet any definitive study to show that such screening programs actually result in a longer life expectancy for women who actually have ovarian cancer. Common sense however, would dictate that this would obviously be the case. The specter of unnecessary surgery in women with relatively small ovarian masses which in fact are totally benign is continually raised. Obviously, knowledge is a good thing, not a bad thing. Knowing that a woman has an enlarged ovary is obviously better than not knowing it. What is then done with this information needs to be individualized, considering all the aspects of each case with informed discussion between a woman and her gynecologist, with the option of a second opinion always a possibility.

Laparoscopy:

Years ago, the decision as to whether to operate or not was much more difficult. Every operation on the ovary was a major operation, involving an abdominal incision, and a commitment to deal definitively with the problem. With the advent of laparoscopy, which is minimally invasive surgery, some fifty years ago, and the continued perfection of laparoscopic technique, it has now become possible on an outpatient basis to make the appropriate diagnosis, and often to treat abnormalities that are found.

Modern laparoscopy involves the insertion of a fiberoptic telescope, the laparoscope, through a tiny incision in the lower margin of the belly button (the umbilicus). Under direct vision, fine operating instruments are inserted through other tiny incisions, usually down near the pubic area. The laparoscope is connected to a small television camera which is then hooked to a color television monitor and the various reproductive organs as well as the abdominal organs are directly seen. Appropriate biopsies can be taken, and if necessary, entire ovaries can be removed intact, without disturbing their inner contents. Frozen section can then be obtained in the laboratory for initial diagnosis. Nowadays it is possible to sample lymph nodes by this technique. In the case of ovary removal through the laparoscope, it is possible for a woman to go home the same day, without even an overnight stay in the hospital.

Gynecologist and patient should discuss beforehand the implications of finding ovarian cancer during this procedure. They may elect to proceed directly to full scale definitive major surgery at that point, or they may elect to wait for the permanent pathologic diagnosis, and to defer major surgery until that point. Of course, if the diagnosis is clear cut on an examination and imaging studies, then laparoscopy may not be necessary at all prior to major surgery.

Insurance programs, including Medicare, are quite averse to paying for routine ultrasonographic screening in women in the pre-menopausal and post-menopausal age groups. The fact that mass screening programs by this modality can have relatively low pick up rates of cancer, and that most ovarian enlargements are benign, and that surgical interventions are increased, serves as a basis for this reluctance. This reluctance may save money for insurers in the short run, but a heavy price is paid inevitably in the eventual need for high cost, complex, and often futile therapy in cases that have been discovered too late, not to mention the price that is paid in sickness and even death by the women who these insurance plans serve.

Ovarian tumors have varying sensitivities to different forms of chemotherapy. The chemotherapy is tailored to experience with similar tumors in other women in the past.

The monoclonal antibody Avastin (bevacizumab) that targets the VEGF/VEGFR pathway, inhibiting tumor blood vessel growth may be used in certain cases of advanced ovarian cancer.

Postoperative follow up may involve advanced imaging techniques including PET scan (positron emission tomography), which utilizes the uptake of glucose (sugar) by the tumor to identify its location.

Ovarian cancer can also be secondary, meaning that the original site of the cancer is elsewhere, often the breast. As well, if the ovaries are still functioning and producing estrogen, this can have an adverse effect on breast cancer. Breast cancers have estrogen receptors. Removal of the ovaries is still sometimes advocated in women who have breast cancer, but this is done on an individualized basis, and must be seriously discussed with the oncologist, as well as the breast surgeon and the gynecologist.

Fibroids

Fibroids are benign tumors that arise in the wall of the uterus. They are composed of muscle and fibrous tissue. They are common, and very often produce no symptoms whatsoever. Fibroids were usually diagnosed in women in their forties and fifties, but with advanced imaging techniques and laparoscopy, their beginnings can be seen in much younger women. They tend to be slow growing except under the influence of pregnancy, when growth can be accelerated. When the growth of fibroids outstrips their blood supply, various forms of degeneration can occur within them. The classic symptoms of fibroids are periods that become heavier and prolonged, often with the passage of blood clots. Pain with periods, called dysmenorrhea, is often associated with significant fibroid formation. Fibroids are usually multiple and vary in their location in the uterine wall. Fibroids that impinge on the lining of the uterus, or endometrium, tend to be the most troublesome. If fibroids grow, the enlarging mass of the uterus will press on surrounding organs, including bladder and bowel, and the mass will rise into the abdominal cavity. Rapid growth in a fibroid raises the concern that sarcomatous degeneration may be present.

The natural withdrawal of hormonal stimulation to fibroids at the time of menopause can result in the regression of these benign tumors and the symptoms that go along with them. Unfortunately however, with significant fibroids, it is often found that abnormal bleeding continues well into the fifties and that without treatment symptoms tend to persist indefinitely.

Fibroids can be made to regress by injection of a gonadotropin (GnRH) releasing hormone agonist known as Lupron (leuprolide acetate). The drug acts by suppressing pituitary gonadotrophic hormones, leading to decreased release of estradiol (an estrogen) by the ovaries. The giving of this medication usually results in the cessation of menses temporarily. It can be most effective when used preoperatively to make surgery technically more feasible, with a tendency to reduced blood loss during surgery. Use of this drug can lead to a decrease in bone mineral density. Like many other drugs, it should not be used in pregnancy.

Hysteroscopy:

Submucous fibroids which impinge on the lining of the womb can be approached with a hysteroscope. This fiberoptic instrument is inserted through the cervix. The uterine lining is visualized in color on a television monitor, and by means of a resectoscope the fibroid is shaved down, and partially or totally eliminated. Operative video-hysteroscopy most often can be accomplished on an outpatient basis, and the patient can go home the same day.

Various techniques have been tried during removal of fibroids from the uterus, a procedure called myomectomy, by the abdominal approach to cut down on the blood loss often associated with removal of fibroids from the uterus. Fibroids can be removed from the uterus with laparoscopic technique, using either a laser technique which can be time consuming and often not effective in controlling blood loss, or electrocautery.

Ultrasonic coagulation cutting (the harmonic scalpel) can be utilized. Tumors of any significant size then have to be removed by a secondary incision at the top of the vagina, a procedure called colpotomy.

Uterine Artery Embolization:

It is possible to largely cut off the blood supply to fibroids by stopping the blood flow through the uterine artery. Under radiologic guidance, the artery is embolized (occluded). Bleeding symptoms are often then improved. A possible complication that has occurred is diffuse (widespread) necrosis (tissue death) of the uterus, requiring hysterectomy.

Image Guided Therapy:

In this available technique, an MRI scanner takes three-dimensional images of the fibroid to be destroyed. Focused ultrasound waves are precisely aimed at the fibroid, raising its temperature and destroying it.

Myomectomy:

The key to myomectomy is proper patient selection. Fibroids are most usually multiple, and myomectomy often tends to be a temporary solution. Most fibroids do not require surgery, but only careful observation. Fibroids that are large enough or causing enough symptoms to warrant removal in women who are in the reproductive age group often need to be approached by open laparotomy, with incision in the abdominal wall, with some days of hospitalization following the procedure.

Hysterectomy:

The ultimate cure for significant fibroids causing debilitating problems is hysterectomy, or removal of the uterus. It often becomes the answer in women who have had all the children they wish to have and women who are in the menopausal years or beyond. Removal of the uterus can be accomplished vaginally in a significant proportion of women, without any abdominal incision. Laparoscopic assisted vaginal hysterectomy (LAVH) can be utilized to separate the ovaries, the blood supply and the upper attachments of the uterus prior to completing the procedure vaginally. It is still often elected for various technical reasons to perform a hysterectomy in an open fashion through an abdominal incision.

Vulvar Tumors

Tumors of the vulva classically are seen in a more senior age group, starting in the sixties and seventies. However, chronic disease conditions, such as diabetes, may make a woman more prone to tumors in this area at an earlier age.

Human Papillomavirus (HPV) causes a significant percentage of vulvar and vaginal cancers, as well as the benign vulvar (VIN) and vaginal intraepithelial neoplasia that precede the onset of cancer. HPV vaccines such as Gardasil reduce the incidence of these premalignant conditions of the vulva and vagina.

The most common vulvar tumors arise in the outer skin of the vulva. Benign skin change in this area can be quite common and can be associated with simple mechanical irritation by exercise, tight clothing that does not 'breathe' properly, harsh soaps or other products, or by simple infection, such as monilia (yeast).

It is important that a gynecologist or other qualified physician, such as a dermatologist, diagnose the condition. It is often not possible to be totally certain of the cause without taking cultures, looking at smears under a microscope, or simple biopsy (a small piece of tissue removed with use of local anesthesia), which is usually, of course, a minor office procedure.

The first symptom of precancerous or true malignant change may be itching, or 'rawness' that does not subside quickly with simple treatment.

With more significant chronic change, the examining physician will see a whitened, often thickened area of skin. Biopsy in cases of 'white' vulva should be done, as accurate diagnosis can only be made by observation by a pathologist of the biopsied tissue under a microscope.

The microscopic overgrowth of tissue, if benign, is usually called hyperplasia or dysplasia, and can be precancerous. The treatment is to remove the area of affected tissue completely, with a clear margin of normal tissue around it. If a predisposing factor, such as diabetes, is present, it is obviously important to get the disease process (diabetes) under proper control.

Actual malignant change in the biopsy is usually squamous carcinoma of the vulva. 'Squamous' refers to the skinlike nature of the cells. The front line, effective treatment is surgery to remove the affected area widely (vulvectomy), coupled with removal of surrounding lymph nodes, if the grade and the stage of the tumor warrant it.

The relative advantage of vulvar tumors is that they are external, and accessible to early diagnosis and treatment. Success rates are good if the tumors are found early.

The Prostate Gland

The prostate gland encircles the male urethra as it exits the urinary bladder and before it becomes the penile urethra. The prostate lies anterior to the rectum, enabling the classic evaluation of prostatic size, symmetry, and consistency by digital rectal examination.

Prostatic fluid is part of the ejaculate, along with sperm originating from the testes, and fluid from the seminal vesicles.

Benign Prostatic Hypertrophy (BPH):

Benign enlargement of the prostate gland becomes quite common as men age and can lead to difficulty in urination, small stream, and urinary retention, necessitating catheterization of the bladder to evacuate urine, and eventually transurethral prostatectomy (TUPR),other surgical approaches, or other treatments using laser or microwave.

Transrectal ultrasonography is used to evaluate the size and characteristics of the prostate.

Urodynamic and pressure flow studies are utilized as well.

Specific drug therapy includes alpha1 adrenoreceptor (AR) blocking agents which cause relaxation of bladder neck and prostate muscle fibers. Tamsulosin (Flomax), doxazosin (Cardura) and alfuzosin (Uroxatral) are such agents. Finasteride (Proscar) and dutasteride (Avodart) inhibit the enzyme 5-alpha reductase, thus inhibiting the conversion of testosterone to dihydrotestosterone (DHT), resulting in eventual prostate shrinkage.

Interestingly, Tadalafil (Cialis), which is primarily used to increase blood flow to the penis and facilitate erection, has been shown to lower the incidence and severity of benign prostatic hypertrophy.

Prostate Cancer

The incidence of prostate cancer increases as men age. Although, particularly when it occurs in younger men, it can be virulent, in older men it tends to be slower growing. This makes mass testing for prostate specific antigen (PSA) controversial, as positive tests are followed up by needle biopsies to confirm the presence of cancer.

The Gleason score is a number that reflects the grade that correlates to the aggressiveness of the prostate cancer. Magnetic resonance imaging (MRI) may be employed to help define the extent of the tumor.

When cancer is found, surgical treatment by prostatectomy often follows, with possible postoperative complications including urinary incontinence and impotence. Radiation treatment also can have deleterious side effects. As it has long been known that older men who are diagnosed with prostate cancer can often live with it, individual judgments have to be made by the treating urologist and the patient as to what route to take. The most conservative route is active surveillance.

The classic surgery for cancer of the prostate has been radical prostatectomy, which was gradually modified to be nerve sparing, in an attempt to maintain urinary continence and sexual potency.

Other treatment modalities include radiation in various forms such as stereotactic high -precision radiosurgery (including Cyberknife), and radioactive seed implants.

Depending on the individual case, hormonal therapy or anti-androgens to suppress testosterone levels, chemotherapy, or surgical castration (removal of the testes) may be advised.

There is now an approved dendritic cell vaccine for use in advanced prostate cancer: sipuleucil-T.

Testicular Cancer

Testicular cancer tends to be a disease of young men. As the testicles are outside the body cavity, enlargements of the testes tend to be evident early on. Thankfully, most are benign conditions and relatively easily treatable. Even testicular cancer itself is now often quite treatable, with long term disappearance of the disease in a significant number of cases. Treatment can involve orchiectomy (removal of the affected testicle) as well as chemotherapy. Depending on the characteristics of the tumor, radiation may be utilized.

Immune checkpoint inhibitors, Opdivo (nivolumab) and Keytruda (pembrolizumab), have been used in advanced testicular germ cell tumors.

Penile Lesions

Penile warts are caused by the sexually transmitted human papilloma virus. Some subtypes of HPV virus do cause penile cancer. Boys as well as girls should be vaccinated against HPV virus , preferably before the onset of sexual activity.

Cancer of the Urinary Bladder

The incidence of bladder cancer increases with age and is more common in men than in women.

If the disease is caught early, careful follow up and adequate therapy, often including local excision of tumor via cystoscopy and chemotherapy directly into the bladder, there is the prospect of long term survival.

Immunotherapy with BCG (Bacillus Calmette Guerin) instillation into the bladder may be used if there is considered to be a significant risk of progression. BCG acts as an immune modulating agent, enhancing the immune response.

More advanced stages of disease may require more aggressive surgery, chemotherapy, and radiation.

Checkpoint inhibitors for advanced bladder cancer include Tecentriq (atezolizumab), Bavencio (avelumab), Imfinzi (duralumab), Opdivo (nivolumab) and Keytruda (pembrolizumab).

Sexual Function

The long term maintenance of adequate sexual function, with the satisfaction and sense of fulfillment it lends to a relationship, is important to a large proportion of adults as they age.

The classic breakthrough on the female side was the development and widespread adoption of the contraceptive pill, a progesterone-like medication usually accompanied by a small amount of estrogen, and with its subsequent gradual decrease in dosage, minimizing side effects while maintaining effectiveness. This was a major factor in giving women control of their bodies and reproductive function. Changes in societal values accompanied by landmark legislation followed.

Changes in attitudes, fitness and lifestyle, along with advances in hormonal replacement therapy (HRT) and other treatments have heightened the ability of women to maintain satisfying sexual function into their later years.

On the male side, and much more recently, the advent of effective treatment for difficulty in achieving and maintaining erection, erectile disfunction (ED), by increasing penile blood flow with the use of sildenafil (Viagra), then tadalafil (Cialis) and similar drugs, has been a major breakthrough.

The early pioneering work in couples therapy by professionals notably including Dr Helen Singer Kaplan at Cornell University preceded the deployment of drugs targeting ED.

Further discussion can be found in the chapter on Menopause.

References

1. Kaplan, Helen Singer MD PhD: Sexual Aversion, Sexual Phobias, and Panic Disorder. Brunner/Mazel 1987
2. https://www.mskcc.org/cancer-care/types/prostate
3. https://www.mskcc.org/cancer-care/types/prostate/risk-factors
4. https://www.mskcc.org/cancer-care/types/prostate/diagnosis
5. https://www.mskcc.org/cancer-care/types/prostate/screening
6. https://www.mskcc.org/cancer-care/types/prostate/screening/screening-guidelines-prostate
7. https://www.mskcc.org/cancer-care/types/prostate/screening/psa-test
8. https://www.mskcc.org/cancer-care/types/prostate/diagnosis/prostate-biopsy
9. https://www.mskcc.org/cancer-care/types/prostate/treatment?utm_source=bing&utm_medium=cpc&utm_campaign=ProstateCancer&utm_term=treatment
10. https://opentextbc.ca/anatomyandphysiology/chapter/27-1-anatomy-and-physiology-of-the-male-reproductive-system

11. https://emedicine.medscape.com/article/437359-overview
12. https://emedicine.medscape.com/article/1923122-overview#a2
13. https://www.mayoclinic.org/diseases-conditions/benign-prostatic-hyperplasia/diagnosis-treatment/drc-20370093
14. https://www.mdanderson.org/cancer-types/testicular-cancer.html
15. https://www.cancer.gov/types/bladder/hp/bladder-treatment-pdq
16. https://www.pcf.org/about-prostate-cancer/prostate-cancer-treatment/immunotherapy-prostate-cancer/
17. https://www.webmd.com/cancer/bladder-cancer/bladder-cancer-immunotherapy-types
18. https://wwww.ncbi.nim.nih.gov/pubmed/30624089
19. https://www.ncbi.nim.nih.gov/pmc/articles/PMC6424849
20. https://www.cancer.org/cancer/cervical-cancer/treating/immunothrapy.html
21. https://www.cancer.gov/about-cancer/causes-prevention/risk/infectious-agents/hpv-vaccine-fact-sheet
22. Bibliography & Supplemental Bibliography: See www.rcaplanmd.com

CHAPTER 7
DIABETES

The Take-Home Message

- Diabetes is a defect in sugar metabolism, along with resistance to insulin
- Obesity is a significant factor
- Diabetes must be carefully controlled in order to prevent, or retard, complications
- Gene therapy shows promise for the definitive treatment of diabetes
- Metabolic Syndrome

Most diabetes is of the adult onset type. This Type 2 diabetes tends to be milder than Type I diabetes that has its onset in childhood and requires rigorous monitoring and therapy.

The discussion here refers to adult onset (Type 2) diabetes.

Diabetes is a defect in the metabolism of sugar. In a diabetic, insulin is not adequately produced in response to a sugar load. As well, there is resistance to the body's own insulin. This results in high blood sugar (hyperglycemia), and a spilling of sugar into the urine, as the concentration of sugar in the blood is too high for the kidneys to handle properly (glycosuria). There is a definite genetic predisposition to this condition. Improper diet and obesity are well known predisposing factors to the condition. As a matter of fact, in an obese individual, it is often possible to restore normal blood sugar levels simply by getting the person to the ideal body weight. This is easier said than done, even in individuals who have great motivation because they are aware of the implications of diabetes.

Diabetics typically may have high triglyceride levels, high LDL (low density lipoprotein) and low HDL (high density lipoprotein).

Long term, diabetes can cause blood vessel changes that shorten the life span, notably in the blood vessels of the heart itself, as well as kidney damage and eye damage. The eye damage occurs in the retina, which is the back of the eye where images are recorded. Blood vessel changes and hemorrhage can be seen in diabetic retinopathy.

It is important to know what comes first. Cause and effect can be confused or overlap. It may be that vascular disease in small blood vessels, microvascular disease, may be part of the cause of diabetes.

Type 2 diabetes may have an immune system component. The body's own immune system can act against the insulin-producing B cells in the pancreas. This abnormal phenomenon is known as autoimmunity.

Inflammation may be another factor playing a role in the development of diabetes.

Prevention of Diabetes

The number of US adults becoming diabetic is increasing, notably in older people.

Obesity is a major factor in diabetes, and of course, obesity is a major problem in North America today. As the matter of fact, some patients with diabetes who lose weight in a controlled fashion under the supervision of a physician revert back to a normal state. Their blood sugars return to normal, and no treatment is needed.

There is an association between arteriosclerotic heart disease and diabetes.

Diabetes in Pregnancy

Approximately forty years ago, I wrote that diabetes can be adversely affected by pregnancy, and that pregnancy is adversely affected by diabetes. I noted that meticulous control of diabetes in pregnancy is important for the wellbeing of both the mother and her baby. I noted the importance of proper diet and rest. I noted that insulin was then the drug of choice to achieve the level of control needed for optimal outcome in mother and child.

Since then, medical technology has greatly advanced. There are now obstetricians who are expert in Maternal-Fetal Medicine, adept at treating diabetes in pregnancy. Human insulin is now made using recombinant DNA technology. The principles, however, remain the same, and insulin by injection is still the treatment of choice for diabetes in pregnancy

Women who have a large number of children have a greater tendency to diabetes. Some women develop abnormal glucose levels in pregnancy, including some women who have a first pregnancy later in life, and then revert to a normal state after the child is born. This is known as gestational diabetes. These women need to be carefully monitored and treated during their pregnancies, both for their own protection and the protection of their babies.

During pregnancy, all women should be given a sugary drink, followed in one hour by a blood test for glucose. This one hour glucose challenge tells the doctor whether the sugar is being metabolized properly. If the glucose level is too high, a full three hour glucose tolerance test is performed, with blood sugar levels taken at regular intervals.

It is now possible to monitor glucose levels in the body continuously, which gives much finer control than the traditional method of spot checking glucose during the day.

With succeeding pregnancies, women with gestational diabetes run the risk of becoming permanently diabetic. A woman's weight at her own birth, whether low or significantly high, can put her at risk for gestational diabetes when she herself is pregnant

Insulin Resistance (Metabolic Syndrome, Syndrome X)

There are people who have excess fat, mainly in the abdominal region. This is called central obesity. As well, they have high blood pressure and are resistant to their bodies' own insulin. They may actually be diabetic or may produce larger amounts of insulin to overcome the resistance and keep blood sugar at a normal level. As well, they have high levels of triglycerides, but low levels of HDL (High Density Lipoprotein Cholesterol).

These people are at increased risk for heart disease because of the multiple risk factors of obesity, hypertension, abnormal cholesterol and triglyceride levels, as well as the propensity towards diabetes.

This distinct combination of problems is known as the Metabolic Syndrome (Syndrome X). It is thought that there may be a genetic basis for this syndrome. A mutation in mitochondria, causing mitochondrial dysfunction, is known to be present in some affected people. Mitochondria are tiny organs (organelles) in the cytoplasm of cells.

The treatment involves proper control of cholesterol and triglycerides, bringing the high blood pressure towards normal, and controlling body weight, as well as dealing with insulin resistance with appropriate oral hypoglycemic agents.

The Mediterranean diet can be helpful in achieving these goals.

Smoking, which is a major factor in the onset of some cancers and arteriosclerotic heart disease, also is associated with insulin resistance. Smoking can cause narrowing in small blood vessels. It is obviously important to stop smoking, or better yet, never to smoke.

Exercise is beneficial. Being physically inactive can promote insulin resistance, which is associated with glucose intolerance.

Surprisingly, drinking alcohol in moderate amounts may improve sensitivity to insulin, lowering risk of diabetes. Of course, alcohol use has negative implications as well, ranging from effects on reaction time and judgment, to deleterious effects on the liver. Alcohol should not be used in pregnancy.

DHEA (dehydroepiandrosterone) is a hormone naturally present in both sexes. Levels of this hormone naturally decline from the mid twenties onward. Replacing this hormone may reduce abdominal obesity by decreasing the accumulation of abdominal fat, and possibly be used in treatment of the metabolic syndrome. However, there are other implications in the use of DHEA in women. DHEA replacement increases testosterone (male sex hormone) levels in women and raises estradiol (a female sex hormone) levels as well. The totality of these effects on women needs to be looked at carefully.

Treating Diabetes

The great discovery of Banting and Best, giving animal derived insulin that literally saved the lives of previously uncontrolled diabetics, revolutionized the treatment of this condition, and changed it from a generally fatal one into a manageable chronic condition, although often with serious long term effects, and a generally shortened life span.

Recombinant DNA technology has allowed the manufacture of human insulin, in both short acting and longer acting forms. Humulin is made in this way.

The side effects of insulin and other blood sugar lowering (hypoglycemic) agents include poor control in both directions: that is, blood sugar that remains too high (hyperglycemia), and blood sugar that is too low (hypoglycemia). A lack of control in either direction can have serious consequences.

Significant strides have been made with the evolution of oral hypoglycemic agents that can return the blood sugar to normal without the diabetic person having to take self-administered injections. Some of these classes of drugs are discussed briefly here. A physician's advice is essential in determining the choice of drug that might be suitable. For example, sulfonylureas have to be used with caution in frail elderly people. Metformin may be one of the possible better choices in that situation.

Metformin hydrochloride, marketed as Glumetza, Fortamet and other trade names, decreases production of glucose in the liver, and decreases the absorption of glucose by the intestine. Insulin secretion does not change, but glucose use is increased. Metformin therapy is associated with weight loss, which can make it an attractive choice for the overweight diabetic individual. A serious, sometimes fatal complication known as lactic acidosis rarely occurs. The risk is increased in diabetics with poor kidney function. This drug is generally not recommended in pregnancy.

Trulicity (dulaglutide) and Victoza (liraglutide) are examples of GLP-1 (glucagon-like peptide-1) receptor agonists. By activating the GLP-1 receptor, dulaglutide acts on pancreatic beta cells, causing glucose-dependent insulin release. These drugs also decrease appetite.

Jardiance (empagliflozin) and Farxiga (dapagliflozin) are examples of SGLT2 (sodium-glucose transporter) inhibitors that promote renal excretion of glucose by reducing renal reabsorption of glucose.

Januvia (sitagliptin) is an example of a DPP-4 (dipeptidyl peptidase) inhibitor which slows the inactivation of incretin hormones.

Incretin hormone levels are normally increased in response to a meal. Therefore, these drugs promote insulin release.

Avandia (rosiglitazone maleate) is one of a class of oral agents called thiazolidinediones that increase insulin sensitivity. These agents can lower triglyceride levels and increase levels of high-density lipoprotein cholesterol (HDL). Actos Tablets (Pioglitazone) is another agent in this class. All Thiazolidine drugs for Type 2 diabetes can cause or worsen heart failure. Rosiglitazone use in type 2 diabetes is associated with an increased risk of myocardial ischemic events, including angina, heart attack (myocardial infarction) and sudden death. It should not be used in pregnancy.

Glucotrol (glipizide) is an example of an older class of drugs called Sulfonylureas that stimulate the release of insulin from the pancreas.

Computerized small instruments are widely available which allow the diabetic person to check their blood sugar levels several times during the day. This allows them to keep their blood sugars in the normal range at all times, so that they do not experience uncontrolled lows and highs, both of which can be dangerous, leading on the one hand to diabetic coma, and on the other hand to insulin shock

Insulin is normally made in the human body in the pancreas in sites called the Islets of Langerhans. One experimental approach has been to transplant Islet cells to affected people, so that they can produce more insulin on their own. Stem cells from the pancreas can be implanted, creating the insulin-producing cells necessary to control diabetes.

The hope is that, in the future, gene therapy will be able to eradicate diabetes in many people permanently. Some people seem to store fat more efficiently. This works well if they are starving: they have body fat to live off. This may have been a survival mechanism for our ancestors. However, if people with this genetic makeup get too much food, they store it as fat. Such people are said to have a "Thrifty Genotype".

A combination of genes are involved in adult-onset diabetes, although some cases are caused by single gene defects. One particular gene that has been implicated is the calpain-10 gene, which carries three DNA variations associated with diabetes.

References

1. Morais, Jose; Kim, Young-Sang: The Care of the Older Person, Third Edition: How to manage Type 2 diabetes in frail elderly patients. RMC Publishing, LLC 2019
2. https://www.healthline.com/health/diabtes/medications-list#type-2-diabetes
3. www.uspl.lilly.com/trulicity/trulicity.html#pi
4. www.docs.boehringer-ingelheim.com/Prescribing%20Information/Pls/Jardiance/Jardiance.pdf
5. www.merck.com/product/usa/pi_circulars/j/januvia_pi.pdf
6. https://www.pfizermedicalinformation.com/en-us/glucotrol/clinical-pharmacology
7. https://care.diabetesjournals.org/content/early/2019/12/18/dci19-0068
8. Bibliography & Supplemental Bibliography: See www.rcaplanmd.com

CHAPTER 8
DISEASES OF THE JOINTS

The Take-Home Message

- High impact sports have a downside
- Minimally invasive surgery, microsurgery, and joint replacement have been significant advances in the treatment of joint disease
- Autoimmune disease often involves multiple organ systems

Arthritis

The predominant form of arthritis in people as they get older is osteoarthritis. Swelling, which can be painful, develops in the joints, notably the small joints of the fingers and toes. This leads to gradual limitation of motion in the joints, with loss of function. Of course, this can interfere with your occupation, if fine movements are involved, and with your recreation, including the playing of musical instruments, and fine work, such as crocheting and knitting. Conservative treatment includes exercise and physiotherapy, as well as anti-inflammatory drugs, usually taken by mouth.

Celebrex (celecoxib), a Cox – 2 inhibitor, is an example of an effective anti-inflammatory agent (NSAIDS: nonsteroidal anti-inflammatory drugs) Cox – 2 is an inflammatory enzyme. There can be a downside to taking such medications. Celebrex and other NSAIDS may increase the risk of cardiovascular thrombotic events, including heart attack (myocardial infarction) and stroke. Bleeding, ulceration, or even perforation of the stomach or intestines can occur with NSAIDS. Celebrex and other NSAIDS should not be used in pregnancy.

Aleve (naproxen) is a NSAID that can be bought over the counter. It carries the same warnings as other NSAIDS and should not be used in pregnancy. In higher doses, it has been shown to increase the occurrence of heart attack and strokes.

Advil (ibuprofen)is another NSAID that can be purchased over the counter. It carries NSAID warnings, including that it should not be used in conjunction with aspirin, when aspirin is being taken to lessen the chance of heart attack. In this scenario, the Advil may decrease the benefit of aspirin. Advil, like other NSAIDS, should not be used in pregnancy.

Many people get by with classic anti-inflammatory agents such as aspirin. However, taking an over-the-counter medication does not mean the drug has no side effects. Alternatives were sought to aspirin because of side effects including gastric irritation and an increased tendency to bleed, sometimes resulting in severe bleeding from the gastrointestinal tract, and even perforation (a break, or hole, in the stomach or intestine). Aspirin should not be used in pregnancy without the advice of the obstetrician.

As a matter of fact, just as some drugs are Cox – 2 inhibitors, Aspirin itself is a Cox – 1 and Cox – 2 inhibitor. The push for drugs that were primarily Cox – 2 inhibitors was spurred on by the side effects caused by Cox – 1 enzyme suppression.

Every drug has an 'effect' for which it is utilized, and 'side-effects', that are often undesirable. Sometimes, a 'side-effect' can become the most beneficial effect of the drug. Aspirin itself is famously used today for its anti-blood clotting properties, taken by many people at risk for heart attack as a preventative.

There is an entire field of medicine, Rheumatology, that deals with all types of arthritis.

A consultation with a rheumatologist can be a good idea, in order to ascertain what type of arthritis is present, and how to control it.

Inevitably, living a long life leads to wear and tear on the joints, especially the larger joints, including the hips, knees, shoulders, and elbows, as well as the wrists and ankles. This is exacerbated by large and small injuries, including falls, and the trauma of other accidents.

Glucosamine and Chondroitin are naturally occurring substances that were widely used, often together. Taken by mouth, they were said to have a beneficial effect in some cases by reducing the loss of joint cartilage. These claims are not supported by recent studies. Glucosamine is made from the chitin found in shellfish shells. Chondroitin is made from the trachea of cattle, or from shark cartilage.

The popularity of high impact sports, such as running and contact sports, increases the incidence of degenerative, arthritic, and traumatic changes in the joints. Such changes are common in professional athletes and dancers. Ligament injuries, most commonly meniscus injuries in the knees, occur as well. More serious ligament injuries can involve the cruciate and collateral ligaments in the knees, avulsion or tears of the Achilles tendons in the feet, the biceps tendons in the arm, or injuries to the rotator cuff in the shoulders.

Fortunately, arthroscopic techniques are now widely utilized by orthopedic surgeons to correct many of these problems. Incisions are small, and surgery is often done on an out-patient basis, so that hospital stays are minimal.

Joint replacement surgery, most commonly for hips and knees, but increasingly for other joints, is now commonplace.

With age, degenerative and traumatic changes in the discs between the vertebrae in the spinal column are common. Treatment is usually conservative, unless the nerves arising from the spinal cord become involved. Advanced surgical techniques, including microsurgery, are now available to help with these problems in more severe cases. It is important to consult with a rheumatologist, orthopedic surgeon, or neurosurgeon if numbness, tingling, or other symptoms of nerve involvement arise.

Rheumatoid arthritis tends to be more dramatic, with obvious inflammation in the joints leading to a loss of function. Rheumatoid arthritis is one of a class of diseases known as autoimmune diseases. In these conditions, the immune system is inappropriately activated, even though no foreign invader is present.

Treatment is largely symptomatic, with the use of anti-inflammatory agents. Steroid hormones can be used to dampen down the immune response, but these drugs have side effects of their own, and need to be monitored by a qualified physician.

Remicade (infliximab) is one of several monoclonal antibodies now available. It can be used in conjunction with Trexall (methotrexate) in the treatment of rheumatoid arthritis. Other such drugs include Humira (adalimumab) that binds to Tumor Necrosis Factor (TNF). Elevsted levels of TNF are present in the synovial (joint) fluid of rheumatoid arthritis patients. One of the predominant complications of Remicade and Humira is an increased risk of severe infection. It is unknown whether use of this drug in pregnancy can cause fetal harm, aside from the possible severe side effects to the mother. Methotrexate is a chemotherapeutic agent (antimetabolite) that can have serious side effects, including toxicity to the liver and bone marrow. It can be lethal to a developing fetus and cannot be used in an ongoing healthy pregnancy.

When joints are badly damaged, surgical joint replacement, even for finger joints, is now available.

Lupus erythematosus is a multisystem autoimmune disease that affects the joints, as well as other important systems in the body. In this condition, the white blood cells known as B lymphocytes make antibodies that attack the body itself. It may be becoming possible to stifle this disease at its source, by decreasing B lymphocyte stimulator, a protein made in white blood cells.

Sjogren syndrome is an autoimmune disorder that tends to appear in mid adulthood.

Dry eyes and dry mouth are common symptoms.

Autoimmune Disease

Women, more than men, are prone to autoimmune disease. There may be genetic factors involved. This is a class of diseases in which the normal immune response is inappropriately triggered and seems to attack the affected person's own tissues and organs. Systemic lupus erythematosus, rheumatoid arthritis, and multiple sclerosis are prominent examples of autoimmune disease. Dysfunction of the immune system is responsible for Hashimoto's disease, which affects the thyroid gland.

It is thought that the immunologic changes of pregnancy can have a role in triggering these disease states. Certainly, getting pregnant can make some of these states better or worse, likely because of the altered hormonal output of the woman during pregnancy. Rheumatoid arthritis and multiple sclerosis can temporarily improve while a woman is pregnant. Systemic lupus erythematosus may get worse.

It is possible that fetal cells that have entered into the mother can lead to an inappropriate immunologic response, and an attack on maternal cells: that is, on the mother's own tissue. Conversely, maternal cells flowing into the developing fetus can cause an immunologic response in the fetus that can damage it.

A hallmark of autoimmune disease is often the involvement of multiple organ systems. Systemic lupus erythematosus is essentially a connective tissue disease, with inflammation affecting the joints, but with major organs including the heart often involved as well.

The nervous system is protected by myelin, just as an electrical wire is protected by an insulating cover. Multiple sclerosis is a disease in which demyelination occurs, exposing the nerves in the body to progressive damage.

It is now thought that prominent disease conditions such as diabetes may well have an immunologic component.

References

1. www.ghr.nlm.nih.gov/condition/sjogren-syndrome#diagnosis
2. www.mayoclinic.org/diseases-conditions/rheumatoid-arthritis/diagnosis-treatment/drc-20353653
3. https://www.accessdata.fda.gov
4. https://www.humira.com
5. Bibliography & Supplemental Bibliography: See www.rcaplanmd.com

CHAPTER 9

DISEASES OF THE CENTRAL NERVOUS SYSTEM

The Take-Home Message

- Alzheimer's Disease can now be diagnosed more definitively, and treatment is available, although not curative
- Strides are being made in the treatment of Parkinsonism

Alzheimer's Disease

Alzheimer's disease, known as AD, affects approximately four million people in the United States alone. Various genetic mutations have been implicated in the cause of AD. There is an association between apolipoprotein E genotype (APOE) and late onset AD. Genetic testing is available.

Deposition of beta amyloid protein between neurons in the brain is seen in AD. There are biomarkers available for amyloid, as well as for the Tau protein that largely makes up the neurofibrillary tangles found inside brain cells in AD. There are biomarkers for neurodegeneration as well.

With AD there tends to be gradual cognitive decline over at least one year and a normal general physical examination.

Whether other factors are implicated in this condition has not yet been determined. There are other reasons for declining mental function and memory, although AD is the predominant cause in older people. Depression, and the use of various medications, can result in a similar picture which can confuse the diagnosis. A whole range of other disorders, including nutritional disorders, inflammation of the brain, cardiovascular disorders, stroke, brain tumors, and the treatment of brain tumors, notably radiation to the brain, can all affect the ability to think clearly and to remember things. Neurologists and geriatricians are among the specialists who should be consulted to properly make the diagnosis.

Preimplantation Genetic Diagnosis (PGD):

There is a rare early-onset form of AD that can be caused by three different genes located on three different chromosomes.

It is now possible by genetic diagnosis to detect these mutations. In fact, a woman with one of these mutations can undergo preimplantation genetic diagnosis (PGD) to ensure that an egg is selected that does not carry the mutation, so that her child to be born will not risk developing early onset AD.

PGD is now being used for many different genetic conditions.

Imaging:

Advanced imaging studies are used to confirm the diagnosis of AD. These studies include the use of positron emission tomography (PET scan), magnetic resonance imaging (MRI), and computerized axial tomography (CAT scan). The PET scan shows glucose uptake by the brain on the metabolic level. In other words, it shows brain metabolism. People who suffer from AD have abnormalities of glucose metabolism in specific areas of the white matter of the brain located in the parietal and temporal lobes of the brain, essentially on both sides of the brain.

MRI and CAT scan, on the other hand, show actual brain structure, and may show brain atrophy. These studies can be normal in Alzheimer's disease.

Cognition:

Cognition means knowing, and includes recognizing, perceiving, conceiving, judgment, sensing, imagining, reasoning, orientation, memory, and attention. The ability to concentrate,and the ability to perform actions properly are important. The level of language skill is significant.

Older people should regularly be involved in cognitively stimulating activities. There is some indication that stimulating the mind does reduce the risk of AD. This includes activities that most of us would consider to be routine, including listening to radio, watching television, reading newspapers, books, and magazines, playing card games, and doing crossword puzzles.

Physical activity, notably regular walking, is associated with better cognition in older persons.

A simple way to evaluate cognition is a mini mental state examination (MMSE). The person is asked if they have trouble with memory. It is then ascertained if the person is oriented as to time, and if they know the year, month, day, and the current date, as well as the season. Questions are asked concerning orientation as to place: present location, including the state and city, and what part of the city the person is in, in what building, and the person's location within that building,

The person is then asked to repeat three random words, then to subtract seven from one hundred, and then to continue to subtract seven from each remainder. The person being tested is subsequently asked to recall the previously mentioned three random words.

The test subject is then asked to identify common everyday objects by name.

The person is asked to repeat a small sentence. This tests repetition, as opposed to recall which was previously measured, and registration, which was the immediate repetition of the three words.

Performance of a simple task, like taking a piece of paper, holding it in a hand, and then putting it on the floor is assessed. This measures comprehension.

Reading is then tested. The person is asked to silently read, to write a sentence, and to copy a simple diagram.

Of course, this relatively simple test simply points out that there may be a decline in memory and mental function, and by no means is definitively diagnostic for AD.

It is thought that the deposition of the substance called amyloid is a significant feature of AD. It is also thought that people with AD have a reduced level of acetylcholine (ACh) in the brain. Nerve cells in the brain called neurons interact by way of impulses traveling down them. The neuron has a long ending, called an axon, which the nerve impulse travels down to a synapse, or small space between nerve cells, or close to an organ acted upon by the nerve cell. Acetylcholine is a neurotransmitter that is released from the nerve cell ending, passing along the signal to the receiving cell.

Treatment of AD (Alzheimer's Disease):

Drugs that suppress the enzymes that break down acetylcholine (ACh), improving neurotransmission, are available. These drugs include Aricept (donepezil) and Exelon (rivastigmine). These drugs have varying side effects, including nausea and vomiting, and should only be used after consultation with, and a prescription given by, a physician.

The NMDA receptor blocker Namenda (memantine) decreases the activity of the neurotransmitter glutamate. There is no evidence that memantine slows neurodegeneration in AD.

Increased levels of the amino acid precursor homocysteine are a risk factor for the development of Alzheimer's disease. Homocysteine levels tend to be elevated if levels of vitamins B_{10} (folic acid), B_{12}, and B_6 are deficient. Good nutrition with adequate intake of B vitamins may be helpful in the management of AD. Homocysteine levels do get lowered with vitamin B_{10} (folic acid) supplementation. In the United States, all enriched cereal grains are fortified with vitamin B_{10}.

Vitamin A (Alpha-tocopherol) may slow the progression of AD.

Monoamine oxidase (MAO) Inhibitors are a class of antidepressant drugs used for major depressive disorders. These drugs may work by potentiating MAO transmitter activity in the Central Nervous System. It is possible that some drugs in this class can slow the progression of AD. Notable side effects of MAO Inhibitors include increased suicidality, particularly in a younger population.

It is thought that inflammation may play a role in AD. It is possible that NSAIDS (nonsteroidal anti-inflammatory drugs) including Motrin (ibuprofen), Anaprox (naproxen) and Voltaren (diclofenac) when used long term may lower the risk of getting AD. NSAIDS can increase the risk of thrombotic events, including myocardial infarction (heart attack) , and stroke. There is an increased incidence of stomach bleeding.

Cognitive decline tends to be more pronounced in elders who have Metabolic Syndrome, (see Chapter: Diabetes) especially those who show evidence of inflammation. This is not surprising, considering that diabetes, high blood pressure, and high blood lipid levels all can be factors in raising the risk of cognitive decline.

Estrogen replacement therapy (ERT) can help visual perception, construction skills, and short-term visual memory. ERT does carry the increased risk of thromboembolic events, including pulmonary embolism and stroke.

None of these treatments are curative. Inevitably, caregivers have become a fundamental part of the treatment and support of people with AD. Community financial resources, as well as education counseling and support, both to people with AD and their caregivers becomes increasingly important as the disease progresses.

Parkinsonism

Parkinsonism is also known as Parkinson disease. The problem arises in the basal ganglia of the brain. It is a chronic and progressive neurologic condition that is debilitating to many people. The most obvious symptoms include shaking and gross tremors of the limbs. It becomes increasingly difficult with this condition to control muscular movements. In later stages, the face may appear masklike. A particular type of cell, the dopaminergic cell, is gradually lost from the lower part of the brain known as the brainstem. Other neurotransmitters are affected as well.

It is unknown why Parkinsonism develops. There are various other conditions that can mimic it, including the use of various drugs and medications, and these other causes must be ruled out by the neurologist. Everything from viruses to smoking have been implicated. In some cases the condition may have a genetic predisposition. The parkin gene has been implicated in relatively rare early-onset Parkinson disease. It is more likely that multiple genetic factors may be at work in the more common late-onset Parkinson disease.

Current treatment tends to be by medication in the earlier stages. Exciting new neurosurgical techniques are now available to control the condition. Obviously, all treatment should be thoroughly discussed with the treating physician, and carefully monitored.

Medical treatment involves either Levodopa or use of dopamine agonists. An agonist is a drug that combines at receptor sites, in this case creating activity like dopamine.

Stalevo (carbidopa, levodopa,and entacapone) is a combination of levodopa and other drugs that effectively get more levodopa to the brain. Levodopa is a precursor of dopamine: it is converted to dopamine in the brain. The range of side effects can include fainting, diarrhea, hallucinations, and increased dyskinesia (distorted voluntary movements). The drug is generally not used in pregnancy.

Dopamine agonists include Requip (ropinirole), and Mirapex (pramipexole). Side effects can include falling asleep, even while driving a car, low blood pressure, and hallucinations. There can be risks to the fetus in pregnancy

New surgical techniques include precise positioning in three dimension, called stereotactic technique, of an area of the brain called the globus pallidum. Precise surgery is then done to that area. This is known as pallidotomy.

Conversely, by the same precise stereotactic techniques, a wire can be implanted neurosurgically for deep brain stimulation.

An experimental development has been the actual implantation of healthy cells capable of producing dopamine.

As yet, there is no cure for Parkinson's disease, but with modern drug and neurosurgical treatments, the lives of affected individuals can be improved.

References

1. Gauthier, Serge, MD: The Care of the Older Person, Third Edition: Chapters: Update on Alzheimer's disease diagnosis and management; Doctor, my wife is getting forgetful. RMC Publishing, LLC. 2019
2. www.accessdata.fda.gov/drugsatfda_docs/label/2013/021487s010s012s014,021627s008lbl.pdf

3. https://www.nia.nih.gov/health/what-happens-brain-alzheimers-disease
4. https://www.brightfocus.org/alzheimers-disease/article/tau-protein-and-alzheimers-disease-whats-connection
5. Bibliography & Supplemental Bibliography:
See www.rcaplanmd.com

CHAPTER 10

MENOPAUSE, OSTEOPOROSIS, MIGRAINE, SEXUAL DYSFUNCTION, DEPRESSION

The Take-Home Message

- The interplay of female sex hormones is choreographed by a feedback mechanism
- Menopause means the stopping of the menstrual flow
- Abnormal bleeding in a woman in the menopausal age group must always be investigated
- Woman do not normally menstruate beyond the age of 55
- The average age of menopause is approximately 50
- In perimenopause, the periods become shorter, lighter, and farther apart
- It is important that symptoms attributed to PMS (premenstrual syndrome) or PMDD (premenstrual dysphoric disorder), be evaluated before concluding that PMS or PMDD is indeed the explanation
- HRT (hormonal replacement therapy) must be individualized, after the risks and benefits have been explained

as well as the possibility of using other therapy, such as bisphosphonates, Denosumab or SERM's (specific estrogen receptor modulators) and after careful examination

- In most women, after four years of use soon after menopause, the risk of hormonal replacement therapy with estrogen and progesterone outweighs any possible benefits
- Osteoporosis, diagnosed by bone density studies can be counteracted by aerobic exercise, calcium and vitamin D intake, bisphosphonates, SERM's, or HRT. Statins, other drugs, or 'natural' alternatives may be helpful. It is important that risks and benefits are explained, and the choice of therapy is made with a gynecologist.
- Sexual arousal, a complex phenomenon, is recently better understood.
- Therapy for sexual dysfunction arising from a wide variety of causes is now readily available.
- Treatment with triptans has been a breakthrough in the management of migraine

It is only in recent generations that remedies for the menopause have become a popular topic of conversation. Historically, the menopause was not much of a problem to society. Life expectancy was such that many women unfortunately never reached that age. As a matter of fact, primitive women did not menstruate much. Menstruation was uncommon enough that women who menstruated were segregated in separate huts in some societies. In others, they were considered unclean. Shortly after menarche, when periods began, or even before that time, a woman would be married. When she began to ovulate, she would inevitably become pregnant. After having the baby, she would lactate and nurse the baby, often for a prolonged period of time, until she was pregnant again. The cycle would repeat itself through the woman's child-bearing reproductive years. It was necessary for the survival of the human race that she reproduce early and often. Many of her offspring would die, and she herself faced a significant chance of dying in childbirth. In any case, with a life expectancy of 37 years the problems of menopause were not the most pressing ones facing womanhood.

With the advent of preventive antenatal care and scientific medicine, as well as major advances in childbirth, including the introduction of aseptic techniques to minimize infection, and the prevention and treatment of hemorrhage, women could expect to live a healthier life, and to live longer.

Increasing wealth of societies coupled with better nutrition, and better understanding of public health measures along with their implementation, has resulted in the lengthening of the reproductive years.

This by itself, without the use of any treatments, whether so called natural treatments or synthetic replacements, has helped women to stay healthy longer.

The often accepted philosophy that 'if a little is good a lot must be great' can be dangerous. A menstruating woman in her reproductive years will normally produce all the estrogen and progesterone that she needs cyclically from her ovaries, on command from the pituitary gland, which in itself is under the control of the hypothalamus situated at the base of the brain. Gonadotropin Releasing Hormones (GNRH) from the hypothalamus act on the pituitary gland to release FSH, which is Follicle Stimulating Hormone, and LH, which is Luteinizing Hormone in a rhythmic fashion.

Inhibins

Substances called inhibins are peptides made in cells (granulosa cells) of the ovarian follicles. One type, inhibin B, is prominent during the first half of the menstrual cycle, in response to FSH stimulation.

Inhibin then acts to suppress the output of FSH. Inhibin A is more prominent during the second half the menstrual cycle, when release of the egg (ovulation) has occurred.

This is a part of the "feedback" mechanism by which hormones are regulated. In other words, secretion of hormones into the blood stream by the pituitary gland is regulated and turned off by the production of other substances in the 'target' ovary.

The average age of menopause, which in the 1960's was 47 in our society, is now about 50 years of age. Some women normally get the menopause as early as 42 years of age, and some women will not normally get the menopause until 55 years of age. It is very important that women in their 50's who are still menstruating be monitored by qualified physicians to ensure that their bleeding patterns are normal and are physiologic menstrual patterns, as opposed to bleeding problems caused by disease states which may be pre-cancers or cancers.

Diagnosing the Menopause

Women will not normally stop menstruating prior to the age of forty-two. Vaginal bleeding after the age of fifty-five should be regarded with great suspicion and always be investigated by a qualified gynecologist. The defining feature of menopause is cessation of menstrual flow, permanently. Essentially, the normal function of the ovaries is lost. The actual microscopic structure of the ovaries is changed. There is a high density of nerve fibers in postmenopausal ovaries, which infers altered communication. There is diminished output of estrogen and progesterone by the post menopausal ovary. The pituitary gland puts out increased amounts of follicle stimulating hormone (FSH), and luteinizing hormone (LH). The physician can detect these hormonal changes by blood tests. It is necessary to rule out pregnancy at the same time, as the hallmark of pregnancy is, of course, a missed period.

Symptoms are variable, and in some cases severe. Commonly, women will experience hot flashes, which are the sudden onset feeling of heat and flushing of short duration. There may be night sweats as well. Other symptoms may include sleeplessness, irritability, lack of concentration, changes in appetite, and headache. There may be a change in libido, or sexual desire and satisfaction. It may be noted that the hair is less lustrous and that the skin has lost some of it smoothness and glow.

Later changes may include bone loss and osteoporosis. Postural changes may result, as well as vertebral compression, and the so-called dowager's hump. The tendency to bone fracture increases. Cardiovascular changes can occur as well.

Menopause means the stopping of the menstrual flow. As the menopause approaches, the periods will get shorter, lighter, and farther apart, and eventually or abruptly stop altogether. Unfortunately, many people seem to think that any abnormality in the menstrual flow in the 40's or 50's is related to the menopause. Nothing could be farther from the truth. Abnormal bleeding in this age group represents a major warning sign of disease and should be properly investigated. This is especially true of any woman who is taking any kind of hormonal replacement therapy, whether she believes it to be natural or not. The same age group of women who are in the menopausal years are also an age group who are vulnerable to various benign and malignant diseases of the reproductive system. A woman who wants to live a long and healthful life should regularly see a gynecologist for evaluation and preventive care.

The normal pattern of slowing menstruation must not be confused with periods that are either getting heavier, longer in duration, or closer together. Such changes in menstrual pattern are suspicious in nature and should be reported to the gynecologist. The passage of blood clots with the periods is another warning sign. The endometrial lining of the womb that is shed with each menstrual period contains substances that prevent blood clotting. When this mechanism is overwhelmed by excessive blood loss, the excess blood will clot. Bleeding, spotting or staining between the periods is another suspicious sign. Early tumors that start as polyps in the uterine lining can present in this way. It is important not to ignore bleeding in between the periods just because it is a very small amount. Such bleeding or staining can be an important warning sign of disease that can be treated early. Bleeding, spotting, or staining after intercourse is another very important warning sign of disease in the female reproductive tract. Most often, it points to abnormalities in the region of the cervix, or mouth of the womb. It is a classical symptom of cancer of the cervix.

Periods that are too close together are abnormal. Ovarian disease including ovarian tumors, can cause this symptom. A cyclic hormonal release from the ovaries normally regulates cycle length. Ovarian abnormalities can create a dysfunction in this hormonal release.

Menstrual Pain

Pain with the periods should not be dismissed, especially if it has changed in nature over the years. Diseases of the reproductive tract, including benign and malignant uterine tumors, can declare themselves this way. Some cramping with the periods can be normal, and has been referred to in the past as primary dysmenorrhea.

Dysmenorrhea is simply a Latin word that essentially means "pain with the periods". "Primary" is a word used to signify that the cause is unknown. In other words, tell someone that you have pain with the periods, and they tell you that you have primary dysmenorrhea, which means that you have pain with the periods and they don't know why.

In fact, we now do know why there can be some cramping with the periods. During the normal menstrual cycle, there is prostaglandin release. This substance causes uterine muscle to contract rhythmically. That is why aspirin and aspirin-like substances are generally effective in controlling physiologic, or normal menstrual cramping. Aspirin and similar substances are not painkillers: they are antiprostaglandins. For this reason, aspirin and similar substances work better to relieve normal menstrual cramping if they are given before the onset of pain, to prevent any prostaglandin release. However, no drug, even aspirin, should be taken without the advice of a qualified physician if there is any chance of pregnancy.

Normal menstrual cramping should not be debilitating and does not prevent the majority of women from going on with their normal life pattern, including work and most recreation. Significant pain with the periods, or any change in the pattern, should be evaluated by the gynecologist. There are myriad reasons for abnormal pelvic pain, whether related to the periods or not. These reasons, of course, include diseases of the uterus itself, as well as tumor growth.

Pain in between the periods has been called Mittelschmerz. This is simply a German word which means pain in the middle. Again, if you tell somebody that you have pain in the middle of the cycle, they tell you that you have Mittelschmerz. In other words, they have just told you the same thing, but in German. No diagnosis has been made. In fact, very few women report the slight twinge midcycle that can be associated with actual ovulation. The vast majority of women do not feel it. Pain that occurs in the abdomen or pelvis that is related to, or unrelated to, the menstrual period should be checked out by the gynecologist.

Perimenopause

Prior to the stopping of the menstrual periods, the periods will often become shorter in duration, less in amount, and further apart. This pattern is often referred to as the perimenopause. It can be appropriate in this circumstance to take, with a doctor's advice, low dosage contraceptive pills, which will provide some estrogen and a progestin, while providing contraception at the same time.

There is, however, an increased risk of taking contraceptive pills, in women as they get older, of thrombotic disease. A woman who smokes increases her cardiovascular risk, and that risk is heightened by the addition of the contraceptive pill.

Contraceptive pills should not be taken to mask bleeding abnormalities. Proper diagnosis of the abnormality should be carried out by a gynecologist prior to any treatment.

Hormonally, the onset of menopause is characterized by increasing levels of FSH (follicle stimulating hormone) and LH (luteinizing hormone) from the pituitary gland, as the pituitary gland seemingly attempts to increase stimulation of the ovary, which is putting out lowered amounts of estrogen and progesterone. Elevated levels of FSH are tied to the onset of hot flashes. Levels of inhibin decrease, along with the rise in FSH. The hormonal changes can be detected by blood tests.

There is a hormone called antimullerian hormone, produced by cells (granulosa cells) of follicles developing around ova (eggs) in the ovary. This hormone prevents the depletion of the follicles in the ovary that a woman is born with, protecting her reproductive ability.

A reduction in antimullerian hormone signals that the stock of follicles (and eggs) is decreasing, and that menopause is approaching. It may be possible to detect this change in antimullerian hormone before the classic increase in FSH (follicle stimulating hormone) appears.

PMS (Premenstrual Syndrome)

A wide variety of symptoms normally occur in many women just before or with the onset of the menstrual period. Depression, anxiety, bloating, constipation, diarrhea, breast tenderness, weight gain, headache and other symptoms have been reported. A majority of women who have one or other of these symptoms find them to be mild, not debilitating, and not interfering with lifestyle. Women who have one or more of these symptoms that are severe, or do interfere with lifestyle, should be evaluated by a gynecologist, to ensure that no generalized disease process or problems in the reproductive organs are present that are really responsible for the symptoms. Such symptoms generally are a wake-up call by the body that something might be wrong, and this possibility has to be properly addressed.

Changing the diet may be of some help to women with PMS. A high protein diet, with salt restriction, may help mild fluid retention. Calcium may be supplemented. Aerobic exercise may be of value.

A wide variety of treatments are available for PMS. After significant disease processes have been ruled out, treatment is targeted to the presenting symptoms, so that they are properly taken care of. It is important to rule out early pregnancy before taking any medications. Symptoms such as breast tenderness are classically associated with early pregnancy.

PMDD (Premenstrual Dysphoric Disorder)

A relatively small percentage of women experience severe mood and behavioral changes premenstrually. The range of symptoms include anxiety, depression, irritability and anger.

Management includes the use of antidepressants. Sarafem (fluoxetine) which is Prozac, a selective serotonin reuptake inhibitor (SSRI) is one of the medications that is used. SSRI side effects can include an increase in suicidality. Zoloft (sertraline) is another SSRI antidepressant approved for PMDD use. It is important to rule out pregnancy prior to the use of these drugs, because of potential damage to the baby.

Fertilization of the egg, that is the beginning of pregnancy, occurs before a menstrual period is missed. If the chance of pregnancy exists, drugs and medications should generally be avoided, except with the concurrence of a qualified treating physician who is aware of the situation. The same is true for the nursing mother. Many drugs can cross in breast milk to the baby, with potential for harm.

Postmenopausal Bleeding

Post menopausal bleeding, that is bleeding in any fashion after the menopause, is one of the most important early warning signs of medical problems in the female reproductive tract, including precancerous and cancerous conditions, especially endometrial carcinoma. Endometrial carcinoma is cancer of the uterine (womb) lining.

Gynecological pelvic examination, ultrasonography of the pelvic organs, and actual biopsy of the lining of the womb are valuable tools in early diagnosis.

More modern techniques include videohysteroscopy, where a fiberoptic telescope is placed vaginally through the opened cervix, which is the mouth of the uterus. This instrument, which has an operative capability, is then attached to a small television camera, which in turn is hooked up to a color television monitor. The womb lining is visualized, magnified, on color television, and direct biopsies of areas of the womb lining are taken. Abnormal growths within the womb can be removed by this technique. This is most usually outpatient surgery and the woman does not have to stay in the hospital.

Migraine

Migraine headaches have been a debilitating scourge for men as well as women. Until recently, there have been no easy answers. Migraine headaches are vascular headaches involving the blood vessels of the brain. The trigeminal nerve, which is the fifth and largest cranial nerve, is stimulated. The trigeminal nerve is the major sensory nerve of the face. One if its branches, the ophthalmic nerve, gives sensation to the eye, eyelids, forehead, and the mucous membrane of the nose. It is easy to see from this nerve distribution why facial pain and pain around the eye, which is so common in classic migraine, arises. Serotonin (5HT) is released at nerve endings. Pain signals are sent up to higher brain centers. Blood vessels in the brain and the dura, which is the sheath that covers the brain itself, dilate. Dilation means that the blood vessel enlarges. This can be painful. Fluid is released, with inflammation and irritation.

Migraine headaches are often related to the menstrual cycle. Magnesium deficiency may have a role in menstrual migraine. In some women, the headaches do diminish by themselves after the menopause, although this is not something that can be relied upon. In some women, taking birth control pills, or taking hormonal replacement therapy with estrogen at the menopause can be a trigger for migraine.

A migraine headache will often start with some aura, or warning, such as a visual disturbance. The visual disturbance may persist throughout the headache. Migraine headaches tend to be one-sided, often over the area of an eye. They can be throbbing and are often accompanied by other symptoms such as nausea and vomiting. For many, they result in an inability to perform normal activities. Any person with these dramatic symptoms must be evaluated by a physician in order to rule out other causes of headache. These can range from simple tension to sinusitis, middle ear problems, and problems in the brain itself, including tumors and infarcts. An infarct, which may be tiny, is an area of tissue death due to a sudden lack of blood flow.

It is important for a person affected with migraine to know what can trigger attacks. Various foods, such as aged cheese or processed meats containing nitrites can be the precipitating cause. Hot dogs and sausage are in this category. Beware of MSG (monosodium glutamate) added to food as seasoning. Red wine and beer are common culprits. Caffeine and chocolate may be implicated. Even foods often thought of as healthful, including some fruits and beans, may trigger migraine in some people. Bread and other baked goods in which yeast is used may not be well tolerated by some affected with migraine.

Many people find that altering their lifestyle somewhat can reduce the frequency of migraine attacks. Eating regular meals and getting enough sleep is a good idea. Avoiding anxiety and stress can be easier said than done.

It can be important to avoid unnatural chemical odors and fumes. Commonly used sprays, deodorizers, and so-called air fresheners used in the home, especially bathrooms and kitchens, and hung on the rearview mirrors of cars, often taxicabs, can be a trigger.

Some migraine sufferers cite temperature and weather change, or time zone or altitude change. Such triggers can impact significantly on lifestyle, impeding travel and vacations.

Migraine Prevention:

The prevention of migraine, or at least reducing the frequency and severity of headaches, is a goal that is being worked towards. Topamax (topiramate) an antiepileptic drug, has been shown to be effective for migraine prevention. Side effects include a loss of bicarbonate by the kidneys, resulting in a potentially severe medical condition know as metabolic acidosis. The drug is generally not used in pregnancy, as it can be harmful to the fetus.

The classic treatment for migraine headache has been ergot alkaloids. One such drug is Migranal (dihydroergotamine mesylate). As with similar medications, caffeine is included in the drug, which in this case is given as a nasal spray. There can be serious drug interactions with other medications, and other serious side effects, including heart attack. The drug should not be used in pregnancy.

Triptans:

A major breakthrough in controlling migraine has been the development of a class of drugs called triptans. Triptans are serotonin (5 HT) receptor agonists. Serotonin causes blood vessels to contract. An agonist is a drug that combines with a receptor in a body cell and mimics the action of a naturally occurring substance, in this case serotonin. The triptans cause blood vessels to constrict, and fluid does not leak out. There is less pain transmission via the trigeminal nerve. These drugs can be used either to prevent migraine, or to treat it during an episode of headache. The results tend to be quick and efficacious. Such drugs include Imitrex (sumatriptan). This medication is provided either as tablets, nasal spray, or subcutaneous injection, which can be self administered. Amerge (naratriptan) and Zomig (zolmitriptan) are similar drugs.

These medications can have significant side effects, including increased blood pressure and heart attack. A physician should be consulted prior to their use. These drugs are generally not used in pregnancy, as there is a potential of harm to the fetus.

Calcitonin Gene-Related Peptide (CGRP) Monoclonal Antibodies:
More recently Aimovig (erenumab-aooe), a human monoclonal antibody, has been introduced.

It prevents migraine by binding to the calcitonin gene-related peptide (CGRP) receptor, antagonizing CGRP receptor function. It is injected once monthly. Similar drugs are Ajovy (fremanezumab-vfrm) and Emgality (galcanezumab-gnim)

Hormonal Replacement Therapy (HRT)

In the earlier years of my gynecologic practice, I looked askance as estrogen replacement therapy for menopause symptoms was being touted as a boon for women, to be used indefinitely. A significant part of my practice was performing surgery on patients sent to me for cancer of the lining of the womb (endometrium). It was evident that much of this cancer was due to stimulation of the womb lining by the estrogen. A backlash developed among many women and their gynecologists, and estrogen replacement became less popular.

It then became routine to add progesterone to stop the unremitting stimulation by unopposed estrogen.

HRT again became very popular and widely used, with many supposed benefits, aside from the obvious relief of hot flashes. It was again being touted by a wide variety of physicians, non-physicians, and self-proclaimed menopause experts.

Sobering recent studies, however, reveal a significant risk of heart disease, cardiovascular disease, thrombosis (blood clots) and stroke with the use of this replacement therapy. The pendulum has again swung. Women and their gynecologists are once again wary of the wholesale use of HRT.

HRT should not be used in pregnancy.

Once the menopausal state is diagnosed, an informed discussion should take place to decide whether or not medication is appropriate for each woman on an individual basis, taking into account her health status and family history. There are several options. One obvious option is to simply wait, watch, and see how life is progressing. Assuming that a woman is not having any symptoms such as very bothersome hot flashes, that she eats a healthful diet rich in nutrients especially calcium, that she exercises aerobically regularly, and that parameters such as her bone scan are normal, no hormonal supplementation is needed. However, it has been shown that intake of calcium and vitamin D alone is usually not sufficient to stop bone loss. Hormone levels can actually be checked by blood tests, if necessary. Bone density testing is now commonly done.

Hormonal replacement, whether so-called natural hormonal replacement or hormonal replacement by medication, carries an increased risk of breast cancer. There is also a significant increased risk of cancer of the lining of the womb, the endometrium, if insufficient progesterone is taken along with estrogen replacement. As well, there appears to be an increased risk of ovarian cancer in women taking HRT, whether estrogen alone, or estrogen along with progestins added at the end of each cycle, especially with long term use.

Most importantly, large well controlled recent studies show that women who take estrogen replacement for more than four years past the menopause, face a significantly increased risk of severe heart and cardiovascular disease, as well as strokes.

This has caused a sea change in the thinking about estrogen replacement therapy, both by women and their doctors. Many had previously thought, and some less definitive previous studies even seemed to show, that hormone replacement therapy might be good for the cardiovascular system.

This is one of the pitfalls of research. If a scientist starts from the false premise that estrogen is 'good' for the cardiovascular system, then does experiments to show how this 'benefit' might occur, the result can be a rather elegant explanation of the 'good' effect. Ideally, scientists try to be unbiased in their research, and let the facts lead where they may.

If estrogen must be used, the dose should be as low as possible. Hot flashes are still controlled with these lower doses. Protection against bone loss is still provided, but with fewer side effects. The incidence of bleeding and breast soreness is reduced. High - density lipoprotein (HDL), is still increased, which may or may not be a beneficial effect (see section on hypercholesterolemia). LDL (low-density lipoprotein), "bad cholesterol", is still decreased. Atrophy or thinning of the vaginal mucus or lining, which occurs in postmenopausal women, is still significantly improved with lower dosages of estrogen. Progesterone should still be added.

The estrogen replacement therapy with which there has been the most experience is Premarin (conjugated equine estrogens). 'Equine', of course, refers to a horse. These estrogens are naturally made by pregnant mares, and excreted in their urine, which is then collected. Traditionally, this pill, taken once a day, is given cyclically.

Premarin and progesterone have been combined into one pill, Prempro, taken daily.

Premphase contains Premarin to be taken daily for fourteen days, followed by combined conjugated estrogen and progesterone for the next two weeks.

Other such preparations include Enjuvia (synthetic congugated estrogen). Angeliq contains estradiol (an estrogen) and a synthetic progestational compound , drospirenone. Drospirenone can have the potentially adverse side effect of increased potassium levels.

With estrogen replacement therapy, Progesterone (medroxyprogesterone) is given at the end of each cycle, or every day throughout the cycle, to obviate any risk of overstimulation of the womb lining (endometrium), which could lead to endometrial cancer. Micronized progesterone (Prometrium) is another form of progesterone that may be used.

Both estrogen alone, and estrogen coupled with progestin use, increase the eventual risk of getting breast cancer.

Estrogen and progesterone can be delivered by patch. The medication is absorbed through the skin. Climara delivers estrogen in the form of estradiol. Climara PRO contains estradiol and the progestin levonorgestrel.. The patch is placed on the lower abdomen, and a new one applied every three to four days.

The Estring Vaginal Ring contains estradiol, as does Vagifem which is in the form of vaginal tablets.

Estrogen replacement takes away the most distressing symptoms of the menopause, most notably hot flushes and irritability. The estrogen probably works by raising the sweating threshold: body temperature still goes up, but sweating doesn't start until a higher temperature is reached.

It was previously thought by some that mental sharpness and memory might be helped by hormone replacement therapy (HRT). However, it is now known that estrogen replacement therapy increases the risk of stroke in postmenopausal women. Furthermore, there is now evidence that postmenopausal women who take estrogen replacement may increase their risk of getting dementia and impairment of thinking (cognition).

Dry eye syndrome is seen more frequently in women who take estrogen. There is an increased risk of gallbladder disease with hormonal replacement therapy.

Estrogen does have beneficial effects upon the skin, increasing its luster. The lining of the vagina becomes more lubricated, facilitating pleasurable intercourse. Hair may be more lustrous and less subject to loss. All in all, there may be a feeling of well-being. Some women report that sexual activity is enhanced and more pleasurable.

Progesterone must be added in order to reduce the risk of cancer of the uterine lining. However, this addition does not take away the risk of breast cancer, which in fact is increased by the hormonal supplementation with estrogen and increased further by the addition of progestins.

A gynecologist should be advised of any history of phlebitis or thrombophlebitis (blood clots in vessels). Such clots can occur anywhere in the body, but more commonly in the legs, female pelvis and brain. If there is such a history, estrogen replacement should not be used. Even a family history of such events is significant and should be part of the physician's thinking before starting any hormonal replacement regimen.

A thromboembolic phenomenon refers to the formation of a blood clot somewhere in the body, with the breaking off of part of that clot (embolism) and that broken off portion of the clot traveling to a distant part of the body, where it lodges and can do life-threatening harm. A common place for such emboli to travel is the lungs. Pulmonary (lung) embolism is dangerous and can be fatal.

Diminished libido (sex drive) in some women at the age of menopause can be enhanced by the addition of small amounts of male sex hormone (androgen), testosterone. After menopause, there is a decrease in androgen production from the ovaries, and from the adrenal glands which are located above the kidneys. The androgens dehydroepiandrosterone (DHEA), DHEA sulphate (DHEAS), androstenedione, and testosterone are all decreased. The giving of estrogen replacement therapy to women further decreases bioavailable free testosterone because of an increase in sex hormone - binding globulin (SHBG). Decreased testosterone can possibly lead to muscle wasting, depression, loss of energy, and decreased libido, as well as osteoporosis. Giving this hormone to women is not without hazard. Irreversible changes in the voice and permanent hair growth in places in which a woman would rather not have hair growth can occur with testosterone supplementation. The clitoris can enlarge. Acne can be a problem. Oral methyltestosterone may also cause toxicity to the liver.

One preparation that combines testosterone with estrogen is Estratest (esterified estrogens and methyltestosterone). Side effects can include estrogenic side effects, including an increased incidence of endometrial cancer.

DHEA itself has been proposed as a possible hormonal replacement treatment in postmenopausal women, although it is not an accepted treatment at this time.

It does not usually matter if estrogen is taken orally or by a skin patch. Oral estrogen is processed in the liver, which can lead to problems in women with liver disease. On the other hand, because of passage of oral estrogen through the liver, there can be beneficial effects on cholesterol levels, with LDL (low density lipoprotein) cholesterol being lowered, and HDL (high density lipoprotein) cholesterol being raised. On the other hand, levels of C-reactive protein are raised. This protein is associated with inflammation, and inflammation can be a contributing factor in heart disease.

With estrogen, with or without progesterone replacement, bleeding can result, sporadically or cyclically. A woman should never take bleeding after the menopause for granted, whether it happens with hormonal replacement, or without it.

SERM's:

SERM's are a good alternative to estrogen replacement therapy for many women. Acronyms are a popular way to talk about things, and this particular one stands for specific estrogen receptor modulators. Soltamox (tamoxifen citrate) is such a substance. It was originally used successfully in the treatment of some breast cancers. Subsequently, it has been shown to actually decrease the incidence of breast cancer if taken as a preventative. Unfortunately however, it does increase the incidence of endometrial cancer. Like estrogen, tamoxifen helps prevent osteoporosis, and the dreaded dowager's hump as well as the increased tendency to bone fracture, which can be so deadly in more senior women. The drug generally is not used in pregnancy because of the risk of fetal harm.

Evista (Raloxifene) which is also a specific estrogen receptor modulator (SERM) that binds to estrogen receptors, has the advantage of not increasing the incidence of endometrial cancer. Raloxifene prevents osteoporosis, reducing the risk of fractures of the spine (vertebrae). It may also decrease the size of fibroids that are present in the uterus. Raloxifene use can reduce the risk of breast cancer in women past the menopause. Side effects include an increased risk of venous thromboembolism. The drug should not be used in pregnancy.

The estrogen receptor modulators to this point have not been as widely accepted as one might expect for the very simple reason that they do not take away symptoms of the menopause, including hot flashes.

Osteoporosis

Osteoporosis refers to a reduction in bone quantity. The supporting fibers of the interior of the bone, called trabeculae, become scanty and thin. This leaves the bones much more susceptible to fracture. A similar process in the spinal column can result in compression fractures of the vertebrae. A woman can actually end up being shorter as she ages.

It is probable that many women have a gene that makes them susceptible to osteoporosis. A test for that gene should soon be available.

Osteoporosis has serious implications for a woman's longevity and wellbeing. As a woman ages, it is increasingly important for her to remain mobile. A hip fracture in a senior woman can be particularly devastating. She is temporarily immobilized. The fracture may not heal well because of the osteoporosis. As well, she is subject to blood clots that can travel through her circulation, and be life threatening.

In normal bone, the activity of cells called osteoblasts, which form bone, and cells called osteoclasts, which absorb and remove bone, are in balance. If bone resorption can be inhibited, then bone density increases, and the bones are stronger.

In general, fair, slim women are more at risk for osteoporosis, although all women should be on guard against it as they approach the menopausal years. A healthy life style, including regular aerobic and weight bearing exercise, as well as sports activities, are important from early adult life onward. Lean muscle mass is important in itself, and for its impact on bone density. These active skeletal muscles are attached to bone. When the muscle contracts, the bone moves.

Cigarettes should be avoided. Alcoholism is a risk factor for osteoporosis. The diet should be healthful and be rich in calcium. Milk, and milk products, are most important in achieving this end. This can be done without adding a lot of calories, by the use of skim milk and skim milk products. Ideally, three glasses of skim milk a day or their equivalent should be included in the diet. A calcium pill is roughly equivalent to the calcium in one glass of milk. This means that women who take in no milk generally need three 500 mg calcium tablets each day. It is also important not to take in too much calcium, as there is a possible danger of kidney stones.

Vitamin D is important in bone metabolism. An adequate diet will generally supply enough vitamin D, but especially in the elderly when the diet may be deficient, daily supplementation with 800 IU (international units) of vitamin D can be helpful.

However, with the menopause, simply taking in calcium along with a proper diet and exercise is not enough to prevent osteoporosis in large numbers of women.

It is important for women in the menopausal years to undergo bone density testing. The testing, known as DXA (Dual-Energy X-ray Absorptiometry), is now widely available in the United States, and can be ordered by a gynecologist or other physician. For simple bone loss screening, this test and other imaging techniques can be done even on the fingers.

Estrogen works by inhibiting bone resorption. Bone mineral density is therefore increased, strengthening the bones. Estrogen can be replaced either orally or by skin patch. It is important to discuss the dosage with a gynecologist, in order to ensure that an adequate level of this female sex hormone is attained, without creating side effects. Progesterone, which is another female sex hormone, will be prescribed along with the estrogen in order to limit the possibility of developing uterine cancer from overstimulation of the endometrium, or womb, lining.

However, hormone replacement therapy carries a significantly increased risk of heart disease, cardiovascular disease, and strokes. Long term HRT beyond three years often does not give the benefit of a further gain in bone density. If a woman on hormone replacement therapy (HRT) stops it, she usually does not experience a fast rate of bone loss. Nowadays, there are other efficient medications that combat osteoporosis.

Bisphosphonates:

Fosamax (alendronate sodium)is a nonhormonal drug taken by mouth which is specifically used to combat osteoporosis. A similar drug called Actonel (risedronate sodium) is available. Taking these drugs significantly reduces the risk of hip and vertebral fractures in older women. These medications are a valuable addition to the options available for treatment of osteoporosis. However, they can irritate the esophagus (the passage leading to the stomach). Both Fosamax and Actonel are now available in pills that need to be taken only once a week. The bisphosphonates act at the level of the cells known as osteoclasts, which resorb bone, inhibiting their activity. Less bone is absorbed, so bone remains dense and strong. These drugs are not advisable in pregnancy due to the risk of harm to the mother and to her developing fetus.

Denosumab:

Denosumab is a human monoclonal IgG2 antibody. "Monoclonal" refers to the fact that the antibody protein is derived from one clone of cells, all of which are identical. The antibody goes to a receptor site on the cell surface. It inhibits bone resorption by impairing the development, activation, and survival of osteoclasts, which are cells that resdorb bone. Denosumab has become, along with bisphosphonates, a widely used osteoporosis treatment. Its effect on bone turnover is quickly reversible. However, stoppage may result in an increased propensity to fracture, and usage may impact response to infection.

Calcitonin:

Miacalcin (calcitonin) which is administered by nasal spray, can have some effect more than ten years after menopause in increasing bone mineral density, although it tends to be ineffective in early menopause. This hormone acts by inhibiting bone resorption. Nasal symptoms can be among the possible side effects. It is not advisable to use this drug in pregnancy.

Parathyroid Hormone:

The parathyroid glands are tiny glands situated very close to the thyroid gland in the neck.

It is known that parathyroid hormone promotes bone growth and can be used in the prevention of osteoporosis. There is now genetically engineered parathyroid hormone available.

Growth Hormone:

Growth hormone output decreases as a woman ages. Theoretically, giving growth hormone to women approximately seventy years of age can lessen the decline in their bone mass, as well as the decline in their muscular strength. At the same time, the tendency would be to gain less abdominal fat. At the present time, this is not an approved treatment.

Statins:

A group of drugs called Statins can reduce the risk of bone fracture. Atorvastatin, known as Lipitor, Zocor (simvastatin) and Mevacor (lovastatin) are included in this class of drugs. Statins increase bone formation and bone density and may also inhibit bone resorption. The recognized use for Statins, which influence the metabolism of cholesterol, is to reduce the risk of cardiovascular disease. Statins also can reduce the risk of thrombosis in the veins.

People who have heart disease or are likely to develop it because of risk factors including smoking or diabetes, are candidates for statins, which lower cholesterol. However, like all drugs, their use should be carefully discussed with a doctor, as side effects, including liver and muscle damage, can occur. Statins effectively inhibit cholesterol production in liver cells, causing liver cell receptors to remove low density lipoprotein, or LDL cholesterol from the blood stream, so that the liver cells get the cholesterol they need for cell function. Statins may also relax blood vessel walls, promote growth of new blood vessels, and prevent blood clotting.

Cholesterol itself, in normal quantities, is necessary for life. However, high concentrations of cholesterol in the blood lead to cholesterol deposits in the walls of blood vessels. Immune cells feed in this cholesterol, creating foam cells, named for their fatty appearance, that create plaques that can rupture. Platelets, which are clotting elements present in the blood, then stick to the plaque so that a blood clot is formed. This cuts down on the size of the blood vessel opening. The blood vessel can then no longer deliver adequate oxygen-carrying blood to the muscle or organ the vessel supplies. In the case of heart muscle itself, this is a mechanism of heart attack. Heart muscle actually dies because it is deprived of oxygen.

Because cholesterol biosynthesis is necessary for fetal development, statins should not be taken in pregnancy.

Phytoestrogens:

Natural alternatives include foods and herbs containing phytoestrogens which are derived from plants. The problem with taking such supplements is that the dosage actually ingested into the human body is often unregulated and unknown. As well, there is no progesterone taken to counteract the increased incidence of cancer of uterine lining. Some manufacturers of such substances in pill form and some women themselves unfortunately think that if a little supplementation is good than a lot must be great. This can lead to overdosing with health risks including cancer.

No supplement should be taken in pregnancy without consultation with an obstetrician, who knows which supplements are indeed important in that situation.

Recent studies suggest that phytoestrogens do not improve symptoms of menopause, and do not alleviate hot flushes.

Soy contains isoflavones, which are a phytoestrogen. As with any estrogen, cholesterol may be lowered. However, it has recently been shown that the lowering of cholesterol in and of itself may not be of the benefit once thought. The cholesterol level may have much to do with genetic makeup. In other words, it is inherited. There may be no strict correlation between cholesterol levels and the incidence of arteriosclerotic heart disease. Soy intake may not reduce hot flashes. It is possible that eating soy throughout life could have a preventive effect on breast cancer because breast cells mature faster when stimulated in this way. This is pure theory and it is unproven. Some studies show that these substances may actually increase the incidence of some breast tumors. A cautionary note is that soy supplements tend to have high levels of isoflavones and may increase the incidence of cancer.

Contrary to some popular beliefs, rubbing yam cream on the body will do nothing for menopausal symptoms. Moderate doses of vitamin E may help somewhat with hot flashes. Black cohosh, a herb used by native Americans, may relieve various menopausal symptoms including hot flashes. It is unknown how it works.

Possibly the most important thing anyone could say to women, including women in the menopausal years, is "Don't smoke!". It is now widely known that smoking, which is addictive, has bad effects on the cardiovascular system. As well, there are cosmetic effects on the skin, not to mention bad breath. Lung cancer used to be rare in women. The advent of generalized smoking led to a huge rise in the incidence of lung cancer in women. This is a particularly lethal disease and is now one of the leading causes of cancer deaths in women. Unfortunately, too many teenage girls think of smoking as some sort of rite of passage, and as a way to reduce their normal appetite so that they can more closely achieve an often unrealistic body image. Too many of them pay a terrible price for this in adulthood.

Depression

Depression, of course, is not confined to women in the menopausal years. It is a common problem that can occur in any age group. It is appropriate to be depressed in certain circumstances. Illness, or illness of a loved one, can bring on a depressed feeling. Financial uncertainty, including the loss of a job, may bring on similar feelings. Most people confronted with such situations manage to cope by taking appropriate action to improve the underlying problem. For example, treating and hopefully curing illness can alleviate much of the stress and uncertainty involved. Taking positive steps to secure one's financial future, such as retraining, seeking more education, or securing an even better position, can turn the negatives of losing employment into a positive situation. The breakup of an emotional and loving relationship can precipitate feelings of inadequacy and depression. Divorce proceedings are almost inevitably linked to such feelings in many people. It may take a great deal of effort to go forward with a social life and forging relationships. A loss of a loved one is particularly devastating.

In all such circumstances, the closeness of family, friends, and institutions, particularly religious institutions, can be of great help.

Many people in trying times of great stress seek professional counseling, which fortunately is readily available in today's society.

The stigma of seeing psychologists and psychiatrists has, fortunately, long disappeared. There is a widespread general understanding in society now that depression is an illness that can and must be treated. Otherwise, there can be debilitating and serious consequences, up to and including suicide.

It has long been recognized that, when there is an appropriate underlying cause, depression can be short lived and easily treated. With the advanced understanding of the condition and the increased efficacy of modern antidepressant medications, most people with depression can be brought back to their full functioning normal state with little difficulty. The relatively recent advent of specialists in using these treatments, psychopharmacologists, has increased the knowledge of, and general acceptance of, newer antidepressant medications.

Older people, who have seen more than their share of life's vicissitudes and may themselves have a combination of various minor or major illnesses or disease states, coupled with a perceived loss of attractiveness, or general usefulness in society, can be particularly prone to depression. In fact, the incidence of suicide in the senior population may be under recorded.

There is an inherited predisposition to depression. In many cases of depression, the depth of depression being experienced may seem to be out of proportion to any precipitating event, or may come on with apparently no precipitating event. Timely intervention with antidepressant medication is very important in such cases. Obviously, such treatment should be monitored by highly qualified individuals, notably psychopharmacologists and psychiatrists.

SSRI's:

A group of drugs called selective serotonin reuptake inhibitors (SSRI) are now widely available and have to a large extent taken over the treatment of depression. These well known agents include Prozac (fluoxetine hydrochloride), Zoloft (sertraline hydrochloride), Paxil (paroxetine hydrochloride) and Celexa (citalopram hydrobromide). As their name suggests, these medications tend to prevent the neurons, which are the cells of the central nervous system, from taking up serotonin. Serotonin (5 HT) is a substance that is present in high concentrations in areas of the central nervous system and can act as a neurotransmitter.

Side effects of these drugs include an increase in suicide risk. It is important to rule out pregnancy prior to the use of these drugs, because of potential damage to the baby.

Prozac may improve hot flashes as well.

Older antidepressant drugs include the monoamine oxidase inhibitors (MAO Inhibitors). These drugs should not be used when selective serotonin reuptake inhibitors are being used, as dangerous consequences, including death, can occur. Tricyclic antidepressants are another class of drug. As with all other medications, these should be monitored by an appropriately qualified physician.

Women with flushing (hot flashes) along with depressive symptoms may be helped by hormonal replacement with estrogen and progesterone, but the increased risks of heart disease, cardiovascular disease, and stroke must be taken into account.

In an individual case, the psychiatrist may well suggest combining psychologic support and treatment along with drug therapy.

In mild depression, St. John's Wort may have some value, although not when depression is more severe.

Endorphins:

It has been well publicized and found to be true that regular exercise helps to improve mild depression. The exercise works naturally to enhance mood by stimulating the release of endorphins from the brain. Endorphins are naturally occurring compounds that in many ways resemble opiate drugs and bind to the same cell receptors as opiate drugs. Again, it is most important that people with depressive symptoms do not seek to treat themselves but get appropriate professional help early in order to guide them into the best approach for their individual case and to get them better quickly.

Anxiety can become a prominent problem in older people, although it is by no means confined to the senior age group. Some people actually get panic attacks. There are now effective medications available to control these problems as well. Niravam (alprazolam) is one of the class of drugs called benzodiazepines. The medication binds specific receptor sites in the central nervous system. Another drug of this class used in panic disorder is Klonopin (clonazepam). Side effects can include withdrawal symptoms of varying severity. These drugs should not be used in pregnancy due to possible damage to the baby, as well as withdrawal symptoms after birth.

It is important that anyone who suffers from anxiety, depression, or both take the appropriate steps and seeks the appropriate professional guidance needed to correct the problem, just as they would with any other disease state. We are much too enlightened a society at this point to neglect the proper treatment of such a widespread and potentially debilitating problem.

Insomnia

Sleeplessness can become a frequent problem as one becomes older. There may be difficulty in falling asleep. Early waking is common. Sleep itself may not be satisfying, and a person may find that she or he is tired and irritable during the day and is inefficient because she or he cannot concentrate and has no energy. Like any abnormal condition, it is important that these symptoms be reported to the doctor, so that possible underlying causes can be ascertained. Depression and anxiety, although commonly associated with insomnia, are by no means the only reasons for sleeplessness.

In fact, sleeplessness may result from a lack of comfort due to other medical conditions, such as sinus congestion, headache, arthritis pain, or backache arising from disc protrusions. In these circumstances, treatment should be directed at correcting the underlying disorder.

Attention should be given to the sleep environment. Mattress and pillows should be properly supportive, yet comfortable. If allergies are identified, hypoallergenic materials should be used. Sheets and pillowcases should be soft and supple when they are bought and should be kept that way by careful laundering. The same is true of nightgowns and pajamas. Extraneous noise and light should be removed as much as possible from the sleep environment. Humidity in the air should be properly controlled. Humidity needs to be added to the air during winter heating and needs to be removed from the air on humid summer nights. A good air conditioning system will take care of this, provided it is properly maintained and the filters cleaned.

It is important to maintain a regular sleeping time. Afternoon naps, or siestas, although beneficial for many people, may interfere with night time sleeping for others. Someone who has trouble sleeping at night should not be napping during the day.

Caffeine can be a significant factor in causing sleeplessness. Coffee is the obvious source, but colas, tea, and chocolate contain caffeine as well. If insomnia is a problem, caffeine should be eliminated from the diet, especially in the evening after dinner.

Nicotine can similarly cause sleeplessness. This is just another bad effect of smoking, which should be eliminated from the lifestyle.

A doctor should be consulted concerning other medications that can cause difficulty in sleeping as a side effect.

If depression and anxiety are diagnosed, these conditions should obviously be treated by a competent professional. The symptoms of insomnia, or sleeplessness, should abate as the underlying depression or anxiety improves.

A sleeping pill, or hypnotic agent, will, of course, put a person to sleep. However, the underlying cause of the problem is not addressed, but often masked. Such medications can be habit forming or even addictive and may require increasing doses to achieve the desired effect. As well, there may be side effects including respiratory depression which can be dangerous in older people.

The result may be a hangover effect, with a greater likelihood of lack of concentration and physical stability, so that the possibility of falling and fracture of bones increases, especially in the elderly.

Sedatives are now available that tend to limit some of the adverse side effects of classic sleeping medications, but side effects can still occur, including a reduction in mental alertness. These medications include Sonata (zaleplon), Ambien (zolpidem) and Lunesta (eszopiclone). These medications work by interacting with a cell receptor known as GABA. When hypnotic agents are used, they should be monitored by a physician.

These drugs should generally not be used in pregnancy.

Sexual Function

Women are staying in their reproductive years and having normal menstrual periods, on average, longer in our society. The average age of menopause, that is the cessation of menstrual periods, has gradually increased from forty-seven to fifty. Although menopause can occur normally as early as the age of forty-two, in some women it does not occur naturally until the age of fifty five. A woman who is still menstruating naturally is automatically putting out adequate amounts of estrogen and progesterone in a cyclic fashion. If this was not the case, she would not be menstruating. Along with that, the vagina remains normally lubricated, and secretions from the cervix, which is the mouth of the womb, remain normal. If indeed, some extra vaginal lubrication is needed for intercourse, readily available non- prescription lubricants such as Astroglide and K-Y jelly can be used. Replens is widely available for vaginal insertion. It has the advantage of not having to be used prior to intercourse but can be used on a regular basis as needed twice weekly. Modern tampons tend to be extra absorbent, and while this is efficient for absorbing menstrual flow, tampons can also unnaturally soak up normal vaginal secretions which are the normal lubricants for pleasurable sexual intercourse, and cause vaginal dryness.

Undergoing the menopause and the cessation of menses (menstrual period) should not in this modern age interfere with sexual intercourse or sexual pleasure. It has been said that sexuality is more in the mind than in the body. Of course, it is a combination of both. A woman should not be afraid of "using it up". Contrary to a lot of popular beliefs, women who are sexually active early and often tend to be sexually active much later into their lives than women who become sexually active relatively late in their lives and have infrequent sexual encounters. If a woman has been brought up to believe that sexual intercourse is a natural function, she is more likely to derive pleasure from it throughout her life than if she was sexually repressed.

Humans tend to be visual, but virtually all of the senses come into play in sexual arousal. It has long been known that olfactory cues, dependent on the sense of smell, are important This fact is not lost on perfume and scent manufacturers, who are constantly in search of "come hither" aromas.

Pheromones:

A gene, VIRL1, is responsible for a pheromone receptor that is found in the mucous membrane lining the nose. Pheromones are molecules that actually have no odor, but stimulate instinctual areas of the human brain, setting off the sex urge. Humans may communicate on a very basic sexual level via pheromones.

Male Sexual Dysfunction:

There are a few physical barriers to pleasurable sexual intercourse in older women past the menopause. Not the least of these is the fact that the male partner may be losing sex drive, having erectile problems, and may be incapable of having intercourse and orgasm. There have been major breakthroughs in correcting these conditions.

Psychological evaluation and behavior modification are used in couple therapy, with specific attention being paid to arousal techniques that enables the man to achieve erection and orgasm. Along with physical stimulation to the penis itself and mutual physical stimulation by the couple to each other, these techniques are basically rooted in trust, time, relaxation, and most importantly in a nonjudgmental approach in order to get rid of performance anxiety in the male. Performance anxiety leads to the inability to attain erection.

Penile injections have been developed which can cause erection of the penis. The penis is erect when it becomes engorged with blood.

The biggest breakthrough to date occurred when Viagra (sildenafil citrate) was developed. Cialis (tadalafil) and Levitra (Vardenafil Hcl) are available as well. These drugs cause penile engorgement and erection in approximately two thirds of the men who take them.

Vaginal Difficulties:

The woman past menopause who has infrequent or no sexual intercourse may find that the vagina will gradually tighten. The vagina will lose its elasticity, and much of its lubrication. When she tries to resume intercourse, she will find that it is painful or impossible. This becomes a vicious cycle, as attempted intercourse causes pain, so intercourse gets less frequent, and the vagina tightens even more. As well, the area of the opening of the vagina, called the vulva, most commonly at its lower end, which is called the fourchette, can tear and bleed. There can also be tears with penile penetration further up in the vagina. With regular intercourse and the use of vaginal lubrication when needed, these problems generally do not occur.

In severe cases of vaginal tightening, the gynecologist can prescribe the use of vaginal dilators. These smooth objects, in graduated sizes, if properly used, will gradually stretch the vagina back to its normal state, allowing normal intercourse.

Hormonal replacement therapy (HRT) may be prescribed, keeping in mind the increased risk of heart disease, cardiovascular disease, and stroke. Giving estrogen or progesterone either cyclically, or in combination by mouth once daily, or by means of a patch placed on the skin, can keep the vagina supple and lubricated.

Sometimes these measures alone are not enough for a woman to achieve orgasm. It can become necessary to add a little testosterone, or male sex hormone, to the mix in order to increase libido, or sexual desire. Some women are concerned that their sexual appetites are diminished after the menopause. Addition of a small amount of testosterone to hormonal replacement therapy is often beneficial to these women. It goes without saying that it is very important for this type of therapy to be given with medical supervision. Improper dosage of testosterone can lead to permanent changes such as hair growth and deepening of the voice. These changes can be permanent and irreversible.

Increasing genital blood flow in a woman may have a role, if genital engorgement is absent, but studies of medication for this purpose have, so far, been disappointing.

Drugs are probably not of value when genital engorgement does occur but is not attended to in the sexual relationship. Emotional intimacy and sexual stimuli initiate arousal. Sexual stimulation of the breasts, clitoris, vulva and vaginal areas then lead to orgasm. Emotional and physical satisfaction are achieved, leading to emotional intimacy, which again motivates the couple toward using sexual stimulation and achieving arousal.

This cycle of intimacy, arousal, desire, and emotional and physical satisfaction is fragile. It can be negatively influenced by disappointing or failed sexual encounters, and by physical discomfort.

A lot of women report a new freedom in sexual relations after the menopause. They no longer have to protect themselves against unplanned childbearing. They tend to be alone more with their mate, and unexpected intrusions, like the patter of little feet, are no longer a problem. They tend to be more relaxed and have the time to care for themselves. Many couples find themselves able to take trips and vacations in an unhurried way to beautiful places where they can spend languorous afternoons and evenings. Partners can spend the time and effort to keep themselves fit and attractive, so that sexual arousal becomes natural.

Hysterectomy

In spite of all the recent developments in gynecology, including minimally invasive surgery and the ability to treat various diseases of the reproductive tract both medically and surgically without actually removing the uterus and the ovaries, there are still a significant number of women who at some time in their lives will have to undergo hysterectomy. Hysterectomy is the removal of the uterus. Total hysterectomy means removal of the uterus including the cervix, which is the mouth of the womb. Total hysterectomy with bilateral salpingo-oophorectomy refers to the removal of the uterus complete with the cervix and with removal of both ovaries and fallopian tubes. Some women tend to think that if they have to undergo such an operative procedure, that they will become obese, hairy, sexually uninteresting, and sexually uninterested. Nothing could be farther from the truth. A woman who is fit and attractive can stay fit and attractive whether or not she has a uterus and ovaries.

The hallmark of the menopause is ovarian failure. The ovaries cease to effectively function and put out adequate levels of the sex hormones estrogen and progesterone. The uterus is no longer induced to build its lining of endometrium every month in preparation for a pregnancy. Because the lining is not built, and is not shed every month, there is no longer a menstrual period. Especially after menopause, removal of the uterus and ovaries, which should only be done out of medical necessity, does not lead to any profound physiologic change in a woman. If needed, women should still be able to get one of the several therapies available for menopausal symptoms. She will not grow excess hair any more than she normally would have.

Much attention has been paid to the role of the cervix in female sexuality. It was shown years ago by Masters and Johnson that during sexual intercourse, in the majority of cases, the cervix is not touched but actually pulled out of the way by tenting of the vagina. The cervix itself is not well supplied with sensory nerves. Sensitive areas of the female for sexual pleasure include the clitoris and the vulvar area around the opening of the vagina. During intercourse and orgasm, the vaginal muscles contract around the penis, heightening sexual pleasure for both partners. It has not been scientifically shown that removal of the cervix for medical reasons interferes physically with sexual pleasure. On the contrary, if a woman has disease of the reproductive tract, which is causing pain, abnormal bleeding, cramps, or other physical discomfort, it is usually found that removal of the disease process takes away the symptoms including the pain, makes the woman healthier, and sexually more interested, because she is no longer ill and in discomfort.

Healthy women, even at the advanced age of ninety to one hundred who are used to a lifetime of sexual pleasure are often still capable of deriving pleasure and satisfaction from sexual activity. Often, they are abstinent, not because of inability to be sexually active, or because of a lack of libido, but because their partner is incapable of maintaining an erection. Statistically, women in our society tend to outlive men, and so there are a significant number of older women without partners, through no choice of their own.

References

1. Caplan, Ronald MD: The Care of the Older Person, Third Edition: Chapter: After Menopause. RMC Publishing, LLC 2019 www.careoftheolderperson.com
2. https://www.aimovighcp.com/?gclid=Cj0KCQiA6IHwBRC-JARIsALNjViVEk2i-kXujUDg6WfQN1wHZZVXIizfM-HoOff8cK1o0gQVE243MfF2waAjAWEALw_wcB&gclsrc=aw.ds
3. https://www.mayoclinic.org/diseases-conditions/migraine-headache/diagnosis-treatment/drc-20360207
4. Bibliography & Supplemental Bibliography: See www.rcaplanmd.com

CHAPTER 11
DISEASES RELATED TO CHILDBEARING

The Take-Home Message

- One of the great hallmarks of modern medicine is the prevention and effective treatment of diseases related to childbearing
- Prenatal (antenatal) care has probably been the pre-eminent success story in preventative medicine
- Effective medical and surgical treatments are available for a variety of dysfunctions of the urinary bladder and bowel
- Reproductive technology has revolutionized the treatment of the couple having difficulty in achieving pregnancy
- The biologic 'clock' still exists
- Immunologic interplay between a mother and her fetus is important in protecting the growing fetus, and has contributed to our knowledge of organ transplantation, and to our knowledge of the aging process.

Historically, many of the debilitating conditions women were forced to live with were directly related to childbearing. One of the best- kept secrets of many of the royal houses of Europe for centuries past was that queens and princesses often were confined to their palaces due to pelvic injuries that caused urinary and fecal incontinence. In other words, they had poor or no control of their bowel movements, and either leaked urine or could not control their bladder function until they could discreetly relieve themselves.

The inability of women to protect themselves against unplanned pregnancy, coupled with the real dangers of physical damage and even death in childbirth, were some of the factors responsible in the past for women's inability to attain equal rights in society. It is only in recent years, and in highly industrialized societies, that women have been able to largely free themselves of these real concerns and fears and enter modern society as equals. In much of the world even today, the goals of properly monitored pregnancy and safe childbirth without injury to mother and child have not yet been realized.

Fortunately, the most debilitating and talked about consequences of obstructed labor and traumatic delivery are only rarely seen today in advanced societies although they are unfortunately still present in underdeveloped nations. These conditions are called fistulas. Fistulas are abnormal openings or passages between the urinary bladder and the vagina, or between the rectum and the vagina. Other types of fistulas can also occur, but these two types tend to be the most devastating. If a woman has a hole communicating between her bladder and her vagina, urine will leak from the vagina. If there is a communication between the rectum and the vagina, the woman will pass flatus and feces through her vagina. The obvious answer to most of these problems lies in their prevention. Great advances in modern obstetrical care have been keyed to the prevention of long obstructive labors that led to abnormal pressure and trauma to the bladder and the rectum. The prevention of such injuries has altered the fate of countless women in our society. Advances in modern obstetrical care have also led to the expectation by parents that they will have normal healthy offspring. This, in and of itself, is a great way for a newborn to start on the road to longevity.

The other great advance came in the development of gynecologic operative techniques by which tissue repair, layer by layer, of these holes or fistulas was accomplished, allowing the affected women again to be continent of urine and feces, and to again be able to have normal sexual relations and to live a normal life.

Obstetrical damage does not actually have to tear into the bladder or rectum in order to produce incontinence, a loss of urine, or loss of control of bowel movements. The rectal sphincter muscle mechanism which normally keeps the rectum closed until a woman desires to have a bowel movement can be damaged. Good obstetrical care can often, but not always, prevent such damage. Good obstetrical practice includes properly controlled delivery. Judicious use of a surgical cut called an episiotomy, at the time of delivery, made in such a way as to prevent tearing of the rectal sphincter mechanism, can be employed. Nowadays, when damage to the rectal sphincter does occur, the muscles of the sphincter can most often be adequately repaired by modern gynecologic surgical techniques, usually immediately after delivery, while the mother is still in the delivery or birthing room. Thus, the great untalked about and unsightly scourge of women, fecal incontinence, has largely been eradicated.

The dropping of the urinary bladder is another matter. Contributing factors to this condition are age, heredity, and childbearing. With the downward pressure of the enlarging uterus during pregnancy, and the pushing efforts required in the second stage of labor while the baby is being moved down the birth canal and subsequently is born, great pressure is put on the supports to the bladder, the uterus, the vagina, and rectum.

Bulging of the back wall of the bladder into the front wall of the vagina is called a cystocele. Conversely, bulging of the front wall of the rectum into the back wall of the vagina is called a rectocele. A true hernia of the abdominal contents, including small bowel, within a sac bulging into the top of the vagina is called an enterocele. A dropping down of the uterus into the vagina is called uterine descensus or prolapse. It is commonly called a fallen womb. All of these conditions can exist singly or together. Each of them can cause distressing symptoms.

Depending on the amount of childbearing a woman has done, these conditions can become obvious quite early in life, but usually are not distressful until a woman has reached her forties, and often much later. A woman may not complain of significant symptoms until she is in her postmenopausal years.

A bulging of the urinary bladder into the vagina, or cystocele, most often does not cause any symptoms. The urethra is the passage through which a woman urinates, and leads from the bladder to the outside. If the urethra is falling down, the condition is called a urethrocele.

Urinary Stress Incontinence

There are various types of urinary incontinence that a woman can have. The type of incontinence of urine that a woman gets from the bladder and urethra being pushed downwards, and loss of the normal anatomy that results, is called stress incontinence. When the woman coughs, laughs, lifts something heavy, or exercises she loses urine.

There have been many gynecologic operations devised to restore the proper anatomy of the bladder and urethra. Some of these operations are done through the vagina, some are done through an abdominal incision, and some are done laparoscopically. Various types of sutures or slings are used to support the urethra and bladder in these procedures. The procedure should be done by an experienced gynecologic surgeon, or in some cases by a urologist and the approach individualized for the best chance of success in each case. There are now gynecologists specifically trained in urogynecology who tend to confine their practices to the treatment of these conditions.

As with any medical condition, women considering medications to treat these conditions must ensure that pregnancy is not present, or an issue. Nursing women must be vigilant as well, as many medications can cross into breast milk and potentially harm the baby.

Cymbalta (Duloxetine) is a newer serotonin/ norepinephrine reuptake inhibitor for treating depression that seems to improve closing of the urethra, reducing the severity of stress incontinence. However, the drug is not approved for that use at this time. As well, there is a cautionary note on this type of antidepressant concerning suicide risk in depressed users. The drug should generally not be used in pregnancy.

Urgency Incontinence

Another form of incontinence frequently encountered by women is called urgency incontinence. The woman feels the urge to urinate but cannot hold her urine until she reaches a bathroom. Most commonly, this type of incontinence is due to some type of irritation within the bladder. This can occur when a woman gets a urinary tract infection. Urinary tract infections are quite common in women. This is usually ascribed to the fact that the length of the passage from the urinary bladder to the outside in women is generally about 3.5 cm, or less than an inch and a half. Therefore, it is quite easy for germs to ascend from the outside world and the vagina into the urinary tract. The treatment of a urinary tract infection should be tailored to the underlying cause. A urinalysis and a urine culture and sensitivity should be obtained. The causative germ is cultured and identified. Furthermore, it is tested against various antibiotics to see which antibiotic will most effectively kill the germ.

Interstitial Cystitis

In their forties and beyond, women are subject to bladder irritation that does not seem to have any specific known bacteria causing it. This condition is called interstitial cystitis. This is, as yet, a poorly understood condition, and tends to be chronic. Interstitial cystitis is currently treated by urologists with bladder lavage with analgesic substances, and antispasmodics.

Ditropan (Oxybutynin Chloride), has an antispasmodic effect on the smooth muscle of the bladder, relaxing it. Drowsiness and decreased tolerance to higher temperature are among possible side effects. The drug should not be used if there is urinary retention (inability to empty the bladder properly). A qualified physician has to ensure that benefits outweigh the possible risks prior to this (or any) drug being given in pregnancy.

Detrol (Tolterodine tartrate), works in the same way. Side effects may include electrocardiographic changes. The drug is generally not used in pregnancy.

Elmiron (Pentosan polysulfate), may protect the bladder lining (epithelium). Side effects can include rectal hemorrhage and liver function abnormalties. There is the possibility of fetal harm if the drug is used in pregnancy.

One answer in a postmenopausal woman seems to be the administration of estrogen by mouth, or by skin patch, which restores the health of the inner lining of the vagina, the vaginal mucosa, and probably helps the bladder mucosa as well. All the precautions with estrogen use should be observed.

Overactivity of the detrusor muscle of the bladder is a hallmark of urgency incontinence. The overactivity tends to respond to treatment with antispasmodic (anticholinergic) drugs, including Ditropan and Detrol.

Urologists, while examining the inside of the bladder with a cystoscope, have actually injected Botox (Botulinum A toxin) into this muscle to quell the overactivity, but this use of Botulinum A toxin is not approved as yet. This drug is a neurotoxin, with potentially severe side effects, and should never be used without consultation with a qualified physician. The drug should not be used in pregnancy.

Neurogenic Incontinence

The third relatively common form of urinary incontinence encountered in women is the neurogenic type. As its name suggests, the nervous system control of the sphincter muscles of the bladder is damaged. This is predominantly seen in older women and can be extremely difficult to treat.

The root causes of incontinence in any individual woman are often complex, leading to misdiagnosis and inappropriate treatment. Fortunately, there are sophisticated techniques involving pressure studies of urethra and bladder, as well as voiding studies of the bladder that have been evolved. Cystoscopy is a technique in which a fiberoptic telescope is inserted through the urethra into the bladder so that the bladder lining itself, as well as the entrance of the ureters, which are the passages from the kidneys to the bladder are seen. It is now possible to fine tune the diagnosis in each individual case. Treatments can then be tailored to each woman, with a good probability of success, and the restoration of adequate bladder control, and therefore a normal life.

The bulging of the rectal wall into the back wall of the vagina in and of itself rarely causes any symptoms, provided that the sphincter mechanism of the rectum remains intact, and therefore the woman has good control of her bowel movements. However, laxity in that area is often coupled with laxity and widening of the perineal body, which is the area between the vagina and the rectum. Some women complain of a loss of pleasurable sensation with intercourse when the opening of the vagina has been widened in this way. In well selected cases, a surgical tightening of this area by a gynecologic surgeon may give good results. Because the front wall of the vagina rests on the back wall of the vagina, repair of this region, so-called rectocele repair, is often coupled with the anatomic repair of the supports of the bladder, in order to complement the bladder repair.

The fallen womb was a very well known condition historically. In its most dramatic and severe form, the uterus can actually protrude through the vaginal opening. The mouth of the womb, the cervix, then can easily become ulcerated. The woman can have a constant feeling of pressure, have difficulty in walking, and of course be extremely limited in her sexual function. In extreme cases, an older woman may find that she must physically, with her hand, push the uterus back up the vagina so that she can urinate. Uterine prolapse can be more common in people with uncontrolled diabetes.

In any such case it is essential that the treating doctor ensure that there is no enlarging tumor inside the abdominal cavity, which is causing increased pressure and therefore forcing the uterus, along with the bladder and rectum, downwards.

The classic treatment for this condition was the pessary, which is one of the oldest medical devices known to womankind. This device, which comes in various shapes, configurations and sizes, is an object that is placed in the vagina so that the uterus cannot descend. With long term use, infection often occurs, and the vaginal walls erode from the constant pressure of the foreign object, no matter how soft it is.

Advances in gynecologic surgery have led to the development of various gynecologic procedures to recreate and fix the supports of the uterus, with or without the removal of the uterus itself. Again, the approach to be used should be individualized for each patient, and the case discussed with the gynecologic surgeon.

The same is true for enterocele, where the intestinal contents are forced downwards, bulging into the top of the vagina. After appropriate tests are taken, and the presence of any underlying cause or tumor has been ruled out, the appropriate operative approach is determined on an individual case basis.

The longevity of the human race is inextricably bound up in the reproductive role of women. Unlike the male, the human female does not simply contribute fifty percent of the genetic material and one half of each chromosomal pair to the developing fetus. Beyond that, she creates the all important intrauterine environment in which the fetus will develop over a crucial nine month period.

The nine month gestation period in women is probably influenced by relatively "new" genes found in humans that have the code for producing specific pregnancy hormones (beta-1- glycoprotein and choriogonadotropin beta proteins).

The conduct of the labor process, and the stresses placed on the fetus during labor, are all important to the future wellbeing of the child. The delivery of the baby is a critical time during which great care must be taken that no harm comes to either mother or baby.

Even in developed countries today, one to three mothers die in childbirth for every ten thousand live births. It goes without saying that for every mother who is actually lost in the labor and delivery process, many more are dangerously ill with conditions that can have impact upon their future lives. The passage of the baby through the birth canal during the labor and delivery process has been called a perilous journey. It is only in the most recent of times and in the most developed countries that women have rightfully come to expect that they will pass through this landmark event healthfully, with little danger to themselves or to their baby. Women in our society have come to expect that every pregnancy will result in a baby delivered in optimum condition, although regrettably even today this is not always the case.

Rapidly advancing knowledge and techniques in reproductive medicine continue to make childbearing a safer experience with less danger to both mother and child. However, medicine is practiced within the context of society. The problems confronted by obstetricians are directly related to the shifting values and practices in our society. This phenomenon is seen in the gradually advancing age at which motherhood is undertaken in large segments of our urban society, and the smaller number of children many women expect to have. Many women in our society tend to delay childbearing until later in their reproductive years while they pursue other goals and interests. Strong bias against so-called teenaged pregnancy is now present in our society. It is true that pregnancy from a purely physiologic point of view is dangerous before the female pelvic architecture is properly formed. However, most women have achieved this stage by approximately the age of seventeen years. From eighteen years of age into the early twenties, a woman is physiologically at the height of her reproductive power. From a purely physiologic point of view, it is then probably most likely that she can undergo pregnancy with a minimal risk of any complications either to herself or to her developing child.

However, societal factors come heavily into play. In our society today, huge numbers of women in that age group have not yet completed their education or entered into a stable monogamous relationship with an emotionally mature partner who is ready to take on the responsibilities of fatherhood. Powerful economic forces come into play. Appropriate health insurance coverage, access to quality obstetrical facilities, family support, a stable physical environment in the form of a sheltering home, and the sophistication to deal with a pregnancy healthfully are not yet present in many young women's lives. The diet is often not healthy. The use of tobacco products, alcohol, and so-called recreational, or illegal drugs during pregnancy all take their toll disproportionately among young mothers, especially if they are unwed. Any or all of these factors may not be present in other societies that are more geared toward marriage and childbearing by younger women. That was common even in our own society less than two generations ago. Stable homes were established by younger people and childbearing in the late teens and early twenties was considered the norm. Biblically, a generation is twenty years, and in most of the world today, this has not changed.

The tendency towards delayed childbearing, with a consequent increase in incidence of disease of the reproductive tract and generalized diseases that can interfere with pregnancy labor and delivery, including hypertension, heart disease, renal disease, and diabetes, has been largely offset by major advances in the understanding of these diseases and their treatment, coupled with advances in the conduct of prenatal care, labor, delivery, and neonatal care of the newborn. It is also now possible through reproductive technology for women who naturally would not have been able to conceive to get pregnant and have babies. Many of these women are in a significantly older age group.

Fertility

Women who delay childbearing later into their reproductive years face the prospect of declining fertility, especially beyond the age thirty five. This decline in fertility may be related to the onset of various conditions within the reproductive system which can interfere with the ability to achieve a successful pregnancy. As well, more generalized conditions that have an impact on reproduction may be more prevalent, or have progressed to a more significant stage, in older women. Advances in reproductive technology increasingly allow large numbers of couples who previously would have been unable to achieve pregnancy to successfully have children in spite of such conditions.

It had been thought that a woman, at her own birth had all the eggs in her ovaries that she would ever have. That thinking is changing. It is likely that ovaries have active cells that continuously restock eggs in fluid - filled follicles.

The vast majority of couples who have natural unprotected intercourse over a period of one year will achieve pregnancy. In fact, worldwide, there is a population explosion. However, in modern industrialized society, difficulty in achieving pregnancy has become a major concern for many couples.

Proper diagnosis begins with an evaluation of the male partner, an evaluation of the female partner, and an evaluation of the interaction between them. Evaluation of the male involves physical examination with attention to his general health status as well as a specific examination of his reproductive organs. A microscopic sperm evaluation is carried out. Cultures are taken to insure that there is no infection present in the sperm.

A history is taken to document the frequency and adequacy of intercourse, to ensure that coitus results in ejaculation and proper deposition of sperm within the vagina. This is followed by post- coital testing, in which the mucus from the female cervix is evaluated under the microscope some hours after sexual intercourse in order to ascertain that the sperm are properly living and motile within the mucus.

The woman is checked to ensure that she has none of the general diseases that can interfere with fertility, including diabetes, thyroid disorders, and tuberculosis. Her hormonal status is evaluated to make sure that her endocrine organs are functioning adequately. Specifically, attention is paid to the output of Follicle Stimulating

Hormone (FSH) and Luteinizing Hormone (LH) from the pituitary gland, as well as the cyclic output of estrogen and progesterone from the ovary itself. If there is an abnormal output of the hormone prolactin from the pituitary gland, then the pituitary gland itself is evaluated by MRI(magnetic resonance imaging), or CAT scan (computerized axial tomography).

The output of androgens by the woman, including delta T androstenedione, dehydroepiandrosterone (DHEAS) and testosterone are checked to ensure that there is no abnormal output of these substances from either the adrenal glands or the ovaries themselves.

Attention is given to all of the female reproductive organs. Cultures are taken from the vagina and cervix to ensure that there are no sexually transmitted organisms or other significant bacteria that can interfere with conception or an ongoing pregnancy. The uterus itself is checked, as are the ovaries and the fallopian tubes. Pelvic examination is followed by ultrasonography to evaluate these organs. A hysterosalpingogram may be done. A radio-opaque dye is introduced through the cervix and flows through the uterus to the fallopian tubes. This older, fluoroscopic Xray technique, can show deformities of the uterus, as well as blockage of the tubes.

In many cases, videohysteroscopy and videolaparoscopy are used for direct visualization of the reproductive organs to ensure that they are functioning and without disease process. The lining of the womb, the endometrium, is biopsied and dated to the time of the cycle, to ensure that the woman is ovulating properly. Developing follicles containing the maturing eggs, can be actually seen on the ovaries. This process of ovum development can be easily checked by sonography as well.

Actual ovulation can be anticipated by readily available urine tests, which show color change at the time of the LH (Luteinizing Hormone) surge that occurs prior to actual ovulation.

The basal body temperature can be charted daily. When a woman is ovulating, the chart will show a biphasic pattern, with a sustained rise in temperature in the luteal, or postovulation, phase of the cycle.

When the problem areas have been identified by proper diagnosis, a treatment plan is formulated. Depending on the circumstances, this can vary from education and advice on proper coital technique, enhancement of the cervical mucus, targeted antibiotic therapy to clear up existing infection, all the way to advanced surgical techniques and assisted reproductive technology.

Fallopian tubes that are blocked can be opened, often by laparoscopic techniques that are minimally invasive. However, the fallopian tube is a living structure that is not merely a pipe or conduit. Frequently, tubes that are blocked are damaged in their endothelium, or lining, with the disappearance of cilia, the microscopic hairlike projections on the cells, as well as damage to secreting cells. The mobility of the tube may be impaired. Thus, the successful reopening of fallopian tubes often leads to disappointing results in the quest for a successful pregnancy. A much higher pregnancy success rate is achieved with microsurgical reanastomosis (relinking) of tubes that have been previously interrupted for sterilization purposes. In such cases, of course, the fallopian tubes are inherently healthy.

Advanced Assisted Reproductive Technology (ART)

Advanced assisted reproductive technology (ART) has been responsible for major breakthroughs in the number of couples who are now capable of having successful pregnancies, and in the numbers of women in the later reproductive years who successfully conceive and bear children.

Ovulation, the release of eggs by the ovary, is induced by means of various agents. Clomid (Clomiphene-citrate) was one of the first drugs to actually achieve this. Clomiphene interacts with estrogen receptor containing tissues at several levels .Side effects can include ovarian enlargement, up to the level of Ovarian Hyperstimulation Syndrome with marked ovarian enlargement and abdominal (intra-peritoneal) fluid collection. The drug should not be used where there is an existing pregnancy.

Follistim (Follitropin beta) is a recombinant human follicle stimulating hormone (hFSH) manufactured by recombinant DNA technology. FSH acts on the ovary to induce ovulation. Ovarian Hyperstimulation Syndrome can occur. The drug should not be used in pregnancy.

Egg retrieval from the ovaries is carried out under ultrasonographic guidance through an aspirating needle introduced into the abdominal cavity through the vault, or top, of the vagina.

The retrieved eggs are then fertilized by sperm in the laboratory, so-called in vitro fertilization. Maturing fertilized eggs are then introduced into the woman's uterus, through the cervix, some forty-eight hours later.

In cases where the sperm is suboptimal, with microscopic guidance, a single sperm can actually be inserted under microscopic vision directly into the egg, fertilizing it. This technique, now commonly used in advanced A.R.T. settings, is known as ICSI (intracytoplasmic sperm injection). Even if the male partner has no sperm in his ejaculate (the fluid he releases at orgasm), sperm can now be retrieved by advanced microsurgical technique from the testis, or the epididymis, which is an organ surrounding the testis. ICSI is then utilized to microscopically to insert one fertilizing sperm into the egg cell.

It is now even possible, in a woman in danger of losing ovarian function, to preserve her own ovarian tissue by freezing it, and then reimplanting it in her body so that she can produce eggs again.

Even with such advanced techniques, success rates, measured in actual numbers of babies born, drop off markedly with advancing maternal age. It is still difficult to achieve successful pregnancies by ART (assisted reproductive technology) in women in their late forties and older.

Most pregnancies that are well publicized in women in their fifties or even sixties are presently achieved with donor eggs from another woman implanted in the womb. The pregnancy is then supported by the administration of female sex hormones until delivery.

Endometriosis

Endometriosis is a relatively common condition often discovered in women in their thirties and forties who have delayed childbearing. With advanced diagnostic techniques, the beginning of this condition can be seen in much younger women. Actual deposits of womb lining, or endometrium, are seen in abnormal sites, most commonly in the lower part of the abdominal cavity behind the uterus, which is known as the cul de sac, which roughly translates from the French as "bottom of the bag". When laparoscopy is performed at the time of menstruation, it can be seen that retrograde menstruation actually does often occur. In other words, the womb lining mixed with blood that is the normal component of menstrual flow (that normally comes out of the vagina) can be seen laparoscopically to be flowing backwards from the uterus through the fallopian tubes and actually exiting from the fimbriated ends of the tubes into the area behind the uterus called the cul de sac. These deposits of womb lining or endometrium can then persist in this abnormal location. Each time the woman menstruates, these deposits bleed, causing scarring, especially along the ligaments behind the uterus, resulting in decreased mobility of the pelvic organs and increasing difficulty with achieving pregnancy.

More rarely, deposits of womb lining can occur in many other parts of the body. This phenomenon, of course, cannot be explained by retrograde flow through the fallopian tubes.

Ordinarily, foreign invaders into the body are managed by the body's own immune system. However, the endometriotic tissue involved in endometriosis is not foreign: it derives from the woman's own uterus. It is also becoming apparent that women who have endometriosis may have some defect in their immunologic system. There can be an enhanced inflammatory reaction with endometriosis involving inflammatory proteins from the deposits of endometriosis themselves.

There may be a genetic aspect to endometriosis as well.

Intron A (Interferon alpha - 2B), an immune cytokine, on an experimental basis, can inhibit the growth of endometrioma cells. This may hold some promise for future treatments. It is not presently approved for this purpose. The drug can cause a wide range of life-threatening, even fatal, disorders.It should not be used in pregnancy.

Endometriotic deposits and the adhesion formation associated with them can be readily diagnosed during videolaparoscopy. At the same time as they are recognized, they can be removed by the use of electrocautery or laser. At the same time, adhesion removal can be achieved with the use of small scissor-like instruments specifically designed for the purpose that are introduced at the time of laparoscopy. The patient most usually goes home the same day she undergoes this minimally invasive surgery.

Lupron (Leuprolide Acetate) does induce endometriosis to regress. Lupron is a GnRh (gonadotropin releasing factor) analogue. GnRh derives from the hypothalamus, located at the base of the brain. This hormone acts on the pituitary gland to release Luteinizing Hormone. (LH). FSH (Follicle Stimulating Hormone) and LH cyclically act on the ovary to secrete estrogen and progesterone.

By binding at receptor sites, Lupron can effectively stop menstruation for a period of months, and endometriotic deposits regress.

Various side effects of Lupron can include hot flashes and hirsutism (hair growth). The drug should not be used in pregnancy.

Immunology of Childbearing

Complex and fascinating interactions between the mother and her developing fetus impact directly on the life and health of the developing child. At the same time, these interactions have effects on the mother and her own health.

The developing fetus can in many ways be thought of as a homograft. The fetus derives half of its genetic material from the father. In that sense, it is a living foreign organism accommodated within the mother, without being immunologically rejected.

Transplanted organs, including kidneys, lungs, heart and liver, must be tissue-matched to the recipient as closely as possible. Even then, medication must be taken by the woman receiving the transplant throughout her life in order to counter rejection. However, transplanted organs unfortunately do get rejected in spite of all attempts to dampen down the process.

It is obvious, therefore, that natural accommodations are made by the mother in order to protect the fetus growing inside her from being recognized and immunologically attacked as an invader.

The fetus, in order to survive, has to interface with the mother on a very basic level. The fetus must receive vital oxygen and nutrients from the mother. Carbon dioxide and waste products of metabolism must be removed from the fetal blood supply by the mother and then disposed of by the mother. In order to achieve this, the placenta develops as an organ of exchange. The fetal placental tissue, which is called trophoblast, implants into the wall of the mother's uterus, or womb. As the placenta enlarges and grows, characteristics can be seen that are similar to an invading tumor, yet under normal circumstances and in the vast majority of cases the growth is limited and there is a clear definition microscopically at which the placenta will detach after the baby is born. Fetal blood vessels, which carry blood circulating from the fetus through the umbilical cord to the fetal side of the placenta, come into close microscopic contact with maternal blood in the uterine wall. The fetal blood vessels are contained within villi, which are microscopic finger-like projections. These villi are constantly bathed in a stream of maternal blood coming from the blood vessels of the uterus. Exchange of oxygen, carbon dioxide, nutrients, and waste products occurs between these two blood supplies which are in fact separated only by a very thin microscopic membrane.

This is a key point in the immunologic protection of both mother and fetus. Technically, the fetus is not a vascularized allograft. That means it is not directly connected to the mother's blood supply. In the transplantation of organs such as kidneys and hearts, these organs are directly attached to the blood supply of the recipient. Otherwise these organs could not survive. At the same time, it makes them very vulnerable to immunologic onslaught by the host. In the more subtle and elegant arrangement of mother and fetus, the fetus is protected from this direct pathway.

However, because of the huge expanse of chorionic villi that make up the placenta, and their fragility, it is very possible for small breaks to occur. This leads to an actual intermingling of maternal and fetal blood cells. In fact, this is known to occur.

During pregnancy, various changes occur in the pregnant woman that are consistent with dampening down of her immunologic responsivity, so that she can better tolerate her growing fetus.

The lymph nodes lose their germinal centers. The thymus gland atrophies. Lymphocytes, a particular form of white blood cell, are decreased in number.

Human chorionic gonadotropin (HCG), which is a hormone produced in great supply during pregnancy by the placenta, tends to reduce the uptake of antigen by macrophages, which are cells that are prominent in combating invaders. The hormones of pregnancy, including chorionic gonadotropin, estrogen, and progesterone tend to depress the mother's reticuloendothelial system. The reticulo-endothelial system is a widespread system in the body that forms antibodies to counteract foreign antigens. Generally speaking, the mother develops immunologic tolerance.

Immunity which the mother does develop can even be advantageous. It is well known that inbreeding reduces the viability of offspring. Therefore, immunologic difference between mother and fetus is not necessarily a bad thing. The exposure of the mother to small amounts of fetal antigen can possibly result in the development of immunologic tolerance of the fetus. A woman who has had several children tends to have a wide range of antibodies.

A fertilized egg (ovum) is itself protected from immunologic attack from the mother by a covering which is called the zona pellucida. The histocompatibility antigens within the egg probably do not provoke the same type of immunologic response that would occur in adult tissue.

Early Pregnancy Factor (EPF) is produced by the fertilized egg and appears in the mother's blood serum. EPF suppresses lymphocytic activity, suppressing the maternal immune response. The level of EPF falls prior to delivery.

The invading fetal trophoblast tissue of the placenta itself has low immunogenicity. It is protected by a barrier of sialomucin at the juncture with the maternal uterus.

In spite of all these elegant protections, immunocytes from the mother can enter the fetal circulation via minute breaks in the tiny vessels. Such mechanisms have been implicated in spontaneous miscarriage and stillbirth.

The breaks in the blood vessels of the villi, resulting in fetal blood cells escaping into a mother's blood circulation, can result in damage by the mother to her fetus. The classical example of this is Rh isoimmunization. In this condition, fetal blood cells are actually detected in the maternal blood circulation. The mother immunologically reacts to this by creating Rh antibodies to the fetus. This occurs in an Rh negative mother who is carrying an Rh positive fetus, in whom the Rh factor has been derived from the baby's father. The major break between the fetal and the maternal circulations, of course, occurs when the placenta separates at birth. Therefore, the first Rh positive child of an Rh negative mother is usually not affected by maternal antibodies. However, with the subsequent buildup of antibody levels in the mother, the next child comes under immunologic attack, and can develop anemia, jaundice, and heart failure while still in the uterus. This condition is preventable by giving Rhogam, which is essentially anti-D (Rh) antibody, to the mother. The Rhogam eliminates the fetal Rh positive red cells as they cross into the mother's circulation, so that the mother never develops her own antibodies to the Rh factor (D).

It is fascinating that, while the growing fetus is progressing towards birth, the fetal-derived trophoblastic tissue of the placenta noticeably shows characteristics of progressive aging and senescence. Thrombi (clots) in the blood vessels, areas of infarction (death of tissue from lack of blood supply), areas of calcification and deposition of fibrin may all be seen in the 'aging' placenta just prior to the birth of a child.

CHAPTER 12
LIFE EXPECTANCY

The Take-Home Message

- No matter how old you are, you have a life expectancy
- Theoretically, we should all be able to live healthfully to an age well beyond our current experience
- Early diagnosis and state of the art management of conditions can significantly prolong life span, with good quality of life
- This is one important aspect of 'prevention'
- Organ transplantation, and the development of techniques to grow new organ tissue, can greatly prolong lifespan

The longer a person lives, the longer they can expect to live. Everybody, no matter how old, has a statistical life expectancy. Obviously, that life expectancy gets shorter as the person ages.

The first major obstacle to a long life expectancy is genetic background. If family members are long lived, there is a better statistical chance of enjoying a long life. As genetic therapies become more available and prevalent, many of the genetically predisposed life threatening and life shortening conditions that we all are heir to in varying respects will become less and less important factors.

The next barrier encountered on the road to longevity is the intrauterine environment of the developing fetus. A healthy mother provides optimal blood flow to the placenta (afterbirth), so that the fetus is properly oxygenated and nourished. Harmful substances that can pass the barrier from the placenta into the fetus have to be avoided. Such substances include alcohol, illegal or so-called recreational drugs including opioids, marijuana, cocaine, and many prescription drugs, which should not be used in pregnancy unless there are proper medical considerations. Smoking constricts the blood vessels leading to the placenta causing intrauterine growth retardation, as the fetus is not adequately nourished or oxygenated.

The next major roadblock on the way to longevity is the labor and birth process itself. This process should be supervised and handled in a professional and sophisticated way so that the newborn baby enters the world without being abnormally stressed or subjected to oxygen deprivation.

The next great hurdle is getting through the first two years of life. Although we almost take it for granted in our society today that we can keep our children safe and free of life-threatening disease during their infancy, regrettably, this is not true in a large part of the world even today. Myriad risks facing small children include everything from sudden instant death syndrome, which may be partly genetically based, partly due to lung immaturity, and often due to poor positioning of infants in cribs, to a wide range of infectious diseases. Accidents, including car accidents and household accidents, also play a large part. Leaving a small child unattended can lead to disaster even in a matter of seconds. There is also a serious threat of violence to infants, including baby shaking syndrome. Other problems that can be life threatening to small children include developmental problems and even malignant tumors. Bacterial and viral infectious processes that may be relatively innocuous in adults, can be extremely damaging and life threatening to babies and conversely to the older, senior, population. Examples of this are the emergence of West Nile and chikungunya viruses, as yet incurable mosquito borne illnesses that can be lethal, especially to infants and seniors.

Failure to properly immunize children has become an increasing problem. The resurgence of measles is a prominent threat.

Surviving age two is a significant milestone.

Subsequent growing up can also be hazardous to your health and life. One of the predominant causes of death in children and young adults is accidents. These accidents include auto accidents, and violence, especially gun violence. Older people are definitely not immune to these problems either. Pre-teenage children, teenagers and young adults, are particularly susceptible to the illegal and inappropriate use of street drugs and improperly obtained prescription drugs including opioids. This can lead to overdose and death. Alcohol abuse by young people is responsible for illness and death in a startling number of cases.

People in the reproductive age group, starting in their early teens or even earlier, are susceptible to a whole host of sexually transmitted diseases, most of which are not fatal today if properly treated. A glaring exception to that is Acquired Immunodeficiency Syndrome. This disease process, which is caused by a virus that is overwhelmingly spread by sexual contact, is presently decimating the populations of some countries, most of which are in the developing or third worlds. There is a large population of AIDS victims in our society. Recent significant advances in drug therapy of the condition have now made it possible to transform many people with HIV syndrome to survivors, with a chronic condition, and even the possibility of cure. The HIV virus compromises the immune system of the host person, thereby leaving the affected person open to a plethora of life-threatening infectious disease processes, including tuberculosis and pneumonia. Beyond strengthening the immune system, treatment is targeted at treating specific infections. One of the major problems in our society with the control of this virus is that it is very difficult to develop a vaccine against it. As the cause is a slow virus, it can take a long time to discover if any particular vaccine preparation is going to be efficacious. As well, the virus has the ability to mutate and scientists are trying to hit a moving target.

Another problem with controlling the immunodeficiency virus in our society is a political one. Consistently in the past and today, life threatening infectious diseases that are rampant in the society are reportable. Health authorities must by law made be aware of infected cases, so that they can accurately plot the spread of the disease and be able to alert contacts of infected persons. However, just the opposite has occurred with this one single major life-threatening disease, Human Immunodeficiency Syndrome. The test results of any given person must be held in the utmost secrecy. Even at the point when a patient requests their doctor to release their records to another doctor in writing, the doctor can release all other records with the one exception of HIV test results, even if those results are negative, unless the doctor has received a separate, special consent. This flies in the face of any rational concept of long evolved commonsense public health measures. The rationale for this is that knowing the HIV status of people would lead to discrimination. Hopefully, our society is getting beyond this type of discrimination, and there are better ways to handle illegal discrimination in the workplace or elsewhere.

It was presumed that the virus was spread mainly through homosexual contact and anal intercourse. In actuality, heterosexual transmission through vaginal intercourse occurs with great frequency and indeed is probably the prime mode for the disease transmission in many underdeveloped countries. It is also probable that the type of AIDS virus that causes Kaposi's Sarcoma can be transferred by oral kissing, in the saliva. Obviously, the world AIDS pandemic has been responsible for a downward slide in the life expectancy of young women.

It is interesting how various threats to our longevity interact with our thinking and our political processes. The so-called sexual revolution is not spoken about so much anymore. Sexually active people of every age in our society tend to think twice before having casual sex with partners they do not know well. It is interesting that although doctors cannot easily share HIV status information with other doctors, even with the patient's consent, unless that consent specifically relates to HIV information, insurance companies certainly do demand HIV testing in people, and demand results of that testing, before they issue life insurance policies. This is perfectly legal: there is money involved.

Our politicians now tend to speak in terms of morality, monogamy, and renewed religious values. A rethinking of the way in which we conduct our lives sexually can have a great impact on the spread of Human Immunodeficiency Virus (HIV). Condom use, of course, helps, but it is by no means the final answer. Medical workers who have been directly exposed to HIV through breaks in their skin (often, inadvertent needle puncture) are offered access to HIV treating drugs. Similar post exposure treatment can now be offered to sexual contacts of infected individuals, although the efficacy of this post exposure treatment has not yet been fully established.

For women, the great hurdle to achieving longevity was the danger associated with childbearing. Women classically died in childbirth of hemorrhage, infection, and a disease condition called toxemia. Toxemia is now classified as a group of diseases called the hypertensive disorders of pregnancy. These conditions tend to be among the leading causes of death in women in childbearing. The ability to prevent and treat these conditions has now risen to the level where only a small number of women in our society die in childbirth.

With the advent of increasingly successful treatment of congenital heart disease, that is, defects in the heart that women are born with, large groups of women who previously would not have lived to reproductive age, or would have not been able to reproduce, became able to bear children. Thus, heart disease became a significant factor in the death of women during the childbearing process. Rheumatic heart disease, which damages the heart valves, has thankfully been largely reduced in incidence by the effective use of antibiotics. However, women with heart valve problems still can and do get pregnant and are in danger. As well, as the proportion of women in an older age group in our society who get pregnant becomes larger, there is an increasing incidence of actual myocardial infarction, or heart attack, during labor and delivery. Along with the growing pregnancy, there is a great increase in the circulating fluid volume in the cardiovascular system. As well, the enlarging uterus exerts upward pressure on the lungs, as well as the mediastinum, which is the area between the lungs where the heart is located. During the labor process, there is an increased workload on the heart because of the uterine contractions. This is greatly exacerbated in the second stage of labor when the mother is actually exerting downward force, or pushing, to help send the baby downwards through the birth canal. Instances of true heart attack in the second stage of labor, particularly in older mothers, are well known.

Diabetes is another condition which is impacted on by pregnancy, and which in turn impacts on the pregnancy. Pregnancy is a diabetogenic state. That means pregnancy increases the likelihood of a woman becoming hyperglycemic, and spilling sugar into her urine. There is a state known as gestational diabetes. The woman who is not ordinarily diabetic develops the manifestations of diabetes during her pregnancy, and after the pregnancy reverts to a normal state. Theoretically, if such a woman has repeated pregnancies, she eventually will become a full-blown diabetic. This, of course, can impact on her longevity, as diabetes, especially if it is not properly controlled, leads to blood vessel changes and cardiovascular complications, as well as eye changes (retinopathy) and kidney changes (nephropathy) which can be irreversible.

The concept of high risk pregnancy has evolved. Every pregnancy, of course, carries some low degree of risk. As the woman gets older, she faces a greater degree of risk of disease conditions and harm either to herself or to her developing fetus, or both. The cutoff age of high risk pregnancy is described as thirty-five years. Of course, this is not a magic number. The woman of age thirty-five has statistically more risk than a woman of age thirty-four, and less risk than a woman of age thirty-six. Round numbers are easy to use statistically when looking at large populations to see how they fare in given situations. It is evident that older women do not fare as well in pregnancy as women in a younger age group, provided that the younger age group is not socioeconomically deprived and in their early teenage years.

The vast majority of women in our society today pass through their childbearing period unscathed. Indeed, childbearing is a totally normal process. Most women come through that period in their lives emotionally fulfilled and physically healthy. They can than look forward to watching future generations of children, grandchildren and great grandchildren grow. There are now large numbers of women in our society who are still fit, active, and able to enjoy, and keep up with, their great grandchildren.

Gradually, in the reproductive years and thereafter, women start to experience the various diseases and conditions associated with a more mature population. Some of these diseases are characterized as degenerative processes. Many new and exciting therapies now exist and are being formulated to counteract the effects of these processes, or to obviate them altogether. A healthful lifestyle certainly helps in retardation and diminution of these processes. Such disease conditions include arteriosclerotic heart and blood vessel disease, diabetes, various forms of arthritis, and neurologic diseases such as Parkinson's disease, Alzheimer's disease and stroke, and of course various cancers.

The immune system which protects all of us from infection and the invasion of organisms does change as we get older. An important type of white blood cell, the lymphocyte, no longer divides as effectively when challenged. The thymus gland in the neck, which produces thymic hormone, that is necessary for the normal maturation of T- lymphocytes, ceases to be present in people over age sixty.

Certain antibody responses also decrease with age.

The neutrophil, which is the predominant form of white blood cell, is a most important defense against bacterial and fungal infection. However, older people tend to have decreased bone marrow reserves. As neutrophils are made in the bone marrow, older people may have a deficiency of these cells as well. It is well known that sickness and even death due to infectious disease increase in people over sixty-five years of age. That is why it is advocated that people in their senior years get an influenza vaccination, commonly known as a flu shot, each year. It is important for seniors to discuss getting these shots, as well as pneumonia vaccine, with their doctor, in spite of the fact that a person over the age of sixty five does not have as good an antibody response to the vaccines as a younger person would.

Fortunately, antiviral drugs, such as Tamiflu (oseltamivir), Relenza (zanamivir), Rapivab (peramivir), Xofluza (baloxavir marboxil), Symmetrel (amantadine), and Flumadine (rimantadine) are now available that can combat influenza. Effective antibiotic regimens are used to prevent and combat secondary bacterial infection. It is important to contact your doctor even when you have a so-called 'cold' prior to using any medications, especially in pregnancy, or when nursing.

Upper respiratory infections are usually viral in nature, but can be bacterial, and can spread to the rest of the respiratory tract, resulting in bronchitis and pneumonia. It is even more vital to contact your doctor at the onset of symptoms in this age of potential and real bioterrorism: anthrax infection can present with upper respiratory symptoms. Nowadays, your doctor will advise appropriate treatment suited to your individual case.

The COVID19 pandemic is a serious threat to older persons. This contagious corona virus has the ability to attack multiple organ systems and causes fatalities particularly among our older population. The well known precautions include social distancing to the point of quarantine, and the use of protective gear including masks and gloves.

If you can reach your seventieth birthday relatively unscathed by these conditions, especially the life-threatening ones, then you are well on your way to longevity. You have by then escaped the threat of once fatal childhood infections, the exuberant risk taking and accident prone years of adolescence, conditions threatening your life and health during childbearing, and many of the risks associated with diseases of mature people such as sudden death with a first heart attack.

Theoretically at least, it may be possible to survive to the age of one hundred and thirty-five years. Beyond that, we can only speculate. There are large numbers of people in America today who are well past the age of one hundred, and furthermore are fit and active.

Merely to achieve a long life span, if you are severely physically, mentally or emotionally impaired, does not seem to be a very attractive goal. However, it is becoming increasingly obvious that it is realistic to expect to be able to live beyond the age of one hundred, and have a useful, meaningful, productive, and fulfilling life at a great age.

Even for the vast numbers of us who have encountered one of a wide range of life-threatening diseases, if we are in relatively good health past the age of seventy, chances are good that our long term life expectancy has been increased measurably. For example, appendicitis, which was potentially lethal in children, young adults and older adults, probably now has a lowered incidence due to antibiotic use. When actual appendicitis does occur, it is of course most often successfully treated surgically. Minimally invasive surgery with a laparoscope can be used in selected cases to remove the appendix. That life-threatening ailment is now generally thought of as a condition that can be treated definitively and successfully.

Minimally invasive surgery is now starting to be enhanced and replaced by robotic surgery. The surgeon works at a console, or computer terminal, and manipulates controls that send orders to fine robotic instruments that have been placed within the body near the organ being operated on. These techniques allow for greater flexibility and precision, with smaller instruments, and smaller incisions.

Another exciting new field in medicine is cybernetics. This is, to be dramatic, essentially the melding of person and machine. Computer chips may be implanted in the body in various disease states so that appropriate commands can be sent to various muscles.

Work is progressing to repair the spinal cord, and other areas where there are gaps in nerve transmission. It is now possible to grow human central nervous system cells, and to stretch out their axons, which are the elongated connecting parts of the nerve cells that carry signals.

It is often possible to overcome certain cases of deafness with cochlear implants. Computerized devices that effectively allow certain people with visual handicaps to discern their surroundings are also becoming available.

The long term prognoses for chronic conditions such as diabetes improves as diagnostic techniques, allowing efficient and easy monitoring of blood sugar, evolve. As more efficient treatments become available degenerative changes are less likely.

Organ transplantation is now performed almost routinely in major medical centers for 'end stage' disease of various organs. Corneal transplants were done relatively early. The first major vital organ to be transplanted was the kidney. Heart, lung, and liver transplants are now being performed. The donor may be a relative, but more often the organ comes from a donor who has just died. Tissue matching is performed to lower the risk of rejection of the organ by the new host. Drugs that lower the incidence of rejection have much improved over the years, so that many people now survive successfully with donated organs.

Animal tissues may become increasingly important in transplantation. One example is the current use of pig heart valves to replace defective heart valves in humans. Animals are being selectively bred and immunologically altered so that their organs may be used in humans with a lessened chance of organ rejection.

People in times past who would have died early of coronary artery disease and arteriosclerotic cardiovascular disease are treated with blood pressure lowering medications if they are hypertensive, and with cholesterol lowering medications if their cholesterol levels are abnormally high. Coronary artery bypass operations have been successful in achieving efficient new blood supply to the heart. Minimally invasive procedures to open blocked blood vessels have been and continue to be a major advance. Damaged arteries in the body can often be replaced with grafts. Abnormal blood vessel formations in the brain can be clipped off or treated with radial surgery.

There is a reluctance to pronounce anybody cured of cancer, because of the nature of the disease process in its ability to resurface many years after initial treatment and long, ostensibly disease-free periods. However, there are now uncounted numbers of people who seem to have achieved cure. As a cautionary matter, such people are usually called disease free rather than cured.

Precancerous conditions, and early cancerous conditions of the uterine cervix, which is the mouth of the womb, are definitively treated now with a high degree of success and by relatively simple means. The same is true for early cancer of the uterus itself. Huge numbers of women with breast cancer, especially if it was detected at an early stage, are now well past their seventies and beyond, even if their initial disease occurred relatively early in their forties. To such women, their disease is a memory, although a singularly unpleasant one. They know that they must remain vigilant. There are even significant numbers of women who have had ovarian cancer who are alive and well with absolutely no evidence of disease twenty years and more after initial diagnosis and definitive treatment.

Such people are survivors. They are toughened and shaped by the stark experiences that they have been through. They have much wisdom to pass on to succeeding generations. They know how to survive. Then again, all of us at a certain age are survivors. We have made it through life's vagaries with varying amounts of physical, mental, and emotional scarring. What we have to tell about those experiences that shaped us used to be called wisdom.

In ages past, only a few of us survived to the prescribed three score and ten years. Families were close knit and did not often venture far from their roots. Not too many generations ago, most people had rarely been beyond the confines of their own village. Astoundingly, this is still true in much of the world today. Elders in such communities were usually revered. Even the term "elder", connotes reverence; a person whose opinions should be respected.

As something becomes more common, it becomes demystified. In our society, advanced old age is becoming increasingly common. Therefore, those of us of a certain age can no longer expect to be on a somewhat mystical level. However, in the natural scheme of things, the older generations can rightfully expect respect and love from their family members. Happily, this is most usually the case.

Native Americans, historically, tended to be mobile peoples. The earliest Americans, the Native Americans, probably migrated to this continent across what is now the Bering Strait, and gradually traveled and settled across the American continents. All the rest of us have had ancestors who crossed mighty oceans on flimsy craft to reach these shores. This was followed by a great migration westward.

Constant travel has had a great impact on the traditional family structure and the role of older persons. People are often separated by great distances from their children, grandchildren, and great grandchildren. Now that a large proportion of the Americas is effectively settled, a lot of this dislocation has stopped. Furthermore, many families are seeing the advantages of keeping the generations relatively close together for mutual physical, emotional, and economic support. The availability of easy and quick travel opportunities to just about everybody in the population allows the different generations of a family to visit each other on a far more frequent basis, more than could ever have been thought possible. This brings up problems of its own, as we now face a domestic airline situation that seems to have been stretched to its limit for the near term, with major security concerns, delays, cancellations of flights, and commonplace general frustration. Rapid and efficient screening techniques, including encoded identification cards, fingerprint, eye, and facial recognition devices, and much more sophisticated screening of all baggage items for banned items including weapons and explosives will have to be instituted. Airport scheduling will have to become more efficient, and airport capacity will have to be increased. Alternative methods of travel in the busiest urban corridors, such as efficient high speed trains that already exist in Europe and Asia, are already functioning in some locales.

A dramatic explosion in our ability to communicate has strengthened the bonds of far flung families. Most of us now routinely carry cell phones, so that we can be in instant communication with businesses and loved ones. Not only is this convenient, but it can contribute greatly to safety in the event of an emergency, an attack, a car breakdown, or if there are sudden symptoms of sickness. The most advanced automobiles now have satellite positioning systems coupled with emergency cell phone communication, which instantly activates in case of an accident, pinpointing the location to a central station so that help can be immediately dispatched. Unless a vehicle is stopped, drivers should not use a cell phone unless it is hands free and voice activated. We are now in an age where you can simply state to your telephone who you want to call, and the telephone does the rest. Voice activated calling is probably also available for a small fee on you wired home telephone through your local telephone company. It is a great boon to people who are busy, forgetful of telephone numbers, or somewhat vision impaired. It is simple to program the telephone numbers you usually use into the telephone. This part is easy, as the telephone voice prompts you through the procedure.

People now routinely communicate with their families by e-mail, text messaging, and similar online methods. This is one way to obviate the anxiety of dealing with traditional mail that is possibly contaminated. Just because you are older does not mean you do not have the computer skills to do this. As a matter of fact, many older people find that their computers give them great freedom and even entertainment. Shopping of all types is increasingly done efficiently by computer. The frustration of being constantly put on hold on the telephone has largely been obviated by switching to the computer instead, to do everything from buying airline tickets to making and confirming reservations. Cameras are now digital, so the pictures taken can instantly be displayed on the computer screen, and instantly sent to loved ones no matter where they are.

References

1. cdc.gov/coronavirus/2019-ncov/index.html
2. thelancet.com/pdfs/journals/lancet/PllSO140-6736(20)30558-4.pdf

CHAPTER 13
DIET

The Take-Home Message

- We are not what we eat
- Fat does not (necessarily) make a person fat
- Fat intake is necessary, to a degree
- Calcium is important
- Chances are good that most of us eat too much
- Many of the dietary rules we traditionally follow are arbitrary, and do not have much relation to our body physiology
- We should be critical of words that seem to suggest health benefits
- Vitamins are necessary, but except in pregnancy, adequate amounts are usually contained within a varied diet
- A vitamin and mineral supplement should usually contain some trace elements such as zinc and chromium. I was once asked how one gets chromium – I said off the bumper of a '58 Buick – but I should not be facetious.
- The best meals tend to be made by master chefs, not by a committee

"You Are What You Eat"- this is one of the greatest bits of misinformation ever foisted upon the human race. It is at best, a platitude. In fact, we are NOT what we eat. The body is adept in turning foodstuffs into what it needs for energy, namely simple sugar or glucose. What is eaten in excess of energy needs is converted into fat stored in places where people would rather not see it. There are certain things that must be taken in which the body cannot manufacture. These include essential amino acids which are obtained from protein, and most efficiently, probably, from animal protein, contrary to some popular politically correct beliefs. If a varied diet is eaten including fruits and vegetables, with an intake of green vegetables, as well as natural dairy products, protein, and eggs including the yolk, in most cases necessary amounts of minerals and vitamins automatically will be obtained. There can be a tendency to excess in our society. Some people think that if some is good, then a lot is better. However, overdosing on certain vitamins, which are normally present in the diet in only trace amounts and serve as organic catalysts expediting chemical reactions within the body, can be dangerous.

Excessive vitamin A intake, in the form of Retinol found in multivitamins and liver, may promote osteoporosis and hip fractures. Beta carotene, on the other hand, does not seem to increase the risk of hip fracture.

A normal healthy person, eating a healthful varied diet, in the absence of any disease state should not need vitamin supplementation. This does not include pregnant women, who do need specific vitamin (folic acid) and iron supplementation. On the other hand, taking a multivitamin supplement once a day should not be harmful and may have a beneficial effect.

What are we supposed to eat? It is now believed that the Neanderthal was a carnivore. Those rugged beings were hunters and ate meat. On the face of it, this would not speak well for longevity, as their life expectancy was probably somewhere in the range of the early thirties. This most likely had much less to do with diet than to the brutal nature of their existence, with encounters with live beasts, and little knowledge of how to protect themselves against disease or fight it. The most frightening encounter any of us is likely to have, on the other hand, is with a diffident maitre d'hotel who is saving the table for a regular.

Many in our society now think we should be herbivores, and point to the good health of some peoples who have very little animal protein in their diets. This, in many instances, may be of necessity, as animal protein is an expensive resource. It is notable in our own society that as the general wealth of the population increases, so does the consumption of animal protein. The steak house is alive and well in America. In actuality, human beings are omnivores. We are capable of eating a wide variety of foodstuffs and converting them to our needs. It is possible to be healthy following a variety of diets.

"Natural" and "Goodness" seem to go together very well. It is a nice fit. This is somewhat in the nature of self-fulfilling prophecy, as we tend to attribute naturalness to the things we think are good, and goodness to the things we think are natural. The natural life expectancy in a primitive society, and quite recently in our own, was approximately thirty-seven years. Children routinely died in infancy and mothers routinely died in childbirth. Wars, strife, disease, pestilence, famine, and natural disasters took care of the rest. Thinking people have dedicated their lives and careers to promoting civilization and science so that we could get away from this naturalness. In the natural order of things, births equal deaths. Until relatively recently, it was a struggle just to keep the human race from disappearing from the face of the earth because we were hard put to keep the birth rate equal to the death rate. A notable example of this was the Black Death in the Middle Ages.

The advent of public health measures and the understanding of infectious disease, the advent of scientific medicine, and the introduction of preventive antenatal care for pregnant women all have contributed to raising expectations that a natural life should be what was prophesied in the Bible, three score and ten years. This age has now been surpassed by the expected span of life in many nations today. It could be argued that to go beyond the seventy or so prophesied years would be unnatural and therefore not good. The whole weight of the civilization we have developed would fly in the face of this interpretation. Clearly, if we can create an environment in which people can live healthfully to a much older age and develop the adaptations in society necessary to accommodate this older population in a meaningful way, then we shall truly have achieved something momentous.

Are Natural Foods Good?

We conveniently fit our definition of natural to that which we think is desirable. Historically, our ancestors were hunters and gatherers. They also may questionably have been scavengers. By this definition, natural food is a wild animal that can be killed or a wild fish that can be caught. The definition would also include wild berries, nuts and other plant products that could be found in the forests and on the plains. Most of us would not consider this the natural way to eat today, and if we tried it we would quickly find that it was not politically correct and create a furor.

The next step was to domesticate plants to create a stable supply of foodstuffs, and to domesticate animals both for their dairy products and for their meat and eggs. Once these steps were taken, we were no longer living naturally. These great advances in the stability of the food supply led to their own problems with epidemics of plant and animal disease leading to human ill health. As well, the unnatural practice of tilling the land led to droughts, soil erosion, and dust bowls. The use of natural organic fertilizers including animal and human waste led to epidemics of disease. The water supply, including lakes, rivers, streams, and the water table were all subject to pollution, further increasing the danger of human disease.

It is possible that the lactose intolerant among us really do not have a disorder. Infants thrive on mother's milk and possess the enzymes to process it. As the baby grows to eat a varied diet, and the mother weans her, the baby may naturally lose the ability to process milk products. It is possible that those herders of domesticated cattle who mutated to retain the ability to process milk products had a survival advantage. Those of us who are not lactose intolerant are their descendants.

As people congregated in villages, towns, and cities, food markets contained aging produce and meat products that were infested with bacteria, insects and vermin. So much for the good old days.

This brings us to the present day and the burning question. "Is a single slice of processed cheddar cheese wrapped in a piece of plastic, or a plastic cup of yogurt with a generous dollop of blueberry jam on the bottom a natural food?"

Certainly, in spite of conflicting claims and clamor for our attention by numerous fad diets, we can make reasonable choices in food selection, in line with the changing, and hopefully advancing, scientific evidence of what our bodies need.

Probably one of the first things to remember in seeking a natural diet is that our body types differ. Many of us have been around long enough to have seen different facts and fancies concerning the ideal human body type. Most recently, there has been a tendency to admire the tall and the thin, which has been a great boon to tall and thin people everywhere.

There is some evidence that being a bit thin, and restricting caloric intake, can have health benefits as we get older. For example, a thin woman may have less of a chance of getting breast cancer than an obese woman. Obesity is linked to the risk of getting high blood pressure (hypertension), coronary heart disease, diabetes and some cancers. Being substantially overweight as a young adult, into middle age, can have health consequences in older age.

It is becoming increasingly evident that a we need to maintain lean muscle mass, especially as we get older. Muscle mass impacts directly on bone density. Menopausal women and older men have a tendency to lose bone density. It is important to maintain calcium levels in the diet. It is also important to remember that diet and exercise go together. Sports and weight bearing exercise done under proper supervision throughout adult life have a beneficial effect. Coupled with continued reasonable exercise, such as walking at a good pace regularly in older age, proper diet goes a long way to maintaining lean muscle mass and good bone density.

It is important to remember that adequate calcium intake is important as we get older. Bone density cannot properly be maintained without it.

There is a significant part of our culture that worships muscle mass, and muscle definition. In the years after World War II, with memories of starvation and emaciation clear in our minds, it was okay to carry extra pounds. Old movies tend to prove the point. There are not too many of us left who can remember the Reubenesque figures of the Gilded Age, when plumpness was equated with wealth and sexuality. The hidden message in this was if you were rich enough you could afford to eat, and eat more than just for sustenance.

This whole philosophy has been turned on its ear in present day America, because just about everyone can now afford to eat. Unfortunately, the tendency is to eat processed foods, which by any stretch of the definition are not natural and can pose a multitude of health risks.

People also eat for instant gratification; often fried 'fast' foods with high fat content. Disquieting reports of acrylamide in French fries and potato chips, among other starchy fried or baked foods, including packaged cereals and even bread, provide another reason for avoiding these foods. Acrylamide may be associated with cancer if taken in large amounts.

The best tasting, most natural foods that are presently available also tend to be very expensive. Sophisticated, self-defined members of the upwardly mobile set increasingly tend to eat smaller portions of fine foods made with natural ingredients. At the same time, the scientific evidence is increasingly showing that such foods have health benefits. Our grandmothers generally said the same thing without the research.

Gene Silencing

It is becoming scientifically evident that common sense caloric restriction may prolong life. Caloric restriction can interact with a gene, called silent information regulator, that causes silent information regulator protein to be made. This effectively protects against activation of genes that could interfere with proper cell function. This process is called gene silencing, and it protects the cell, which, of course, is the basic unit that makes up all the body's organs.

Common sense caloric restriction to a level that maintains a reasonable and healthful body weight will result in less glucose being metabolized. This probably reduces the formation of free radicals, which are a byproduct of glucose metabolism that can damage cells, and therefore decrease longevity.

Of course, it is much easier to talk about caloric restriction than to really make it happen. Appetite gets in the way, making it almost impossible for many people to control their urges and their weight.

Nerve cells, or neurons, in an important area at the base of the brain called the hypothalamus, produce various proteins that are appetite stimulants and appetite suppressants. Fat cells in the body itself produce a protein called leptin. Leptin travels in the blood stream to the brain, activating neurons making appetite suppressant proteins, and inhibiting the brain cells which make appetite stimulants. In other words, leptin suppresses appetite. However, obese people make enough leptin on their own, and supplementation with leptin does not necessarily help them. On the other hand, someone who is dieting will have less natural leptin, so that the brain will put out more appetite stimulant and less appetite suppressant. In other words, the brain will signal the person to eat more.

This knowledge is making it possible to develop real and effective anti-obesity drugs that work at the hormonal level to specifically control appetite. The brain and body will properly sense when food intake has been adequate, and appetite will be appropriately shut down.

Zimulti (rimonabant) is a drug that blocks naturally occurring cannabinoids in the brain from binding to their receptors. This should diminish appetite, as cannabis, essentially marijuana, stimulates appetite.

Fats

Snack foods such as chips are often filled with hydrogenated oils and saturated fats and give very little useful food intake for the calories consumed. So-called diet foods very often are variations on the same theme. If a food has no fat, then it is probably loaded with sugar and possibly salt. Sugar needed for energy will be burned off and the remainder will be converted to fat which will ultimately show itself in embarrassing places. There is the side effect of having clogged coronary arteries. Snack foods with fat substitutes, can result in flatulence and diarrhea. Important fat-soluble vitamins will not be properly absorbed. The best way to deal with snack foods is to get out of the habit and stop eating them.

The great historical no-no to the Gallic farmer was oleomargarine. From the economic point of view, it threatened the existence of the family dairy farmer by depressing the price of natural butter. Even in its most modern incarnations, it is hard to fool sophisticated people that butter is being served when in fact they are getting margarine. Unfortunately, we cook with margarine, put it on bread and we serve it to our children. The problem again is hydrogenated oils. The evidence shows that natural butter is a healthier product. It is also more expensive. Exclusive bakeries and restaurants only use natural butter, and the meal you get on the table reflects that in quality and taste. Of course, food should not be slathered in natural butter. Moderation is a good thing.

Eliminating fat from the diet in the absence of certain specific disease states is not a good idea. Although it is true that eating fat does deliver nine calories per gram consumed, essential oils, fats and fatty acids are an integral part of a healthy diet. It is self-defeating to totally eliminate fat from the diet and load up on diet foods which advertise themselves as no fat or low fat, but in fact are crammed with sugar. Extra sugar does get processed to fat in the body, so this exercise in deprivation is self-defeating.

Protein

Lean meat is a good thing unless one is a committed vegetarian. Meat, especially ground meat, such as hamburger, should be properly cooked at sufficient temperature to kill any bacteria that is there. This brings up the question of the radiating of meat to get rid of bacteria. There is a widely held mistaken belief that a person eating radiated meat gets radiated. This is untrue. The fallback position is that in any case, radiated meat is not natural. Neither is much of anything else we do these days, including wearing clothes. Eradicating the germs in hamburger meat that from time to time devastates our population, especially the older, sicker, and youngest members of our population, would be an important step forward.

It is important to ensure that meat products are disease- free. Mad cow disease (bovine spongiform encephalitis) seen in Europe, and to a much lesser extent in North America, resulted from the unnatural practice of feeding meal contaminated by infected animal carcasses to cows. Humans become infected by eating the contaminated beef, getting a variant of spongiform encephalopathy (Creutzfeldt - Jakob Disease variant).

Meat efficiently provides essential amino acids which are the building blocks of our own protein. At four calories per gram, this is a good way to keep the body fit. Most people agree that it also tastes really good.

Poultry products have become very popular in recent years. The days when a chicken dinner was a delicacy we looked forward to once a week are gone. Poultry tends to be quite cheap and plentiful, and supplies protein in abundance. There are however, concerns about bacterial contamination that continually have to be addressed. As well, there are concerns about the contamination of land and water in various parts of a country where the mass industrialized raising of these birds occurs. The same concerns of course apply to other aspects of the industry, notably the raising of hogs.

Animal protein can be obtained from fish. Fish is thought to be natural and lean. However, it is a good bet that the plump complacent fish eaten at dinner may well have come from a fish farm, and it is about as natural as a commercially raised turkey. As well, if it is bathed in fat-filled sauce or margarine, not much has been achieved. Industrial pollution puts mercury into the water, which is then taken up by fish. Increasingly, there are warnings to women, especially pregnant women not to eat too much of certain types of fish, including canned tuna. Modern ocean fishing methods can be very destructive to whole species. Currently, we are in danger of losing many of the magnificent large fish that inhabit our oceans. Wild salmon have been endangered by water pollution and damage to their traditional nesting grounds. Incidently, farm raised salmon can have a significant percentage of fat. Smoked belly lox is not exactly a health food.

Protein of course can also be obtained from various beans, legumes, and bean products. One must watch for exaggerated claims of power and potency.

Carbohydrate

Bread is known as the staff of life. Eating starches such as bread, potatoes, or pasta, is a good way to take in calories needed for energy. In the body, these substances get reduced to simple sugars and are used for energy. The excess is stored in the body as fat. There was also classically thought to be a protein sparing effect due to intake of starches, so that a person who ate starch was thought to need less of the more expensive protein. Additionally, our ancestors tended to think that black bread was for peasants, and that the more expensive refined white flour should be reserved for the gentry. This somehow developed into the white bread and mayonnaise culture of Fifties America. Pretty bland stuff.

It was thought that whole grain products were beneficial to health. This initially came about because whole grain products obviously increased bowel motility and bowel movements, and it was thought that increased bowel function could be healthful. Later, a lot of evidence seemed to show that eating a lot of roughage, including whole grain products decreased the tendency to intestinal cancer. The latest research shows this is not true. It probably promotes extra trips to the bathroom and is otherwise not helpful. However, diets of this type are still promoted in various spas. If nothing else, the laxative effect makes the customers a few pounds lighter before they go home. They then more cheerfully pay the bill because of some weight loss.

People have discovered that whole grain bread and various ethnic black and brown breads taste much better. This has stood the conventional pattern on its ear, so that ethnic breads made in small bakeries tend to be more expensive than white bread, which is now considered déclassé in a lot of circles. However, there are many delicious forms that refined flour can take, including baguettes and croissants. The key in any good diet is moderation. Eating a lot of bread and pasta can lead to obesity.

Dietary intake in the form of carbohydrates has been advocated. However, there is a developing feeling that many people have some insulin resistance. Increased amounts of carbohydrates, which are essentially simple and complex sugars, require increased insulin production in order to process them. This can lead to increased health risks, such as heart disease, instead of the expected health benefits. The old concept of a balanced diet is probably the better choice.

The Mediterranean diet has become part of our folklore. First of all, if properly prepared using olive oil, the foods associated with the Mediterranean diet, low in saturated fat, including fish, meat, vegetables, grains, nuts and fruit, accompanied by good red wine, have been shown to have significant health benefits. Pigments in red wine, polyphenols, probably reduce the formation of Endothelin I which causes blood vessels to close down (constrict). Tomatoes contain an antioxidant, lycopene, that may be associated with reduced risk for certain types of cancer. Use of olive oil in place of butter, and especially in place of margarine, seems to be of benefit in lowering the incidence of cardiovascular disease. Red wine in moderation seems to have similar beneficial effects. Of course, drinking a whole cheap bottle of wine in a brown paper bag probably doesn't do anybody much good. There is still cirrhosis of the liver, largely caused by alcohol, to deal with.

Shellfish, being bottom dwellers, should be properly cooked to obviate the problems of bacterial contamination.

Older people aged 70 to 90 who don't smoke, have good physical activity levels, drink alcohol moderately, and stick to the Mediterranean diet, can cut their mortality rate (risk of dying) by half.

Obesity

Obesity itself has become one of the great health risks in America today. There is a genetic predisposition to obesity. It is easier for some people to stay fit and trim than it is for many others.

The fact is, we eat too much and we do not exercise enough. We also do not sleep enough. When we are up, we eat. If a person is tired, she or he should go to bed. Animals know enough to go to sleep when they are tired. Humans do not. Our biorhythms show us that the Spaniards are probably right about the late afternoon siesta. Lamentably, with the advent of the global economy, instant communication, and vigorous economic competition between societies, this great institution is being lost, hopefully not entirely.

A tired person should go to bed, and not feel guilty about it. A little appropriate safe sex does not hurt either. It is important to get up refreshed and eat a sensible breakfast. This brings us to the question of cold breakfast cereal. It may be a shock to learn that most people do not eat cold breakfast cereal, and that it is an artificial invention. Cold breakfast cereals largely tend to be refined starch paste of various grains, which is then artificially colored and flavored. Fortunately now, they tend to be fortified with vitamins and minerals which are necessary for metabolism. This is an acceptable way to take in the recommended daily requirement, provided that the diet does not already include foodstuffs that naturally contain them. Oatmeal is probably better. Oat bran may have some beneficial cardiovascular effect. Breakfast cereals do supply caloric intake, and if eaten with skim or low fat milk, there is protein intake as well. Eating breakfast this way has the additional advantage of being relatively cheap. An important component of a healthy breakfast is a glass of orange juice or a citrus fruit. The body cannot efficiently store vitamin C, so it must be supplied every day. Like all good things, fresh pasteurized orange juice and citrus fruits tend to be somewhat expensive. They are worth it. Some studies tend to show that drinking fresh orange juice every day may lower the incidence of certain types of cancer.

One of the more recent phenomena seen among people trying to eat healthfully is the emergence of something called the egg white omelet. This concoction loses a certain amount of je ne sais quoi in taste, but beyond that, the egg yolk has gotten a very bad rap. Traditionally, it was the prized part of the egg, not the part to be thrown away. Recent evidence tends to show that eating the entire egg in moderation can be beneficial. Nutrients in the yolk of an egg for most people are not harmful. As a matter of fact, the yolk is genetically designed to be the nourishment for the emerging embryo. Nature may be trying to tell us something.

Genetic Engineering

This brings us to the extremely controversial topic of genetically engineered foods. The hue and cry against such foods in Europe and to a lesser extent in the Americas is partially economically determined by the fear of competition. The importation of genetically engineered foodstuffs from the United States to Europe could damage the economics of the smaller farms on the European Continent. Some people feel that the genetic manipulation of foodstuffs is inherently wrong, and that the long term effects of human consumption of such foods cannot be known. In fact, since the days of Mendel, the manipulation of plant life to create bigger, hardier, more tasteful, disease resistant foodstuffs has been a prime objective of farmers everywhere. Nowadays the science is simply more elegant. We really do not have much to fear from the Tomato that Ate New York. However, it is important to know whether a protein that can be allergenic has been introduced during the process. The mutations caused in the plants will not be translated into mutations in ourselves or our children. However, there is the potential of damage to natural seed stocks.

The widespread use of antibiotics and hormones in the food chain, especially livestock and poultry, is another matter. There are legitimate concerns that the overuse of antibiotics in the food chain may result in new strains of virulent antibiotic resistant bacteria that can affect humans. The use of growth hormone products in animals in order to promote their rapid growth to age of slaughter can be transmitted to humans and have undesired effects included possible tumor formation.

Some people who are, often with good reason, concerned about additives such as hormones and antibiotics to the food supply, themselves indiscriminately use so called natural products that contain naturally occurring hormones such as the female sex hormone estrogen. Some women believe that taking estrogen in this way in the pre-menopausal and post-menopausal years is a more natural way to increase their body estrogen. In fact, it is well-known that the peri-menopausal and post-menopausal use of estrogen in women in these vulnerable age groups predisposes not only to cancer of the endometrium which is the lining of the uterus, but also to pre-malignant conditions of the womb lining. The increased incidence of breast cancer in these women is also a concern as well as the increased risk of heart disease, cardiovascular disease, and stroke. It is important for any woman taking products containing estrogen, whether they are perceived to be natural or synthetic, to be carefully monitored by a qualified physician in order to insure that each woman understands the risks and benefits involved, and to insure that no untoward effects are occurring. (see chapter on Menopause).

It turns out that coffee, which has been giving a bad rap these past few years can be beneficial in moderation.

It is easy to tell nowadays how upscale a bar is by whether they serve real nuts in those little dishes or substitute cheap processed snack food full of hydrogenated fat and salt. Real quality food is expensive. Try buying pure maple syrup these days. What most people put on their pancakes and waffles is a processed substitute. Read the side of the package some time. Some of us can still hark back to idyllic childhoods, when you could actually see the sap running from the tapped maple trees, and you could venture into the shacks where the sap was boiled down. You could take this stuff, role it on a stick in pure virgin snow to cool it and eat it like candy.

Why do we eat three meals a day? One of the great advantages to being a bit older is that we develop a sense of perspective. We not only know some history, we actually have lived some of it. We have also been around long enough to know that rules can be arbitrary. There is much disinformation about eating and diet based on the inaccurate interpretation of science.

Historically, people lived with feast and famine. If the hunt was good, or if the harvest was good, people tended to eat all they could. Methods for preserving food were primitive and chancy. Even when foodstuffs could be stored, and protected from covetous neighbors and rapacious tyrants, people had not yet solved the problem of retaining essential nutrients and vitamins in preserved foods. Vitamin deficiency diseases like scurvy were rampant, and mineral deficiency diseases like rickets were common.

It was later thought that it was important to eat frequent meals during the day in order to maintain blood sugar levels. This is true in disease states such as diabetes. However, in the normal healthy individual, it is debatable whether someone really has to eat breakfast, lunch, dinner, and partake of four o'clock tea. Because of the constraints of the busy modern world we now live in, the quaint idea of tea time, which was once considered indispensable in polite society, has largely disappeared, except during gracious vacations that hark back to a bygone era. So we are left with the concept of three meals a day. Unfortunately, with the ubiquitous availability of food these days, many of us indulge in snacking during the day and long after dinner time. Most of us would acknowledge that this is not optimal, although it is hard to resist an evening ice-cream on a warm summer night. Many successful mature people, having long ago dispensed with a three Martini lunch, now tend to minimize lunch all together, or limit it to a small salad. Salads are another interesting concept. People who are questioned about their weight often state that all they had for lunch was a salad. This can mean anything up to and including a chef's salad loaded with ham, cheese, hard-boiled eggs and salad dressing high in fat accompanied by buttered rolls, croutons, and various other accoutrements. The word "salad" can cover a multitude of sins.

Some healthy people do just fine eating a sensible small breakfast composed of fresh fruit juice, some carbohydrate in a pleasing form, some milk, tea or coffee. It is then their custom to wait for a satisfying evening dinner that is high in protein. By the way, muffins are not health food. They tend to be high in calories, starch, and fat. In many cities in America, muffins have gradually grown in size and therefore caloric intake.

What is a bagel? This ethnic food, largely eaten for breakfast or "brunch" has gained in popularity. Much has been lost in translation. Ideally, a bagel is eaten fresh and contains no preservatives. It is boiled dough: not fried like a doughnut. The caloric intake varies with its size, which has tended to increase, and the size of the hole, which has tended to decrease, and what you choose to put on it. In its simplest form, it can be chewy and delicious. In its loaded form, it can use up the caloric intake for the entire day.

Probiotics

Fermented milk products, notably yogurt, classically have been associated with longevity and good health, even in biblical times, in various rural societies.

The fermentation process is carried out by Lactobacillus, Acidophilus and Streptococcus Thermophilus. These are some of the beneficial bacteria that live with us. We tend to think of germs, that is bacteria, as pathogenic. This means that they cause disease in humans. There are indeed very many such bacteria which pose significant health risks. Happily, however, there are bacteria that do good things for us. These living microorganisms that exert proven health benefits are known as Probiotics. One of the first scientifically described such organism was Lactobacillus Bulgaricus, because it was originally described in the diets of Bulgarian peasants. These Probiotics can enhance the nutrient bioavailability of vitamins and may increase the beneficial effects of vitamins and minerals.

The gastrointestinal tract, largely composed of the intestines, normally contains a microflora of organisms that live with us. Probiotics can help stabilize this flora, and resist infection of the gastrointestinal tract.

Lactobacillus GG will attach to intestinal cells and live in the intestine. It produces an antimicrobial substance that can suppress harmful pathogenic bacteria. Specifically, this can be used in prevention and treatment of diarrhea.

Lactobacillus GG can increase immunoglobulin A and other immunoglobulin secreting cells in the intestine, thereby raising the infection resistance of the intestine. As well, it stimulates the local release of Interferon, which is a naturally occurring substance that can fight infection. Lactobacillus GG can act to close the permeability gaps in the intestine associated with diarrhea caused by the Rotovirus.

Unfortunately though, there is a great deal of confusion and inaccurate labeling associated with Lactobacillus. It is important to know this when purchasing products containing Lactobacillus and other Probiotics.

Vitamins

Vitamin A (Alpha-Tocopherol) builds cells and tissues - bones, teeth, mucous membranes, eyes. Good sources of Vitamin A are milk, butter, cheese, liver, and egg yolk. Carotene, a component of Vitamin A, occurs in leafy green and stem vegetables such as spinach, lettuce, asparagus, and broccoli, as well as in carrots. Vitamin A may possibly help people with Alzheimer's Disease by slowing its progression.

B vitamins are a complex of various vitamins, including thiamine, riboflavin, niacin, vitamin B12, and folic acid. They aid metabolic (building up and breaking down) changes. Good B-complex vitamin sources are milk, cheese, eggs, leafy green vegetables, yeast, poultry, fish, and whole-grain breads and cereals. In the United States, all enriched cereal grains must now be fortified with folic acid (Vitamin B_{10}) in order to prevent the development of neural tube defects in the developing fetus. Neural tube defects are incomplete closures of the developing spinal cord, resulting in Spina Bifida and Anencephaly (absence of higher brain centers).

Niacin (Nicotinic Acid) helps to lower levels of LDL (low density lipoprotein), which is a significant factor in the formation of arteriosclerotic plaques in blood vessels, including the coronary vessels of the heart itself.

Low levels of vitamin B_{10} (folic acid), B_{12}, and B_6 are associated with increased levels of a substance called homocysteine. Homocysteine is a precursor of the amino acid cysteine. Amino acids are the building blocks of proteins. High homocysteine levels are a risk factor for Alzheimer's disease and dementia, as well as for cardiovascular disease, coronary artery disease, atherosclerosis in the carotid arteries in the neck, and stroke.

Vitamin C (ascorbic acid) prevents scurvy and perhaps also, to some extent, the common cold. Citrus fruits are vitamin C's best-known sources, but others are strawberries, tomatoes, cantaloupe, cranberries, and broccoli and leafy green vegetables when eaten raw. Vitamin C is destroyed when food is cooked.

Vitamin D regulates the absorption of calcium and phosphorus, aiding the formation of bones and teeth. The best source is sunlight (but never to excess, please); milk with added vitamin D and egg yolk. Liver, fish, and fish-liver oils are also fine sources.

Vitamin E may be helpful in reducing fibrocystic breast disease. It is found in whole grains, leafy green vegetables, nuts, dried beans, and animal tissues. Excess vitamin E can be harmful in older people with coronary artery disease.

Vitamin K is essential for blood clotting. It is present in leafy green vegetables, cabbage, and cauliflower.

Minerals

The body uses minerals to construct tissues and blood. Adequate intake of vitamin-rich foods should provide adequate minerals. Following is a list of key minerals, through trace elements of several others, including cobalt and copper, are also important.

Calcium hardens bones and teeth, is a factor in blood and tissue fluids, and aids normal response to nervous stimuli. However, too much calcium can lead to kidney stones. Ideally, all the calcium needed can be obtained by eating a proper diet, which may include three to four glasses of skim milk daily.

Chloride aids acid-base balance and helps maintain osmotic pressure.

Chromium helps the body to metabolize sugar.

Iodine is necessary for proper thyroid function. Using iodized salt protects from goiter, a disease caused by iodine deficiency.

Iron is crucial for blood formation.

Phosphorus, an element of bones and teeth, helps maintain the blood-buffer system.

Potassium and *sodium* are essential elements of body fluids. Correct potassium balance is necessary for proper cardiac function.

Sulfur helps form healthy skin, hair, and nails.

Zinc helps the body utilize vitamin A.

Antioxidants

Antioxidants are substances that prevent the chemical combination of oxygen with various other substances, such as fats. There is no convincing evidence that supplementation of various antioxidants, including vitamin E and flavinoids have an effect on cardiovascular disease. In fact, beta carotene supplements can be harmful. Excess vitamin E may have a harmful effect on coronary artery disease in older people.

It has been suggested that vitamin C and E supplementation may somewhat reduce the risk of ovarian cancer. One theory is that antioxidants may protect cells from turning cancerous by increasing cell resistance to damage by oxidation.

Vitamins C and E may also help relieve pelvic pain in women with endometriosis. These antioxidants probably work by increasing the rate of death (apoptosis) of womb lining (endometrial) cells to a normal level.

Long-maligned chocolate does contain flavinoids. However, flavinoid supplementation has not yet been shown to have any beneficial effect on cardiovascular disease.

Vitamin /Mineral Supplements

Vitamin and mineral supplements ensure that some important nutrients, such as folic acid, iron, and trace elements such as zinc and chromium are taken in, although in the normal course of events, a proper diet will be sufficient.

A few cautionary notes are in order:

* The recommended dosage of any vitamin should not be exceeded. Fat-soluble vitamins (A, D, E and K), when taken in excess, accumulate in the body and may be toxic.
* Vitamin C does the opposite: it is excreted daily, so it must be replenished daily.
* Vitamin /mineral supplements are not a substitute for healthy eating. It is important to eat in sufficient quantity in order to get adequate nourishment and energy.

Some fat is needed for healthy skin and hair, and for processing of fat-soluble vitamins.

There should be adequate intake of fluids. Drinking water aids digestion, helps prevent constipation, helps the kidneys flush out waste products and the urinary tract stay clear of infection, and keeps the skin soft. Water is the essential (and no-calorie) drink, but milk also counts. Milk supplies protein, carbohydrate, and fat (which can be limited by using low-fat milk). Fruit and vegetable juices can be beneficial. Artificially sweetened beverages should be avoided.

Salt should be used in moderation. The motto "Moderation in all things" certainly applies here. Edema tends to occur more in women who eat a low-protein diet. Excessive salt is not good. Salty chips, heavily salted nuts, and sodium-heavy processed meats should be avoided. The overuse of salt in cooking should be discouraged. Salt should be iodized. Individuals with high blood pressure should check with their practitioner about salt intake.

The daily menu can be planned around seven food groups:

Leafy Green and Yellow Vegetables

Baked squash, steamed fresh kale or spinach can add key vitamins and intriguing flavors to the evening meal.

Citrus Fruits, Tomatoes, Cabbage

Orange juice, an orange, or grapefruit are important, and usually eaten at breakfast.

Potatoes and Other Fruits and Vegetables

A salad a day can help keep the skin glowing, bowel movements regular, and eyes sparkling. Salads need not be boring; in fact, they invariably benefit from different ingredients, like mushrooms, or apple. For a protein boost, salads may be topped with cottage cheese, chicken or fish. Potatoes have acquired an undeserved reputation as a fattening food. It is guilt by association. Potatoes and sour cream or butter can be delicious, but potatoes without the fat are highly nutritious. It is better to bake them or boil them.

Milk and Cheese

Calcium is very important, and one way to get it is by drinking milk. Low-fat or skim milk provide the necessary calcium without the extra calories. Calcium, of course, is present in other dairy products such as yogurt and cheese. Plain yogurt can be blended with fresh fruit. Aged cheeses, cultured yogurt, or milk products labeled lactose-reduced or lactose-free can be an option if milk is difficult to digest. Fresh steamed greens and salmon are sources of calcium as well.

Meat, Fish, Poultry, Eggs, Peas, and Beans

Protein builds muscles; the diet should be protein-rich. Animal products provide the most efficiently utilized proteins. Dried beans and peas and tofu and other soy products are also good sources for vegetarians and for meat-eaters who seek variety.

Cereal

Shredded wheat, bran, and other whole-grain cereals are an improvement over highly sweetened processed cereal that masquerade as nutritious breakfasts on supermarket shelves.

Butter

A couple of tablespoons a day of butter, or cooking or salad oils, can be a good idea, unless a physician has restricted the diet. The central nervous system contains a significant amount of fat, and fat is needed for healthy skin, hair, and tissues.

The Balanced Daily Diet

* a citrus fruit or other source of vitamin C
* other fruits
* meat, poultry, or fish
* skim milk, or the equivalent in the form of yogurt, cheese, or other calcium source
* green leafy vegetables and yellow vegetables

* whole-grain bread or cereal
* some fat intake: butter, cream cheese, olive oil
* plenty of water

It can be helpful to keep a list of what is eaten. Nutritionists help many to stay on track.

CHAPTER 14
EXERCISE

The Take-Home Message

- Moderate regular aerobic exercise is of proven value
- High impact exercise can lead to a variety of sports injuries
- Looking good usually makes you feel better. There is such a thing as self image
- Get sufficient sleep (but too much sleep is not necessarily a good thing)
- Maintain bone density and muscle mass

Exercise and diet are inextricably linked: what you do with one has great impact on the other.

You can diet to lose weight, and you can exercise to lose weight. You can exercise and modify diet to gain weight. Or you can exercise and diet to maintain your weight and stay healthy.

Diet and exercise programs can be fads that make their proponents rich, and you lighter in the wallet. On the other hand, good trainers are now at the point where they can sculpt the bodies of serious athletes for a particular function. Hopefully, they don't get carried away and put our children and grandchildren on anabolic steroids. The use of certain of these medications in certain selected people in the aging population, however, has become worthy of discussion.

It is well known that women tend to lose bone density after the menopause. It is not as well known that older women lose muscle mass as well, and that the loss of muscle mass impacts on the loss of bone density. Older men are prone to losing bone density and muscle mass as well. For health reasons alone, it is very important for everyone to maintain muscle mass and bone density. It is best not to wait until old age to address these problems. It has been shown that it is important to participate regularly in sports and weight-bearing exercises throughout adult life in order to reap the benefits in older age. Older people, if they are judged to be physically able, should regularly exercise. Specifically, walking at a fast pace on a regular basis can be very helpful.

Body sculpting for the purpose of looking better is a combination of diet, programmed exercise, and more than a little help from your friendly neighborhood plastic surgeon.

There is a great difference between thinking you are overweight and actually being above your ideal body weight. It has a lot to do with body image - what you think you see and what is actually there when you look in the mirror. Many people today are hypercritical of their body image: they expect to look like the models and actors they see on television, in the movies, in magazines, on the fashion runways, and even walking down the street if they happen to be going down the right street.

We should realize that these idealized icons themselves don't usually look that perfect in their natural state, without hairdressing, massaging, plastic surgery, make up, and airbrushing or computer enhancement of their images, although admittedly some of our ideals come really close, even when they get up in the morning. A lot of them are also in their early teens, and you can't expect to compete with that.

Beauty is only skin deep: that is the ultimate rationalization. The truth is, success breeds confidence, and confident successful people tend to project a beautiful dynamism. They also tend to take better care of themselves because they feel good about themselves. They value their health and their bodies, and they know that the better they look, the more successful they may become. They also can afford good care, including hair care, cosmetics, facials, massages, personal trainers, vacations in the 'right' places (where you see more beautiful people and are therefore more motivated to look like them), good clothes, proper medical and dental care. Like good food, good personal care can be very expensive.

The top of the line is the good personal trainer who is familiar with your medical history, your exercise capacity, and your goals. You can achieve similar results more cheaply by joining a good health club and taking classes in everything from relaxation and yoga to various sports.

Vacations can include bicycle trips, hiking, boating, rafting, canoeing and kayaking. Although these sports can get very pricey depending on how exotic the venue, you can get all the healthful exercise you need, and have a great time, without going to Lhasa or Tibet. There is probably a State Park or National Park closer to you than you may think, not to mention local bicycle paths and hiking trails.

The most user friendly, aerobic, low impact exercises are walking, swimming, and cycling. Try to include at least one of these in your daily routine.

If possible, try to exercise in areas where air pollution is not a factor. Exercise increases the respiratory, or breathing, rate, so that impurities in the air increasingly enter the lungs. In other words, don't run in traffic, where hydrocarbon emissions, including large particle diesel fumes are being emitted. Cyclists and runners are at increased risk of being involved in traffic accidents. They should always wear clothing with fluorescent patches. There should be appropriate lights and fluorescent markers on bicycles.

Leave so-called extreme sports to the kids, unless you are a lifelong super athlete. In winter time, cross country skiing and snowshoeing over groomed trails can be invigorating, but you had better be in shape first.

Try to level the playing field in competitive sports. Your knees will love you much better if you play tennis on Har-True or clay instead of all weather courts. You can frustrate younger opponents by your ability to get to any shot they send your way. You can make up for some loss in power and pace by patience and shotmaking ability learned through long practice. Keep your cool. Your younger opponents will tend to have difficulty in matching this. They get especially frustrated, and tend to make poor shots, when you slow down the pace.

Remember the veteran baseball pitcher, who gets the young hitters out by feeding them a steady diet of junk. The ball curves, spins, and drops. The anxious hitter gets way out in front, ahead of the ball. Do the same thing in racket sports. One of the best squash players we ever met was well past his mid sixties. He would come off the court cool as can be, a winner, while his younger opponents were gasping for air. Use strategy: move them around the court. Make them work for their points.

Golf can be the most frustrating game in the world. It is billiards played on a giant, magnificent grass table. Older players know they cannot match the distance of younger competitors, so they work on precision. It is just as good to hit the green in two, and two putt, then to hit the green in one and three putt. If your younger competitor can hit the green in one and one putt, however, resign yourself to the fact that you are going to lose. You can still have a great day walking the course. The pros do it. If your health allows it, do walk. It is far more healthy than madly dashing around in a cart, breathing gasoline fumes. If your cart is electric, at least you have obviated some of that problem.

Do not be a weekend warrior. It is a great way to invite sports injury. Ideally, you should have a weekly program more or less worked out which will become routine. Start slowly, and gradually evolve into your program, which should be supervised by a competent trainer and agreed to by your doctor.

Statistically, many, if not the majority, of health club memberships are never fully utilized - people sign up in a wave of euphoria, and then lose interest. The most important aspect to any exercise or sports program is your ability and desire to follow through with it and keep it going long term. Pick sports and exercise activities that you will enjoy, and that you will get increasing enjoyment from as you become more adept. This will have the added benefit of making your social world more enjoyable, as you will be coming into contact on a regular basis with other people who have similar sports interests. You will be amazed at how many good times you can have discussing the intricacies of a game and its strategy.

It is important to know your physical limitations. Your doctor, of course, is the best person to ask about your starting level of capability. Certain conditions that are more prevalent in the senior years can limit you. However, great strides have been made both in the treatment of these conditions, and the medical thinking concerning them.

Good posture, is, of course, important and attractive in both sexes. Women in the postmenopausal years who are on estrogen supplementation tend to have better postural balance, and a lessened tendency to fractures.

The advent of the qualified sports medicine physician has been a great boon to first, professional athletes, and now to all the rest of us. These professionals will assess your physical condition and needs. They work closely with trained physical therapists, who are assigned individualized prescribed courses of treatment to give to the patient. Insurance plans should recognize the value of such programs and reimburse medically necessary costs.

Sports related injuries include sprains and tears to muscles and ligaments, joint sprains and fluid collections, and longer term effects such as traumatic arthritis that can obliterate joint spaces, causing pain and decreased mobility.

Rheumatologists are specialized physicians who treat, among other things, various forms of arthritis. The commonest of these is osteoarthritis. The rheumatologist can prescribe various anti-inflammatory medications and programs of treatment, including physical therapy, to minimize the effect of arthritis and related conditions. You should ask your doctor about medications such as Celebrex (celecoxib). Such medications like all medications, should be taken only with proper evaluation, by your physician, with knowledge of your personal medical history and possible propensity for complications.

Orthopedic surgeons have developed joint reconstruction and joint replacement, including hip and knee replacement, to a high art. Rehabilitation specialists then step in to make sure that newly reconstructed joints and ligaments work to their maximum potential. People who have successfully undergone multiple joint replacements, and are back to dancing and sports, often jokingly refer to themselves as bionic, and they are not far from wrong. It is amazing how far the science and technology has come.

The use of good equipment in sports cannot be emphasized enough. This starts with good shoes, which above all else should be comfortable and fit properly. If the shoe hurts when you put it on, don't let anyone tell that you it will be alright after you break it in: it is liable to damage your foot first. Shoes should be of good quality and be compatible with the sport for which you are buying them.

It is not cheating to have sports equipment custom fitted, if you need it and can afford it. Always consult a pro before buying sports equipment. If you belong to a golf club, your pro will advise you, and if you so desire, will even custom fit a set of clubs to your individual swing. This a nice luxury, but you realize its limitations when you watch your same golf pro pick up just about any club and hit the ball exactly where he or she wants it to go.

For tennis, you will probably want a large head racquet with a low vibration frame. Get advice from a teaching pro concerning what equipment is individually best for you.

In tennis, as in all other sports, you should try to be taught by a competent professional. This can be done on a one to one basis or in a group setting. Try to stick with one pro and gradually get better in your sport. People have a tendency to get one lesson here or there, especially when they are on vacation. Unfortunately, some pros tend to be perfectionistic. They will try to get you to effectively start over and build a new swing. This is fine if you are just starting a sport, but can be counter productive and even annoying to the more senior athlete who knows her or his own limitations and is only trying to refine the technique that is already there.

The relatively sudden unaccustomed use of various muscle groups, and unaccustomed turning of the spinal column, can result in strain and sports injury.

A pro who is wise and experienced in dealing with a more senior population will realize that he or she is not building the next Olympic Champion, but is bringing people to a level of competence where they can enjoy and get fulfillment from their chosen sport.

Make sure your gloves fit. This is true in golf, as it is in cycling. The glove should fit snugly, but not be constricting. The finger length should match the length of your finger. Socks are important athletic equipment. They should be comfortable, properly cushioning the foot, and 'breathe'.

Good athletic support bras are now widely available, that among other things, largely get rid of the problem of nipple irritation that female athletes used to have. Sports bras also look good, which is a plus.

Make sure that your clothing is appropriate to the sport. You can now get swim wear that is built for speed. Do not stay in a tight wet bathing suit after your workout. This enhances the chance of irritation in the genital area.

Swimming pools unfortunately can be a breeding ground for germs, despite chlorination. Know where you are swimming, and make sure the pool does not have a history of infection incidence. Good circulation and cleaning, with proper attention to disinfection, chlorination, and pH balance will generally obviate most such problems.

Jacuzzis and hot tubs are even more of a concern, due to the smaller space in which people congregate and the higher temperatures. Meticulous attention must be paid to the cleanliness and antisepsis of these facilities.

Protective gear is a necessity in many, if not most, sports. It is a good idea to use protective eyewear in tennis. If a tennis ball hits you in the eye, it can cause a decompression type of injury, leading to serious harm or even blindness. You should never ride a bicycle without wearing a helmet. There are specific helmets made for bicycle riders that are light weight and really look quite futuristic. Serious bike riders wear tight fitting clothing that cuts wind resistance, and ride in groups, changing the lead, so that each front rider in turn cuts the wind resistance for the others.

For inline skaters and ice skaters, there are knee, shin and elbow guards, and helmets. Inevitably, everyone falls once in awhile.

Horseback riding can be a most enjoyable activity. Unfortunately, there is a high incidence of injury, often serious, among even the best riders. It is essential to wear protective headgear, and to be properly trained. Good athletes 'stay within themselves'; that is they have a reserve of expertise, training, stamina and strength beyond what they ordinarily use, in case the unexpected is encountered.

Lessons are forever. The best athletes are coached on the highest level continuously. You cannot objectively assess the defects in your own game, and neither can your friends. Try to be in contact with a good pro who can continually refine and upgrade your game. You will have the major side benefit of lessening your risk of sports injuries if you play your sports properly, within your limits. Annoyances like tennis elbow, which some golfers get as well, can put you out of action for weeks or months. Prevention with good coaching is the better way to go.

Walking is great aerobic exercise. Dress appropriately for coolness and comfort with clothing that breathes. That includes cotton underpants. Unfortunately, panty hose does not breathe. So-called cotton crotch panty hose tends to have the cotton sewn inside the nylon, which takes away the ability of the cloth to breathe.

Wear shoes with good support that are wide enough for your foot. If you need arch supports, use them. Ideally, have them prescribed by an appropriate professional, such as a qualified podiatrist, and custom fitted. Make sure they are comfortable. Cross training shoes may serve your purposes well.

If you hike in the woods or near wooded areas, wear good hiking boots with socks that cushion and breathe. Make sure the boots are comfortable. Clothing should be snug at the wrists and ankles, and closed at the collar, to prevent insects, especially deer ticks, from getting in. Carry insect repellent. Speak to your doctor about the prevention and treatment of Lyme Disease and other tick borne diseases. Remember that mosquitoes are a vector that carry disease as well, such as the West Nile Virus. Protect yourself and your environment. Get rid of standing water.

While you are hiking, a walking stick is probably a good idea. It should be straight and of a comfortable length. How chic it is, and how expensive it is, is up to you. If you are anywhere close to hunting season, you must wear bright orange, especially an orange hat. An orange vest is a good idea as well. You do not want to be mistaken for a game animal.

Fishing conjures up images of old men in rowboats, or on the end of a pier, with a line floating aimlessly in the water. In its simplest form, fishing can be just that. There is something to be said for being quietly outdoors, thinking serene thoughts. Today, fishing is a huge sport, popular with many, with multiple challenges. These range from battling huge sport fish in the deep sea, to the ultimate challenge and finesse of fly fishing, with delicate rods and light line, and flies tied by hand. In fact, fly tying is a craft and skill all its own, which gives many hours of satisfaction to select people who are adept at it.

Much fishing today is catch and release. If you are not going to eat the fish, let it live to fight another day.

Fishing can get you to magnificent sites: rivers, rapids, lakes, and mountain streams, with like minded friends who enjoy nature and good company. The image of a grandparent and a grandchild spending hours together on a boat or by a stream, easily communing and bonding, while wisdom passes to a younger generation, and love flows, is a real one.

Many couples find this to be an ideal way to spend time together, lovingly, peacefully in glorious settings. Fishing is a learned skill, and an art. The better the teacher, the more you will enjoy it. There are great fishing schools in many places today, as well as clubs. Choice of equipment and clothing, of course, is just as important as in any other sport, for comfort, safety, and enjoyment.

Sleep

We tend to be a sleep deprived society. In our desire to fit work, recreation, and family, not to mention such things as travel and social activities, into our schedules, sleep is often neglected.

Adequate sleep is important for the maintenance of good health. People with disturbed biorhythms, for example airline crews, who frequently change time zones, may become unduly sleep deprived.

If there is time for it in the schedule, an afternoon nap can be a good idea. In some countries the siesta in the late afternoon is an old tradition. On the other hand, undue tiredness and excessive sleeping can be a symptom of depression or other medical disorders. It is important to consult with a physician if the sleeping pattern is abnormal.

Sleep disorders can result from a wide variety of conditions. The lack of sufficient activity and exercise during the day may result in an inability to sleep at night. Other causes of sleep disorders can be local, centered around the nasal passages and palate. Structures in the nose called turbinates may be enlarged and inflamed, obstructing the nasal passages. There are ear, nose and throat doctors today (otorhinolaryngologists) who are skilled in microsurgical techniques for the removal of such obstructions.

Apolipoprotein E (ApoE) is involved in fat metabolism. A variant of this protein, Apolipoprotein E e 4 (Apo E e 4) can occur in some, and is associated with sleep disordered breathing. Apolipoprotein E e 4 is a risk factor for Alzheimer's disease, and increases the risk for cardiovascular disease.

CHAPTER 15
DISEASE PREVENTION

The Take-Home Message

- It is not yet possible to prevent all disease: it is now possible to identify many potentially major disease states before they cause significant trouble, often before there are any symptoms at all
- A regular physical examination, even when coupled with an electrocardiogram and basic blood tests, will pick up some abnormalities, but will not identify many important, potentially dangerous problems
- Advanced imaging techniques can identify a variety of potentially significant problems early
- The arguments against the common use of sophisticated techniques, including imaging and blood tests for cancer markers, generally are twofold: early detection of tiny, asymptomatic lesions (abnormal growths) may lead to unnecessary, often dangerous, interventions; and the techniques are expensive, especially if they are going to be used for mass screening

- Knowledge is a good, not a bad, thing. Ignorance is not bliss. A reasoned, and as much as possible, evidence-based approach to a possibly abnormal finding, however small, should logically reap benefits both for the individual and for the advancement of diagnosis and treatment in the general population. Costs inevitably come down-significantly down – as new techniques gain acceptance, and the practitioners utilizing them become adept in using them efficiently. The ultimate cost saving is in the general health of the population, with a lessened need for the continuous care of debilitated people.

Conventional wisdom leads us to believe that if you live 'right' and have regular 'checkups' you can prevent disease. The reality is that some of the strategies being advocated, such as sensible diet and exercise, do have an overwhelming preponderance of scientific evidence in their favor.

There is a great deal of talk, and writing, about prevention being a better strategy than dealing with disease. On the face of it, this seems like a wonderful idea. The problem is, it is overly simplistic, and not always attainable.

Prenatal care for pregnant women has indeed been shown to be of great benefit in the prevention and early diagnosis of dangerous obstetrical complications.

The Papanicolaou smear, a half-century old technology, definitely gives early diagnosis of precancerous conditions of the cervix (mouth of the womb), and although it does not prevent these conditions, the early diagnosis can lead to effective treatment to eradicate disease before it turns malignant. Testing the stool for occult, or hidden, blood can lead to early pickup of cancer of the large intestine (bowel) while the disease is still resectable (removable). Colonoscopy identifies polypoid growths that can often be easily removed, 'preventing' colon cancer.

However, the widely advocated yearly medical 'checkup' tends to be too cursory and simplistic to pick up very early disease processes. It is, however, a great screening and educational tool, focusing people's attention on their lifestyle and condition. On a statistical basis, it may prevent nothing, unless it is coupled with more sophisticated testing.

Medicine today has increasingly become evidence based. That means we should continue with the strategies that are proven by objective scientific evidence and statistical studies, to promote and maintain health, and discard ideas and strategies that, no matter how well entrenched, are proven to be of no benefit. It also means that we should be open to new methods of diagnosis and treatment that are superior to ones we are currently using, even if the current system does have benefit. 'Evidence', however, varies in quality, and must be carefully evaluated. As well, new diagnostic means and therapeutic breakthroughs may not show much statistical 'evidence' of improved health in the population at large until they become widely used by physicians adept in their application. Thus, there can be a temptation to ignore new technologies, especially when significant cost is involved.

You can never be too rich or too thin. This statement, although tongue in cheek, has virtually become the credo of a good part of urban society. People can certainly be too thin. Eating healthfully and well is necessary in order to keep vital body functions working properly, and to help prevent osteoporosis. Starvation is not chic. Obesity is not healthy either. From the viewpoint of longevity, probably one of the more harmful things is for weight to seesaw back and forth, with periods of overeating interspersed with periods of severe dieting. The ideal, of course, is to have an adequate caloric intake every day, with a proper balance of nutrients. Evidence seems to show that being somewhat lean (within reason) long term can be associated with increased longevity. There is now evidence showing that some fasting can be beneficial for properly selected people. On the other hand, obesity is almost epidemic in North America, and is a major risk factor for heart and cardiovascular disease, stroke, diabetes, and other disease states.

A regular pattern of aerobic exercise is important. It is important for older people to stay mobile and to keep walking in order to keep the bones from demineralizing. Significant osteopenia can thus be avoided. After the menopause, just taking an adequate amount of calcium is usually insufficient. Hormonal replacement therapy (HRT) may be considered, but only under the supervision of a physician who is aware of the risks. Bisphosphonates, Denosumab or SERM's (Specific Estrogen Receptor Modulators) may also be used for this purpose. These drugs are discussed in the chapter on Menopause.

It is not always possible to prevent serious illness no matter how healthfully one lives.

Disease prevention, of course, is the ultimate goal. The next best thing to disease prevention is very early diagnosis and treatment to identify and eradicate serious diseases in their earliest and most easy to treat states.

Obstetricians and gynecologists have historically been in the forefront in this area. The concept and wide use of prenatal care during pregnancy, which women so take for granted in our society, is a relatively recent development. Antenatal care is still not routinely available in much of the world. The advance of modern prenatal diagnosis and care has been responsible for a veritable revolution in the way women are able to think about themselves and their families. Prior to the availability of antenatal care, support was only received during the actual labor and birth process itself. By then, it was often too late to prevent a catastrophic outcome for mother and child.

One of the great milestones of early diagnosis was the development of the Papanicolaou smear for the early detection of disease of the cervix. The widespread use of this relatively simple test has saved the lives of countless women in the last of 50 or 60 years.

The concept of the regular physical examination, and regular pelvic examination, is a good one. However, by itself, it is often not specific enough to identify the early warnings of incipient disease. A dip stick urinalysis will detect protein, sugar, or blood in the urine. However, it will not show the presence of abnormal cells. Microscopic urinalysis should be done. Diabetes will not be detected on routine urinalysis until the disease state is quite advanced. Routine blood chemistries are important, but again, diabetes will not be picked up in this way until it is quite advanced. It is important to know the timing of the blood sugar in relation to a meal, and often necessary for blood sugars to be tested after a loading dose of sugar has been taken orally, in order to see if the body properly metabolizes the sugar.

A blood count should be taken at the time of the regular check up, to ensure, among other things, that anemia is not present. If anemia is found, it should not be simply assumed that this is due to dietary or iron deficiency. Further testing should be carried out to determine the actual cause.

A person who is anemic may be having occult, or hidden bleeding. That could mean that cancer is present in the bowel, uterus or elsewhere. It is obviously important to rule out such disease processes.

Although it is somewhat unpleasant, a rectal examination should preferably be part of every routine physical and gynecological examination. Rectal examination in men is used to delineate the prostate gland: its size, shape and consistency. Rectal examination in women is important in order to ascertain if abnormal masses are present behind the uterus, or in the rectum itself. In both sexes, a sample of stool is taken and checked for the presence of occult blood. If blood is present in the stool, it is imperative that colonoscopy be carried out in order to ascertain the site of the bleeding. A polyp or other abnormal growth found during colonoscopy must be sent to the pathology laboratory for proper microscopic analysis.

Adults at average risk aged forty-five or over should undergo screening for colon cancer on a regular basis, either by advanced testing for blood in the stool or by colonoscopy checking the entire large intestine. Obviously, if blood is found in the stool, colonoscopy needs to be done. In any case, routine colonoscopy should be commenced by age fifty. They should speak to their doctor concerning the regular timing of this test in each individual case.

Women today are well acquainted with mammography. Modern mammography is done with low dose radiation, so that over the period of a lifetime, the cumulative radiation from the test is at an acceptable level. This is still the surest way we have at present to detect early cancer of the breast. The accuracy of mammography is very dependent upon the state of the equipment, and on the expertise of the radiologist who is reading the films. Artificial Intelligence (AI) may be helpful in the future in interpreting the films.

The risk of breast cancer can be reduced in significant numbers of women by the use of specific estrogen receptor modulators (SERM's). A woman should speak to her doctor about the advisability of taking medication of this type. Sonography is often used as a supplement to mammography, to better delineate suspicious areas in the breasts. Of course, no test replaces monthly regular breast self-examination. Make sure that the technique of self-examination is taught by a qualified medical professional.

No matter how astute a physician is, she or he will not pick up early lung cancer simply by listening to, or auscultating, the lungs. Even regular chest X-rays have become obsolete as a means to detect lung cancer. Spiral CT (helical computed tomography) scanning of the chest is the method of choice in picking up early lung cancer. The best hope of successfully treating this often lethal disease is to establish the diagnosis early, and to undergo definitive surgical treatment. Obviously, an ounce of prevention is worth a pound of cure. People should not smoke. Smoking is not a status symbol, or a symbol of empowerment. It tends to be a symbol of poverty, and enslavement. It is an addiction.

There are now cancer markers available, taken by simple blood test. These include the Ca125 and the Ca 19-9 tests. These antigens for ovarian cancer, the CA27 and CA29 antigens for breast cancer, and the CEA antigen which is predominantly a marker for bowel cancer, are all available now. Unfortunately, these markers are not very specific. However, they do give some indication that further testing or treatment is needed.

Probes are available that are very specific. For example, a DNA probe is available to detect human papilloma virus (HPV) and its subtypes. This is the virus that most usually causes cancer of the cervix and penis. The test is currently used in women in conjunction with the Papanicolaou smear. It is far more specific than the Papanicolaou smear itself, which is a low technology test by comparison.

Electrocardiograms are useful, but they cannot predict who is at risk for imminent heart attack. Consultation with a cardiologist can be valuable. Stress testing, which involves getting onto a treadmill to exercise and accelerating the heart rate while a continuous electrocardiogram is running may be utilized. The use of an injected radioisotope, thallium, makes the test more specific in predicting heart attack risk.

Fast spiral CAT scanning has been developed that can actually show arteriosclerotic plaques within the coronary arteries. The coronary arteries are the vessels supplying the heart muscle itself.

There are now tiny implantable heart monitors that continuously record and download to a bedside monitor which in turn is in communication with a station in the cardiac unit of a hospital or clinic.

Women have commonly been relatively neglected in years past in the early screening and detection of heart disease. It is obviously just as important in women as in men to get the appropriate screening. It is important to press insurance organizations to pay for these tests. They may save money in the short run by denying claims, but their subscribers will pay for it terms of severe heart disease, with much costlier and more expensive interventions required in the long term. Early diagnosis is in everyone's interest.

Advanced imaging studies should be used when necessary in the older population in order to rule out the presence of early enlarging masses. Ultrasonography of the pelvis, done with a vaginal probe as well as an abdominal probe, is most useful in detecting early enlargements of the ovaries in women in the postmenopausal age group. This can increase the chance of early diagnosis of ovarian tumors. Again, insurance carriers tend to be loathe to pay for such testing.

The emotional state is very important to longevity. In most cases, it is not wonderful to live long if one does not feel good about oneself. The emotional state, of course, is interdependent with physical health, financial stability, and in the happiness of family and friends. Very few of us get to advanced age without major problems in at least some of those areas. At times, life can seem to be somewhat overwhelming. Those are the times when it is important to have loved ones close by, to make sure there is not a withdrawal inward, but continuance of functioning and vitality. If anxiety or depression supervene, it is quite common to have withdrawal as well. Today, sophisticated professional help is available. Consultation with a psychotherapist, psychiatrist, or psychopharmocologist can be more than helpful, it can be lifesaving. Modern anti-depressant medications have fewer debilitating side effects than anti-depressant drugs had in earlier years.

References

1. https://www.cancer.org/cancer/colon-rectal-cancer/detection-diagnosis-staging/acs-recommendations.html
2. https://www.nature.com/articles/s41586-019-1799-6
3. https://www.nejm.org/doi/full/10.1056/NEJMra1905136
4. Bibliography and Supplemental Bibliography: www.rcaplanmd.com

CHAPTER 16
THE NEW ROLE OF GRANDPARENTS

It is hard for most of us nowadays to think of contemporary older people in the same way that we remember our grandparents. Grandparents of two generations ago did not have our access to technologically advanced health care. Plastic surgery was nowhere near as advanced as it is today and was not commonly employed in our society. Women were generally more burdened by household chores as advanced programmable appliances and other labor saving devices were not yet available. Men were less inclined to do household chores. Furthermore, societal pressures caused women to be more homebound and for the most part less involved in other occupations. There was less emphasis on sports for women and outdoor physical activity. Dental sciences were nowhere near as advanced as they are today so that a significantly higher proportion of adults faced the unappetizing prospect of having false teeth.

Much of this had to do with wealth level. The fortunate few always had other people to do their chores. With the relatively high cost and aristocratic nature of travel at that time, those with money not only traveled by ship and airplane two generations ago, but used it as a visible status symbol of their wealth. People in that fortunate circumstance had masseuses and masseurs, hairdressers, manicurists, cosmeticians, tailors and clothing designers, to help keep them attractive, fit, and good looking.

Luckily today, all these services have evolved to the point where they are no longer available just to the favored few but to a huge proportion of women and men in our society. The mass marketing of everything from airplane travel to designer clothing allows great participation in more of the pleasant luxuries in life. The increasing level of sophistication in the society, coupled with a gradual (although sometimes bumpy) rise in available discretionary spending power in affluent societies, and with the hard won freedom of women to do pretty much anything they wish to in society, has led to a great democratization. Women no longer have to live vicariously by reading about the fancy foibles of the favored few.

There is another reason, however, why we remember our grandparents as being old. Children always think of their grandparents, and even their parents, as being old. Even though your peers may consider you young and glamorous, do not be deceived for a moment. Your children and your grandchildren still think you are old, no matter what they say. What we perceive and remember is not necessarily the reality. If your grandmother was blessed with good health and good fortune, it might be instructive to look at pictures of her when she was your age. You might be surprised to find that she was really young and attractive. Many people are grandparents in their forties. This is hardly old. By the same token, many great grandparents are only in their sixties or seventies. This is an age that is not considerably old either. In your most important interests and concerns, you may not be that far away from your grandparents or even your great grandparents. They were concerned with the life, health and happiness of their children. They were concerned about their life partner. They were concerned about their own advancing age, coupled with some insecurity about what the future might hold. They might have been troubled with various minor aches and pains and wondered what they meant. They might have been worried about a serious illness that could debilitate them and prevent them from functioning on their accustomed level. They might have had deeper philosophical and religious questions that were unanswered.

They probably lived through turbulent and dangerous times. On a very personal level, they had to confront issues such as war, considering implications to themselves and family members. They might have had to face very harsh economic realities, especially if they lived through the Depression. Despite our advanced technology, and our ability generally to attain a higher standard of living, we are not so much different.

The dynamism of our economy has created major shifts in the roles of all family members, notably grandparents. In the traditional 1950's family, there was generally one predominant wage earner, the adult male. Women in great numbers then generally took care of the home. If they did outside work, it was often not remunerative, and certainly not remunerative on the level that a male was capable of earning at that time.

The continuing pressure for women's rights, including the right of women to be able to enter the workforce at any level and assume their rightful place in society led to unintended consequences, which could have been foreseen in retrospect. Huge numbers of households now have two major income earners, both husband and wife. Superficially, one would think this would lead to a much higher standard of living with more disposable income available. To a certain extent, this is true. However, the laws of supply and demand do apply. As the gross income of a couple has significantly increased, the price of certain sought-after assets has risen accordingly. An important example of this has often been increased home prices and decreased affordability especially in the most desirable areas, where people with families want to live. The second income in two income families has now largely become indispensable. This can be a huge problem if one earning partner gets laid off or becomes incapacitated. However, in times of very low unemployment and a burgeoning economy, this does not seem to be much of a concern. As the economy lags, these concerns return to the forefront.

However, there are greater issues, which concern the rearing of the next generation. Traditionally, it was well known that the children who achieved the best, and were generally the best adjusted, came from middle class homes. Unfortunate adults who fell below that living standard were forced to place childrearing secondary to work. Their children of necessity often had to fend for themselves in poor neighborhoods, with bad schooling and companions who were questionable at best. The chances for failure, or even disaster, in that environment were greatly enhanced. At the least, it is and was very difficult for such children to extricate themselves from the cycle of poverty and relative ignorance. On the other hand, traditionally, the children of the very wealthy family were left in the hands of comparative strangers with varying levels of ability, motivation, and training. Even in the best of circumstances, many of these children were deprived of a genuine deep feeling of love. Now that the vast so-called middle class is composed of two income families, these issues in child rearing have come to the fore.

Largely unnoticed, without fanfare, and in great numbers, many grandparents, especially grandmothers, have stepped forward to actively take part in the hands-on, day to day, raising of their grandchildren. This obviates many of the uncertainties and the anxieties faced by parents today concerning strangers being in charge of their children for protracted periods of time. There are many grandparents who are relatively young, fit, and healthy. They tend to take on this reestablished role with great joy. Even if they are still working themselves, they often have more free time than the children's parents do, or at least they may have a somewhat different schedule. It is instructive to speak with adults who were in fact either wholly or partially raised by their grandparents. The depth of love and affection that they hold for those grandparents is heartwarming, to say the least.

A major proportion of marriages in our society now end in divorce. In this unfortunate circumstance, children suffer emotionally. Grandparents again often step in at this unsettling time to provide physical and emotional, not to mention financial, support to their grandchildren, and most of all what is urgently required: love and understanding.

The empty nest syndrome has become almost a misnomer. Dedicated grandparents know that the condition can be quite temporary. Just when you thought the children have moved elsewhere, they may well be back along with their offspring. Grandparents tend to rise to the occasion and help with the situation to the best of their ability.

In some ways, we are returning to the more traditional family roles of our grandparents. More families are now discovering the value of close ties. This interdependence can be mutually beneficial. Grandchildren have another resource of wisdom, strength, and support from their grandparents. Grandparents in turn have the great joy of knowing that they are loved, and will not be abandoned to strangers and bureaucracies if they become infirm.

CHAPTER 17
ECONOMICS: HOW MUCH MONEY DO YOU NEED?

Great questions confront people in their more mature years. One of the most important and often pressing of these is 'How much money is needed for a comfortable and pleasurable retirement?' There is no easy answer to this question for several reasons. First, economic planning ideally should be long range, certainly throughout the active working life of a person or a couple. Unfortunately, far too many of us when we are young do not pay enough attention to long-term goals. Very often, there are far more pressing needs concerning us, including creating a home, raising a family, tuition, and the mundane meeting of everyday expenses on a weekly or monthly basis, not to mention paying federal, state and local taxes, both direct and hidden. If you think about it, you would be amazed at what real percentage of your income is going to pay taxes. For example, there are taxes to just about every step in the creation of a product, from its manufacturing all the way through to the retailers' shelves.

The sophisticated answer to the question 'How much money is needed for retirement?' encompasses several factors. One, of course, is the age at which active income production will cease. Secondly, there is the level of lifestyle you wish to maintain. Then there is the issue of life expectancy. You may already have gathered that the longer you are alive and healthy, the further your life expectancy is pushed into the future. This can only be expected to be compounded as the years go by with the advent of new treatments, cures, technologies, and techniques for life preservation. Therefore, any realistic life expectancy you may plan for today may happily be a gross underestimate.

Even with inflation rates at low levels in North America today, inflation does compound on itself. Despite occasional periods of deflation, prices tend to inexorably rise. A good restaurant steak dinner that cost three or four dollars in the 1950's, now can easily cost over fifty dollars. A decent new car that cost three thousand dollars fifty years ago is now thirty-thousand dollars. In 1970, you could get a way above average house for seventy thousand dollars. Now try half a million. Take those numbers, add another twenty years, and try to figure out what you will need. Federal, state and local governments, of course, know these things, and have the economists at their disposal to figure out taxes and calculate what they really need. So far, the government has refused to pass any legislation to index apparent gains to inflation. This means that older people who have to liquidate assets in order to have the capital they need to generate income, are usually faced with massive tax bills for apparent gains that are not real in terms of buying power.

The government will often come up with acceptable ploys to make legislation pass and to make it palatable for those of us who pay the bills. For example, there is a law which effectively states that the first five hundred thousand dollars in gain on the sale of a primary home is not taxed. As the government has rightly pointed out, this means that a majority of people who now sell their primary home at an apparent profit will not have to pay any tax on the transaction. This is welcome relief. What they do not tell you, is to look at the historical example of the rise of housing prices in this country. It will not take too many years until substantial numbers of us will have passed the five hundred thousand dollar barrier and will be paying tax on the paper gain when we sell our homes, not withstanding the fact that these are not real gains. At the same time that provision was written into law, your government took away your ability to put the money tax free into a larger or more desirable home that costs more money if such was your wish. This is creating problems for some older people who wish to sell their homes in order to relocate to another higher priced area for their retirement years. The problem will hit many of us over the next several years if property values in desirable locations rise again.

An alternative minimum tax was put into effect some years ago in order to prevent the wealthiest among us from sheltering a large part of their income from being taxed. The lack of indexing to account for inflation and the consequent rise in wages and income (without a rise in actual buying power) has now subjected large numbers of us to the 'alternative minimum tax'.

Temporary reductions in the inheritance tax are in place. Unfortunately, the decrease in the federal inheritance tax is not in step with state taxes, so that in high tax states, many people effectively could pay more in total tax. Presently, the estate of an individual is not generally taxed when it is passed to the surviving spouse. The size of the estate that can be passed tax-free to children, grandchildren or other heirs tax free, had been gradually raised, although not by nearly enough to take into account the accumulated inflationary rise over the lifetime of both members of a married couple. So apparent gain in value, which is illusory, is still heavily taxed. The result of these taxes is to leave the family less in true assets than what was actually worked for through a lifetime by a couple.

What has not been publicized is the fact that, after a death, assets in the estate can be stepped up in basis. This means that property, for tax purposes, can be calculated at its true present market value. Less capital gains tax therefore has to be paid on its sale by the estate. Inheritance tax, however, does have to be paid.

Unfortunately, many people do not realize that in a decrease of the inheritance tax, the provision to increase the basis of property in the estate from its original cost to true present day market value could be lost. In order to make any decrease in the inheritance tax meaningful, the increase in basis of assets to true market value should be maintained.

If a person makes a true gain on capital risk, it is fair that tax should be paid, just as most of us who toil with their hands and brains must pay tax to support our society. This is only right. However, to tax somebody on a home they have lived in for a generation or more, or on an asset they have worked hard for and owned for many years, without indexing for inflation, is patently unfair. Such a person is actually being deprived of their assets, because after paying a tax they are no longer capable of buying a house for the exact same value, but must lower their lifestyle in order to shelter themselves. The five hundred thousand dollar exemption may not look so great ten years from now, and don't expect anybody in the government to hurry to your aid and raise the exemption to anything near what would be fair.

The inexorable, albeit slow, rise in prices is ultimately devastating to anybody on a fixed income, if you live long enough. That is why we increasingly see elderly seniors minding their pennies, getting discounts where they can, and often forsaking decent nutrition and the medications they need because they simply do not have the money to pay for these necessities. Many such people, if not the majority, had adequate fixed incomes when they started their retirement years.

One obvious part of answer to this important problem is to change the concept of retirement completely. Besides the economic implications, many people who retire find themselves at a loss concerning how they should spend their time. There is a significant incidence of clinical depression in retired people. People seem to age faster, and to be more infirm. Mental acuity decreases. It was once thought that people reached their intellectual peak by approximately age 12, and thereafter, with the inexorable death of brain cells, the point was inevitably reached where they would intellectually become shadows of their former selves. Nothing could be further from the truth. It has now been proven that neural connections can regenerate and that mental capacity can continue to evolve into much later years. The study of London taxi drivers and their built-in brain maps of that city was very dramatic evidence of this.

The trick is to stay mentally challenged and to continue to perform gratifying tasks. This does not mean that you have to work full time, or even to continue to pursue exactly the same work that you always did. However, it is a shame to leave a lifetime of work in a craft or occupation in which you have built up enormous expertise, and from which over the years you have derived enormous satisfaction, just because you think you can afford to. Of course, if the work you did over your lifetime was not something you enjoyed, and which gave you no great satisfaction, you should think about pursuing other tasks that will give you self gratification and a sense of fulfillment. At the same time, you will have automatically indexed yourself for inflation, because wages and fees for work more or less tend to be realistically aligned to the prevalent economic structure. Obviously, you will also be earning extra income, which is a nice thing to have at your disposal.

Until very recently, there was a great drawback to this strategy. Social Security only kicked in if you earned below a certain minimal income. This led people into forced retirement so that they could get their social security check. It also led to the creation of a vast underground economy, in which capable older people worked only for cash so they could still collect their social security checks. Needless to say, these seniors tended not to pay income tax. In this unintended way, government created a class of senior illegal workers, with the added feature that the tax revenues on the unreported income was lost, leading the rest of us to pay higher taxes.

Now that this barrier to legal work by a most valuable sector of our population, seniors, has been removed, it opens the door for many of us to continue to enjoy being productive and satisfied members of society.

It takes a very long time for a government to turn things around in the usual run of things. When Franklin Roosevelt introduced the Social Security System in the 1930's, it was a breathtaking concept. There would now be an income base beneath which seniors could not fall. What was unsaid, however, was that the concept was based on demographics. A much smaller percentage of the population at that time actually lived to be sixty two or older, and therefore had any hope of ever actually seeing a social security check. In the mid 1930's, there were approximately sixteen workers for each retiree. Therefore, a relatively large pool of workers could contribute to supporting their elders, in the full realization that when they themselves attained the appropriate age, they too would receive the benefits.

This strategy has become much more uncertain in recent years, with many fewer working people for each retiree, and is now a major concern for seniors and the gainfully employed younger population alike. With large numbers of seniors becoming eligible for Social Security every year, and the life expectancy of the population increasing dramatically, there is more uncertainty as to the viability of the system. Thoughtful people are putting forth proposals to maintain the integrity of Social Security. These include such things as gradually increasing the age at which people would be fully entitled to benefits, using government revenues to shore up the system, and allowing individuals to put part of their contributions in other relatively safe economic instruments outside the system, so that they could hopefully build more substantial benefits. It is essential to maintain the integrity of social security system. Approximately sixty-one million people now rely on Social Security in the United States, and that number is only going to get larger.

Most people in our society would now agree that we need something beyond the Social Security safety net in order to retire comfortably. It must also be said that retirement is not always voluntary; some of us unfortunately will develop conditions that in later years will prevent us from earning any active income.

Unemployment rates are currently at low levels. This does not mean that jobs are secure in this global environment. The talents needed in the work force in this dynamic economy are constantly changing. Companies are taken over or merged. Management teams are constantly looking for ways to be more productive and efficient. This often means laying off part of the workforce. At the same time, many people are less loyal to a company, and will change jobs as opportunities arise. All this leads to a lessened sense of security, specifically as to the availability of an adequate pension at the end of the road. There have also been too many incidences of raiding pension funds and the inappropriate use of the moneys contained in them, both legally and illegally. Employees are often encouraged or obligated to keep much of their pension money in the stock of the company they work for, with the possibility of disastrous results if the stock price falls significantly.

One answer, of course, lies in the use of individual tax deferred programs such as the 401 K, and IRA (Individual Retirement Account). Unfortunately, too many of us are not really capable of wisely investing our money in stocks, bonds, and mutual funds on our own, although with computer access, the internet, and heightened interest in business television a lot of us are getting much more sophisticated. The more financially sophisticated you become, the more you tend to realize that professional advice might be a good thing. A bewildering array of possible investments exists. If you do invest, you should consider getting financial advice from a qualified, trustworthy financial planner, or an institution such as an investment bank.

Do your homework to ensure that the individual or firm has the right credentials and a good track record. You should learn what magnitude of funds they already have under management. It is important to know if the person or institution who will be managing your funds is getting a flat fee or is relying upon commissions and therefore activity in your account in order to generate their own income. You should be prepared to clearly outline your specific economic and lifestyle goals to the individual who will be actively investing your money. You should also be aware of what degree of risk is involved. Even the most sophisticated investors often get burned, either by bad investments or by unscrupulous or dishonest advisers, or a combination of both. Most of us have been around long enough to realize that markets can go down as well as up and try to protect ourselves accordingly.

References

1. Altfest, Karen C: The Care of the Older Person, Third Edition: Chapter: Financial guidance for seniors: RMC Publishing, LLC. 2019 www.careoftheolderperson.com
2. https://www.ssa.gov/policy/docs/quickfacts/stat_snapshot/
3. Bibliography & Supplemental Bibliography: See www.rcaplanmd.com

CHAPTER 18
THE POLITICS OF AGE

Seniors in our society have now become a potent political and economic force. The most obvious reason for this development is the rapidly increasing numbers of mature people, predominantly women, in our society. People are healthier now in their later years than they have ever been. They are more vigorous. For generations now, in large numbers, women have entered every aspect of the workforce from the most menial positions to the professions and the executive suite. Large numbers of women are in ownership positions of everything from small businesses, companies, and assets including stocks, bonds and real estate, to sports teams and some of the largest corporations in America. Interestingly enough, only a few of the most major corporations in America have women as their chief executive officers or chief financial officers even today, but this is changing.

Seniors enjoy the demographic power of sheer numbers, and economic power. With increasing levels of sophistication in the complexities of how society, not to mention bureaucracy, works, many people have found their political voice. Women have become a significant force in the major political parties. Women are senators and members of the House of Representatives. They are major figures in the structure of the political parties in the United States. Women are increasingly vying for the Presidency.

Although women today in our society make up an indispensable part of the armed forces, they have not, by and large, managed to rise to the top levels of the military in strategic decision making. Because of the vital role that national defense and security performs, and its interaction with geopolitics, a full role for women in the military impacts upon the political power of women. Women have been the National Security Adviser, and the Secretary of State of the United States.

Women in our society today tend to live longer than men. Inheritance laws tend to allow for the free transfer of assets between spouses when one partner dies, without taxation. These two facts alone are responsible for the substantial holding of assets by senior women in our society. Economic power gives great leverage in the creation of political power. More importantly and ominously, as Hannah Arendt pointed out, economic power without political power is an invitation for disaster. If you put a hundred dollar bill in the street without guarding it, don't expect it to be there when you come back.

It is not only important for seniors to exercise political power, but it is essential for their self interest and for the larger interest of society. After all, seniors are now a large and vital segment of our society. Furthermore, they have the wisdom and knowledge necessary to make the hard decisions in a calm and reasoned manner that will shape our society going into the future. This will be their true legacy to their children, grandchildren, and great grandchildren.

Every nonprofit organization tends to start out idealistically, usually with a single purpose. As the organization thrives and matures, it often achieves its preliminary goal of funding a particular kind of research, or even finding a cure for a particular disease. Somewhere along the way, it may fall into the trap of expanding the definition of a disease or a condition, so that more people will have an interest in funding the organization. This can have the unintended consequence of making relatively healthy people think they have a serious condition.

If it is a political organization, it may find over the years that the demographics of the population it serves has radically changed, and that the needs of the population have changed as well.

At this stage, the primary purpose of an organization tends to become more one of survival, and the self-interest of the organization. The original purpose for which the organization was created may become obscured and lost. It is very rare that you hear of an organization that declares that its purpose is fulfilled, and therefore it will disband, and give its remaining assets to some other entity with a worthy, contemporary cause. It is even more difficult to disband a bureaucracy once it is put into motion, because its self-interest is to stay in place.

It is equally difficult to get any law, whether it be federal, state, city, or town ordinance, off the books once it has been enacted, even though that law may be completely archaic and not relevant to modern society. Many politicians get elected by promising new, high sounding legislation, not by stating that they will get rid of masses of old laws that interfere with our everyday existence. There is nothing interesting or vote getting in poring through books of old statutes.

If you are going to support an organization, probably the first thing you should know about it is whether its stated goals, objectives, and ideals coincide with your own. You should make sure that the organization is honest and cost effective. Your money should not be squandered. Resources should be carefully marshalled to address the issues that you want to be addressed and fix the problems that you want fixed. It is important to know whether the organization has the political clout necessary to get its message to the people who are empowered to make sure the job gets done.

The American Association of Retired People (AARP) has grown immensely in recent years. It has a tremendous membership base and reaches much of the senior population. It has the ear of people at the highest levels of government. It is cheap to join, and there are various membership benefits, including insurance opportunities. It may be well to look at these goals, which primarily concern the empowerment of senior people in our society.

There are many worthwhile societies concerned with health issues that merit support. The National Institutes of Health itself is supported by public funds and does not solicit charitable contributions. The Institutes does an incredible job in coordinating and funding sophisticated research activities into the search for cures of many of the illnesses that afflict us in later years. The NIH maintains a massive database that you can connect to through the internet. Health professionals have access to important data and direction from this most important and necessary organization.

The major nonprofit health-oriented organizations need volunteers on every level. Large numbers of older people readily give their time and money to such organizations. Again, it is very important to make sure that the organizations you are giving your time and money to are bona fide and are spending your money wisely. It is important to know who the top administrators are. There have been scandals involving misuse of funds belonging to major organizations.

For many years the American Cancer Society has been a leader in funding major research programs in the continuing struggle to find better ways to deal with the many types of cancer that we are prone to. As well, the society concentrates on public awareness, teaching the possible early warning signs of cancer and encouraging people to get appropriate diagnostic studies. Many people are involved in helping the organization to do its good works, from the grassroots level, up to the senior level of management.

The American Diabetes Association, and the Juvenile Diabetes Association fund important work in defining better treatments for this major disease and helping diabetics to cope with it.

There are specific organizations dealing with just about every major disease process, with the aim of eradicating the disease. Alzheimer's disease is one such illness.

CHAPTER 19

THE SICKNESS AND LOSS OF A LIFE PARTNER

Women in our society today tend to outlive their husbands and life partners. This is a stunning reversal from ages past, when a man could often be expected to outlive his mate, because of the significant dangers presented to her by the process of repeated childbearing. A woman would not be safe after childbearing either, as the postpartum period, that is, the time immediately after bearing a child, was fraught with danger. Theoretically at least, the female reproductive tract presents a potentially open avenue from the outside into the abdominal, or peritoneal cavity. In the usual scheme of things, a healthy woman is protected from ascending infection through this potential passageway by a variety of mechanisms. First of all, this potential passage is essentially closed. The vagina is a closed structure. The cervix, which is the mouth of the uterus or womb, is normally closed, and is protected by mucus. Secretions from the cervix and the vagina itself tend to have an antibacterial function, and the flow is outward.

The endometrial cavity within the uterus is closed under normal circumstances. The lumen, or tiny inner cavity of each fallopian tube is similarly closed. As well, the lining cells of the fallopian tube have tiny microscopic hairlike projections called cilia. Other cells in this lining have secretions that discourage bacterial entry. Beyond all this, the immunologic system will mount an attack against any invading organism.

Most of these mechanisms are compromised in the immediate period after childbirth. The cervix is open. There are very often minute cuts or lacerations in the vagina and the cervix through which bacteria can enter. The mucus plug is gone. Secretions are bloody, and blood is a wonderful culture medium to grow germs, or bacteria, in. The essential immunologic system of the mother is compromised. The fetus that has been growing inside her is essentially a transplant, with half of its genetic material derived from its father. An alteration of the immunologic mechanisms in the mother during pregnancy is one of the ways by which the fetus has the ability to survive and grow.

Most mothers nurse their babies, and rightfully so, as this provides maximal nutritional benefit to the newborn, as well as transferring valuable immunity from the mother to the baby. It is important that the nursing mother does not take any drug or medication without first consulting a qualified physician, as many medications can pass in the breast milk to the baby.

Nursing also develops a strong emotional bond between the mother and the baby. However, the nursing mother can develop cracks in her nipples. This again allows germs to enter her blood stream and can result in abscesses of the breast. With modern treatment, especially with the advent of powerful antibiotics, this condition is no longer the great concern it was in an earlier time. Mothers did die from overwhelming sepsis caused by breast infection in the bad old days.

With most of these problems largely obviated, or at least reduced to manageable conditions that are not usually life threatening, a great obstacle to women's longevity was removed.

Men, on the other hand, historically, tended to die disproportionately actively fighting in battles, and from trauma associated with so-called sports, many of which seemed to copy warlike activities, as well as street violence, crime, and gun violence.

Rural life on the farm is not as idyllic as most people think. Farming as an occupation can be hazardous, and men can be disproportionately involved in crippling and even fatal farm accidents. Since the industrial revolution, both men and women have all been at risk from industrial accidents, and exposure to toxic substances ranging from asbestos to toxic fumes in mines, factories, and chemical plants. More recently, radiation exposure has become a serious hazard. Over the years, men seem to have borne the brunt of this, although women were by no means protected, especially during war years.

The general stresses of the workplace seemed to take their toll. It used to be thought that people with so-called type A personalities were more at risk of having potentially fatal diseases, such as early heart attacks, and duodenal and stomach ulcers, which could perforate and bleed. Many treatments, including biofeedback and psychiatric counseling were employed in order to lessen the supposed risk of being a type A personality. The type A personality was essentially pictured as being driven and high strung. It is now known that most ulcers of the stomach and the first part of the small intestine known as the duodenum are caused by a bacterium, H. pylori. A relatively simple course of antibiotics generally takes care of the problem before it can do significant harm. Another reason for bleeding from the upper gastrointestinal tract is treatment with anticoagulant drugs. These are often given to lessen the risk of coronary thrombosis, or blood clots in the blood vessels of the heart. One of the more common treatments is taking a baby aspirin once a day. This should never be done without a doctor's specific advice. Although this is an important, and sometimes life saving, regimen in many people, it should be understood that aspirin, like any other drug can be quite dangerous. Just because something is sold over the counter, without a doctor's prescription, does not mean that it does not have potentially serious side effects.

Men tended in years past to have a much higher incidence of potentially lethal diseases such as lung cancer and heart disease because of their high incidence of smoking. They also developed mouth and lip cancers from pipe smoking and tobacco chewing. They developed larynx, or voice box, cancers from tobacco exposure as well. At least in our society, the incidence of tobacco use among men has fallen precipitously. At the same time, the widespread use of cigarettes in women has risen alarmingly for a couple of generations now. It has yet to be seen how this shift in the use of tobacco products in our society between the two sexes will change the disparity and longevity between women and men.

At the present, it is apparent in our society that in the older age groups, there are a significantly greater number of women than men. Inevitably, in a long-term monogamous relationship, one partner will get a serious life-threatening illness.

The onset of serious illness in a long-term partner and helpmate is always unexpected, inopportune, and emotionally traumatic. It is, of course, always best to be prepared in advance. No one can ever be completely prepared for such an eventuality, but it is comforting to know in such a situation that great attention can be brought to bear upon the problem, without the necessity of having your attention drawn to extraneous matters.

As a couple gets older, it is essential that adequate financial plans have been made. This is most important if your spouse is still a fulltime wage earner. Many people do carry disability insurance, but this usually only kicks in after a waiting period, which may be many months. As well, very often it cannot fully supplement the lost earnings. It is important that benefits, such as social security and pension benefits, are properly in order. It goes without saying that health insurance coverage should be present and of an optimal nature so that whatever is necessary medically can be obtained without the added frustration of bureaucratic haggling with personnel at a managed care company. Life insurance should, of course, be in order.

Many people, even today, have only a sketchy understanding of what their financial position would be if their spouse became seriously ill. This has as much to do with avoidance of an unpleasant and threatening subject as it has to do with the fact that we are all busy with our lives and have better things to do than to worry about theoretical eventualities. However, prudent people still take the time to go over their financial position, earning capacity, and asset picture with qualified, proven, and honest financial advisers, estate planners, and will and estate attorneys.

It is important that both husband and wife have a personal and preferably long-term business relationship with various people who help to control financial aspects of their lives, especially their lawyer and accountant. The worst possible time to first meet these professionals is in the midst of a sudden health crisis of your life partner. It is important that you read and understand as much as possible about your tax returns every year so that you have an ongoing understanding of your financial condition. You should also have an updated financial statement that specifically states your asset position and your liabilities. It is important to have trustees in place who are compatible with the family's wishes. Far too many families become embroiled in totally unnecessary financial battles because of insufficient economic planning and proper understanding of the issues involved prior to the onset of sickness in a spouse, parent or grandparent.

With financial issues settled, hopefully satisfactorily and to the best of your ability, it is possible to focus on the needs of your life partner. It is important to recognize your own needs during such a time of crisis.

You must be careful to maintain your own physical and emotional health during extraordinary times. You will not be of much use to your spouse, or to yourself, if you cannot manage to keep yourself in the best possible health. Rest becomes an extremely important issue. It is difficult to get proper sleep when a loved mate is in serious trouble. Do not be afraid to enlist the aid of your physician. Your family should rally around you, and help share the physical burden, to ensure that you get proper rest. Do not feel guilty about getting proper sleep and taking proper care of yourself. This will enable you to be the most supportive you can be to the one you love. It is important not to keep vigil in a hospital room twenty-four hours a day, if you can somehow avoid this. Even short walks in the fresh air will do you much good. Try to keep on a regular eating schedule. If the condition is long term, you will have to attempt to keep up as much of a normal life as possible. Do not neglect your work, your home, your children, or your grandchildren, and keep in touch with your friends. Try to remember that if you hear a lot of meaningless platitudes, that people really do not know what to say in extreme situations. They are only trying to convey to you that they care and are there for you.

You should quickly learn what constitutes sound advice, and what is a lot of pseudoscience and just plain nonsense that can derail you in your purpose of getting the best possible medical care for your spouse. You will hear all kinds of advice from all kinds of people, some of it good, some of it bad, and much of it that you will have heard before. It will be up to you to sort through this and to stay with the best possible opinions from the most qualified people.

We are long past the time when doctors at times of serious medical problems told family members little and made decisions unilaterally. You should understand what treatments are being proposed and why. You should understand what the options are, and what the probabilities of a successful outcome is. You should have a good idea of the time frames involved. You should know about possible complications of the disease, and of the proposed treatments. You should know the qualifications of people treating your loved one, and the level of the medical facility within which she or he is being treated.

There is a lot of information available on the Internet on just about every conceivable medical condition. It is important to know, however, that even the most comprehensive treatise on a disease condition of necessity only deals in generalities and statistics, and cannot specifically cone down on the specific circumstance that an individual patient faces. It essential that you discuss the nature of the particular condition with the treating physicians. They should have the deepest understanding of what is happening in the dynamics of the case.

In this age, you will probably have to get very actively involved with the health maintenance organization, or other health insurance carrier to ensure that there is prompt precertification for all necessary diagnostic and therapeutic procedures, and that all your benefits are in place. You may have to talk to them about length of the hospital stay, as many such insurance organizations now tend to try to push people out of the hospital as quickly as possible. You may well have to deal with the insurers concerning coverage for crucial drugs and medications. These are often extremely expensive nowadays, and insurers can be loathe to pay for them.

The most important thing you can give to your loved one during a medical crisis is your time. He or she will need you to physically be there much of the time, more for comfort and reassurance than for anything else. However, you will quickly find out that while you are there you will be able to make life much more bearable, by making sure that there is access to whatever creature comforts are allowed and that needs are fulfilled. Nursing personnel tend to be extremely busy and spread thin. Help of family members is needed, understood, and appreciated in most major medical facilities today.

Of course, your love and sympathy is important. It is much harder to be empathetic. You cannot really understand what a very sick person is going through unless you have been there yourself. Aside from the physical discomfort and even pain, there is a feeling of helplessness, especially if the person has always felt as if they were in total control of their destiny. In this circumstance they may not even be in control of their body functions and may be incapable of doing such mundane things as feeding themselves, dressing themselves, or going to the bathroom. A sick person is restricted in movement, and there is a limited physical environment. Many hospitals take great care in establishing outdoor areas where patients who are not in crisis can go in order to get at least some change in their environment.

A seriously ill person may often become depressed and hopeless. It is important to detect signs of this and to arrange for proper professional help, including consultation with a psychiatrist, if this is appropriate. As well, as much contact with family and friends as possible should be encouraged in order to provide intellectual stimulation, and to distract from constant focus on the immediate pressing health problem.

Beyond this, your spouse will be downright scared. It is hard to face one's own mortality. Most of us do not think about it or confront it until it is staring us in the face in the form of life- threatening illness. It is at such a time that many of us find that our religious leaders can be very comforting, especially if we have established a long-term association with them, and if they have become our friends, or at least good acquaintances. In the absence of such long-term associations, every hospital has a chaplaincy service that is attuned to the needs of its patients. There are also support departments, including social workers, who can be of great assistance in arranging home nursing, and other necessary help for the transition back to normal life.

CHAPTER 20
RECREATING SOCIAL RELATIONSHIPS

There is probably no bond stronger than that between a woman and a man that has been forged over many decades. They have the ultimate common interest in their children, grandchildren and their totally shared life, with all its vicissitudes. They reach a point where they are almost of one mind. They certainly share many beliefs, values, and goals, whether realized or not.

Inevitably, one partner is eventually lost to the other. Women in our society tend to live approximately six years longer than men, and as women commonly tend to marry men of either the same age or older than themselves, the majority of people who must fend for themselves in this situation are women.

If there has been a long debilitating illness, the person most likely has turned somewhat inward, due to the demands of the care required for the partner, as well as the emotional toll that is taken. Enormous concentration has to be given to getting appropriate medical care, as well as to the marshalling of economic resources to pay for the increased help required. Despite the best intentions of family and friends, there is often a necessary drop off in the amount of time that the stricken couple can devote to recreational activities and to social gatherings that cement social relationships.

Isolation tends to be exacerbated in modern society for a person after the demise of a life partner. This is especially true if the terminal illness has been drawn out over many years and if the couple is in a very senior age group, so that many of their lifelong friends and family members are either already gone, or are themselves too debilitated to be of much meaningful support.

There are no easy answers to these large problems for someone suddenly facing life on their own. In many cases, this is the first time since she or he was barely an adult that they are without their life partner.

As in many other serious situations, the best possible approach is always to recognize the possibility that such circumstances can arise, unpleasant and abhorrent that the prospect may be. Paying attention to the emotional and physical health of your spouse, as well as yourself, is obviously important to prolonging your life together. It is just as important, even in the most trying circumstances, to resist the temptation to focus totally inwards on the health and well being of your spouse. Remember that your other family members need you just as much as you need them. The presence of a severe illness can be a time for greatly strengthening meaningful bonds between family members, and between generations. It may be the first time that the members of the younger generation have been faced with some of the starker realities of life. Some young people can become very frightened and withdrawn. It is a good to time to show your wisdom and your strength. Help them to understand and accept the threat to a loved elder person. Paying attention to your offsprings' well being will help them to grow even closer to you.

It is important to maintain a social relationship with friends. Friends usually want to be of help. It makes them feel better about the situation. Draw them closer instead of shutting them out. If they can help in a small way, they will feel closer to you and feel better about themselves. You should, of course, be aware of the limitations of each friendship, so that you do not put unrealistic demands upon your friends. You will find certain people much more willing and able to help than others.

In your senior years, if you are left to face the world alone, it is more important than ever that you are in the best possible emotional and physical shape. Some people tend to pay untoward attention to what their acquaintances might say behind their backs if they look too attractive. Anyone who would speak ill of one of their friends in such circumstances, while a person is trying their best to live a normal life, is obviously not a true and supportive friend.

The individual who has family and true friends willing to lend help and support at this time is blessed. Difficult as it may be, try not to shun their overtures, but to include people as much as possible. They are only trying to help in their own way.

It goes without saying that a long-term religious affiliation can be of great comfort at such a time. It may be of great help to begin to aid in the charitable works of the institution caring for your loved one and help others with all the wisdom you have gained from your own recent experience.

CHAPTER 21

HOW SOCIETY COULD ADAPT TO ACCOMMODATE LARGE NUMBERS OF HEALTHY "ELDERS"

It is intensely interesting how societal attitudes have changed in reaction to new realities. There is now a large, politically influential, and economically powerful population of mature people in our society. Great advances in medical sciences, along with the underpinnings of public health and safety, as well as a rising economic base have helped to create a society where mature women are often not content to play limited roles. Rising political power and awareness, along with antidiscrimination laws, and antiharassment statutes, have given rise to a climate in which older women and men can thrive.

Significant factors behind the redefinition of the workplace have been a rising economy and a low unemployment rate. Our society is literally starved for experienced workers at every level. This is especially true for people with skills in the new technology.

The concept of a mandatory, arbitrary, retirement age is, and should be, becoming abandoned in more and more industries. In crucial occupations where the public safety is at risk, for example airline pilots, it is right and proper to demand appropriate safety standards for the public, including comprehensive monitoring of physical and mental status of the people involved. However, it should now be clear that large numbers of people beyond the arbitrary age of sixty- two, or sixty-five years are still perfectly capable of performing complex tasks at a high level. Furthermore, they have a level of experience in dealing with rarely confronted situations that is invaluable. Great lessons in this regard became forcibly apparent in World War II, when huge numbers of women filled a vast panoply of jobs, ranging from assembly line work and the building of complex armaments, to piloting high performance aircraft. At the same time, as younger doctors were sent overseas in large numbers to staff field hospitals, older surgeons were called out of retirement in significant numbers to tend the hospitals at home, and to care for the sick, which they did with great distinction.

From sheer economic need, large numbers of corporations and industries are now actively recruiting mature people to fill positions in every sector. It has been found, by and large, that mature workers are a stabilizing influence. They tend to be experienced, and to bring good judgement and wisdom to bear on the tasks assigned to them.

At the same time, we are becoming adept at individualizing more senior people, rather than lumping them into a huge amorphous group. Some people, regrettably, at relatively young ages get medical conditions which make them in some way temporarily or permanently disabled to a greater or lesser extent. Other people are healthy, active, and alert, even into the ages that were, not too long ago, considered to be ancient. The imposition of an arbitrary retirement age, whether desired or not, on such a diverse and heterogenous group is at the very least counterproductive.

It is still vitally important for people who have worked hard and productively for a great proportion of their lives to be able to retire at a defined age, if they wish to do so, with their social security and Medicare benefits intact. A great step forward has been taken in allowing people to receive full benefits at the prescribed age of sixty five, without losing their ability to work in any occupation they choose, either on a full time or part time basis, earning money without being penalized. This has the added advantage of not forcing healthy, active, productive people to give up a career that has given them a lifetime of satisfaction and fulfillment, if they wish to continue it. The choice should be at the option of the individual, not at the option of the employer or the government.

It is interesting that many people in positions of high esteem and power, including judges, and owners of various enterprises, have never been forced to retire at any given age. They tend to work well into their later years, unless they themselves decide to take on other pursuits.

A significant bar to the gainful employment of a significant number of mature people who are disabled has been removed. This has been accomplished by legislation, as well as an increasing awareness that many people with various disabilities have much to contribute to the society. Many physical improvements to their environment have been made in the accessibility to offices and other workplaces. Great strides have been made, especially in the development of new technology, to make the office and workplace environment much more user-friendly, both to people with disabilities and to those of us who are more fortunate so that we can simply work more efficiently with the assistance of technology.

We have come a long way as a society. We no longer mass all our elders into a single category and send them off to a single type of facility even if they can still manage their own lives and finances.

Mature people are a huge and diverse group with multitudinous needs and desires. The ideal living arrangement for anyone is to be in their own home, with access to loving family members.

With technological advances in communication, and its extension to such things as in- home shopping by computer and widely available home health care, more and more people are choosing to stay in their own homes later in life. Many people who are fortunate enough to be affluent, are opting to effectively make their vacation homes into their primary residence.

Large numbers of seniors, with or without spouses, do elect to move into communities that cater to seniors. These range from highly luxurious communities in desirable areas of the country, in which each resident either owns a home or apartment, to shared facilities. Of course, any facility that is selected should be carefully researched, in line with the finances and medical needs of the individual. It is important to know the underlying finances of the company that is running the facility, as well as its reputation. The facility must be capable of giving caring support.

A significant number of seniors, because of their physical or mental capabilities, will still eventually need the care provided by a nursing home. Such a facility should be able to provide a sophisticated level of support, with available medical care. The nursing home should abide by all pertinent health regulations. It is very important to make sure that any such facility that is entered into by a senior relative has been carefully looked at to ensure that it is adequately funded and maintained, and that the level of medical supervision available is of high caliber.

It has been thought that the increasing power of seniors in the labor force, and their increasing voice in the political arena, would inevitably lead to conflict with younger generations who have their own goals and aspirations. In fact, this is not really true, as younger people will inevitably become us. In the dynamic, flexible, innovative, and expanding society, there is more than enough room for talented individuals at every age level. This is clearly brought out by the shortage of workers today in key technology sectors, even at the highest levels. Today a lot of dynamic young entrepreneurs have even seen fit to hire their erstwhile retired parents into their new companies and ventures, in order to get their experience, maturity, wisdom, and stability on board as positive factors.

Accountability of the social security system must be worked out on a sound economic basis, so that money is not only available for the needs of the present senior generation, but that solvency of the system extends far into the future, in order that the young people who are now actively contributing into the system can foresee stable benefits for themselves when they attain senior age. Therefore, the integrity of the system is important to all generations.

All in all, we were once youngsters, and they will become us, hopefully with grace and dignity. We are all working toward the same goals.

CHAPTER 22
COSMETIC SURGERY

The Take-Home Message

- There is nothing wrong with looking good
- Major advances in eye surgery are enabling large numbers of people to see better
- The skin is an important organ that should be properly cared for
- Examination should regularly be done for the early diagnosis, and removal of, potentially dangerous skin lesions (growths or discolored areas)
- Medications are now available that actually do enhance hair growth but beware of a plethora of false claims
- Medications are now available that actually inhibit the growth of facial hair

Plastic surgery used to be the provenance of the rich and famous. It was a well guarded little secret. Movie stars, and movie star wannabes invested in plastic surgery in order to enhance or maintain their careers. People in those days did not admit that they had undergone surgery for purely cosmetic reasons. There was significant danger to undergoing the surgery. The results could be less than perfect. Often, people came out of it with a very artificial look.

Techniques of plastic surgery have evolved and improved over the years. In the hands of skilled plastic surgeons, and maxillofacial surgeons, cosmetic surgery nowadays generally has lower risk, and is more likely to end up with a good, natural looking result. The entire process is now democratized, so that great numbers of women and increasingly men in our society avail themselves of the more common plastic surgical procedures. With the general increase of wealth in our society, more people can afford this luxury, even though there is no insurance that reimburses these cosmetic procedures.

Although people are much more open now about discussing their plastic surgery, many people still consider this a private matter. If a friend has gone away for a while on vacation, and comes back looking vital, well rested and healthy, it is quite possible that she or he has done more than surf and golf.

Ideally, good plastic surgery will make a person look younger, and take years off the face and body, enhancing appearance. There are fashions in what is considered to be good or exotic in looks. Fashions can and do change. It is easy to buy a new wardrobe, but much harder to recreate one's appearance after it has been altered.

Such things as high, exaggerated cheek bones, full lips, and tattooed eyebrows can be made too extreme.

As people age, there is a redistribution of fat in the face. Some areas seem to sink in, while others, notably under the eyes and chin, sag. Careful liposuction can be combined with plastic surgery to alleviate such problems.

A competent and qualified plastic surgeon will usually do photographs prior to any surgical intervention. Those photographs can then be marked up, either manually or by computer in order to give a pretty fair idea of what the final result will look like. Beauty is subjective and in the eyes of the beholder. It is important that the photographs are gone over with the plastic surgeon prior to the procedure, so that it is clear what is trying to be achieved. It is better not to have unrealistic expectations.

It is important to be as fit as possible prior to going for elective cosmetic surgery. It is better to be in the best possible health prior to any surgical procedure to help avoid complications. The plastic surgeon will advise preoperative care. This usually includes abstaining from aspirin and aspirin like products which can interfere with the blood clotting mechanism. Another good reason for being as fit as possible prior to cosmetic surgery, is that the plastic surgeon can evaluate the person in an optimal state. Significant weight loss or weight gain after plastic surgery can alter the result and change the hoped-for appearance.

The nose

One of the earlier widespread uses of plastic surgery was rhinoplasty, or nasal reconstruction. If one is unhappy with the way the nose looks, it is never too late to get it altered. Again, there are fashions in what people consider to be the ideal shape of the nose. It is better not to do anything too extreme. The result should be natural looking, but an improvement over the appearance before surgery.

Eyelids

Blepharoplasty, or surgery to the upper and lower eyelids, is now very commonly done. This easily gets rid of bags under the eyes and drooping eyelids. It takes away that depressed look. Nowadays, these procedures are done with hidden incisions that barely can be seen.

Lines and Wrinkles

Silicone injection used to be given to get rid of frown lines, especially between the eyes. There have been many medical questions raised as to the use of silicone cosmetically, especially if it is not within a contained sac or bag, as it was in breast implants. Even where silicone is contained, the bags can leak or rupture. Untoward side effects have been reported that are not limited just to misshapenness resulting from the leakage.

Fat injections are sometimes now used in the facial areas. Body fat is removed from another area of the body, and small quantities injected into appropriate areas to smooth out wrinkles. As this is one's own tissue, it generally will not cause any untoward reaction in the body. However, because this fat is simply injected without a blood supply, it is not vascularized, and therefore it will gradually dissolve, usually over a period of approximately one year. It is then necessary to repeat the fat injection. This is not usually much of a problem.

Injectable wrinkle fillers, in the form of a gel, are now available. As one ages, the amount of hyaluronic acid in the skin decreases, and wrinkling occurs. Restylane is an injectable hyaluronic acid gel being used by plastic surgeons. Recently available fillers tend to last longer, so that the frequency of injections can be decreased.

Radiesse is a synthetic bulking implant (Calcium Hydroxylapatite) approved for injection into bowed or paralyzed vocal cords.

There are injections available to fill out the lips. Again, this is a fashion issue. It is preferable not to exaggerate the "look" in any area. The cheek bones are another example of this. Prominent cheek bones are now considered to be very attractive. These areas can be enhanced by injection or by implants. Again, it is important not to overdo it. Similarly, chin implants are available and quite commonly used.

Another substance that has been injected to alter the facial contours is collagen. CosmoPlast and CosmoDerm are forms of human collagen. The advantages and disadvantages to all these techniques should be discussed with the plastic surgeon.

It is possible to get rid of fine lines and wrinkles with the careful, judicious use of the laser beam. It is obvious that such a complex instrument should be used by a competent and trained professional. Eyes should always be protected from the laser beam, by wearing special glasses which should be provided.

Botox (Botulinum Toxin Type A)

Another answer to facial wrinkles has been the injection of Botox (Botulinum Toxin Type A). This is botulism toxin. This highly poisonous substance (a neurotoxin) is very dangerous if misused. However, in tiny quantities administered by a qualified physician, side effects tend not to be catastrophic in most cases. Eyelid droop is one such possible side effect. The toxin works by paralyzing the muscle locally, so that the frown disappears. Specifically, when injected into muscle, it enters nerve endings, inhibiting acetylcholine (a neurotransmitter) release. This interference with the nerve control of the muscle results in decreased muscle activity. The drug should not be used in pregnancy.

Some people who use Botox have reported a decrease in frequency of tension headache, and possibly migraine. It should be noted that the drug has not been approved for these uses.

Face Lift

Sagging under the chin can be at least partially eliminated by the careful use of liposuction by a qualified doctor. The ultimate fix, however, is the face lift, which can be either partial or total. This is a relative complex procedure that must be carefully planned and done only by a qualified plastic surgeon. The skin of the face is literally pulled back and upwards in order to eliminate wrinkles, and give a smooth, sleek appearance. The incisions are hidden in the scalp and behind the ears. If the procedure is too extreme, the mouth tends to look lengthened and thin, and the whole appearance can be quite artificial. In the ideal case, it would be hard to know that someone has undergone any surgical procedure after several weeks of healing. The person will just look younger, healthier, happier, and much better than before. It is very important during the postoperative course that proper attention is paid to the instructions given by the plastic surgeon, so that natural and quick healing can occur.

Breast

Cosmetic surgery goes way beyond facial surgery. Women can now undergo cosmetic breast surgery. These procedures are not confined to women who have had breast cancer with partial or total removal of a breast. Women who are dissatisfied by the look and shape of their breasts in their mature years, especially if there is some sagging, can undergo mammoplasty procedures that reshape the breasts, or have saline implants inserted under the actual breast tissue in order to lift the breasts. The saline implants, which are essentially sterile salt water in a flexible sac, have largely supplanted silicone implants in the breast region because of concern about the possible long term effects of having relatively large amounts of silicone in the body.

Liposuction

Liposuction is widely used to sculpt the body. Common areas that are attended to include the waist, to get rid of so-called love handles. The buttocks and the abdomen are other areas where liposuction is used. Removal of large quantities of fat, along with the opening up of the blood vessels under the skin, can be hazardous. This procedure should be carried out only by well qualified physicians under properly controlled circumstances. Patients should be properly looked after postoperatively to make sure that there are no untoward results, especially hemorrhage.

Tissue Engineering

Fat does contain stem cells which can be grown to form other body tissues, including muscle, cartilage and bone. Eventually, a person's own fat may be liposuctioned out and used to grow replacement tissue for such things as new joint cartilage. There would be no rejection of this replacement, because the new tissue would actually be the person's own.

Such tissue engineering will probably become increasingly important in plastic surgery. Work is being done in areas including getting good blood supply to tissue, forming new cartilage, and even the regrowth of nerves.

Elimination of Scarring

The fetus is capable of repairing wounds without scarring. In other words, the fetus can heal wounds by actual regeneration of the tissue, rather than forming a scar. Attention is now being paid to identify the mechanisms by which the fetus does this, with the goal being to have wound healing in adults with much less scarring. It is possible, for example, that VEGF (vascular endothelial growth factor) is important in fetal scarless repair.

Cosmetic Dentistry

The threat of tooth loss can be significant as people age. Supplementation with female sex hormone, estrogen, after the menopause results in lessened tooth loss. The estrogen works by reducing the resorption of bone. Risks of the use of this hormone replacement therapy should be assessed by a qualified physician.

There are still a huge number of people in our society who have partial or complete upper and lower plates, commonly known as false teeth. Inevitably, over a long period of years, teeth can be damaged or break. Gum disease and infection can be present that leads to a loss of teeth. In order to safeguard teeth, prevention of dental disease is extremely important. Calcium intake is important for the teeth, just as it is for the bones. Adequate brushing and flossing, combined with regular dental checkups is most necessary. In spite of all these measures of good dental hygiene, teeth can be lost. Fortunately today, cosmetic dentistry has reached the level of a fine art. Dental specialists are capable of removing the nerve from a tooth root. This is commonly known as root canal work. A supporting post is then implanted into the space, and crowns are then precision fitted over these posts. The result is permanent, good-looking, and pain free teeth that function well.

Other advanced techniques, such as apicoectomy to drain the infected area at the apex of the tooth, are used to salvage natural teeth that otherwise would have been pulled in earlier years. Appropriate use of antibiotics, of course, can control dental infection.

Teeth that are dingy in appearance or not properly aligned can be capped. The color and the size of the teeth can be matched appropriately so that the resulting smile is natural, lustrous, and vibrant. Short of capping the teeth, veneers can be placed or the teeth can be bonded to achieve a similar result. All of these techniques have to be discussed with the dentist, who should be able to advise what procedure would be most beneficial. It is important to be aware of the possible risks of any procedure. As well as risk to the local area of the mouth and jaw bones, dental procedures can lead to the spread of bacteria throughout the body. People with valvular heart disease can develop endocarditis from bacteria that are released into the blood stream from dental procedures. It is important to know whether there is a risk of such a problem, and that appropriate antibiotics are given prophylactically in order to protect the heart at the time of the dental procedure. Even cleaning the teeth in the dentist's office can release bacteria this way, and appropriate antibiotic prophylaxis should be given if there is a risk.

Eye Surgery

Although many people wear them, contact lenses have not made eyeglasses obsolete. Eyeglass technology has improved with time, so that bifocals and even trifocals are no longer heavy, uncomfortable and unattractive. Thin lightweight lenses are now available in which the transition between the reading part of the lens and the distant vision part of the lens is not obvious. Most people quickly adapt to eyeglasses when they need them, and can find combinations of frames and lenses to suit their look and the shape of their faces.

Presently available soft contact lenses that are disposable lessen many of the problems that were associated with earlier contact lenses. However, they can still be irritating to the eye, and of course it is easy to lose them.

There have been significant recent advances in laser surgery to the cornea of the eye. The cornea of the eye is the transparent curved tissue that makes up the front outer wall of the eye. Initially, laser surgery to the cornea was used to change the curvature of the cornea to correct nearsightedness. Now, farsightedness that bothers many older adults can similarly be corrected by a laser that is computer controlled in the hands of a skilled ophthalmologic surgeon. This corrects the relative flatness of the cornea, and allows the treated person to again read without glasses. Usually, the procedure is quick.

Conductive Keratoplasty (CK) uses radio frequency energy to the cornea to change its shape. No incision is needed in the cornea. The procedure tends to be quick, and minimally invasive.

Like any surgical procedures, there are possible side effects with laser surgery and the radio frequency procedure, some of which can be serious. It is important obviously to discuss this with the eye surgeon prior to making any commitment.

Many mature adults are confronted with the clouding of the lens of the eye. It is known that environmental factors, such as smoking and sun exposure can hasten this loss of transparency of the eye lens, which is known as a cataract. Cataract surgery to remove the affected lens is well known and has been practiced for many years. It used to result in the need to wear very thick heavy glasses permanently. However, recent advances have led to the development of implantable lenses, and the restoration of sight. Cataract surgery can be done on an outpatient basis. The lens is removed from its capsule by ultrasonic emulsification and suction. Laser ablation of the lens is a possible alternative. An intraocular lens is then placed. Multifocal intraocular lenses have been developed, so that after surgery glasses are no longer required.

Regular eye examinations are important and should always be accompanied by a determination of the intraocular pressure in the eye. An abnormal increase in the intraocular pressure is a hallmark of glaucoma. Raised intraocular pressure along with damage to the optic nerve which supplies the eye, and progressive loss of peripheral vision are seen in primary open angle glaucoma. It is also possible to have optic nerve damage with normal intraocular pressure. This is another form of glaucoma. It is important to consult an ophthalmologist to get a proper diagnosis of such conditions. It is important to make the diagnosis early in order to prevent blindness. Medications can lower the intraocular pressure by decreasing the production of eye fluid (aqueous humor), or by increasing its outflow from the eye.

There are now innovative surgical treatments available to help glaucoma. These are basically surgical drainage procedures that result in a lowering of the intraocular pressure. A laser may be used to perform trabeculoplasty, or surgical trabeculectomy can be carried out. Trabeculae are essentially supporting fibers in the eye. An opening is made into the anterior (front) chamber of the eye, so that fluid flow can be controlled.

Another threat to vision with aging is macular degeneration. Smoking and high blood pressure increase the risk of this problem. Ultraviolet light exposure may hasten the developing of this condition as well. The use of estrogen replacement therapy may help in retarding the onset of macular degeneration. Ophthalmologists use thermal laser photocoagulation in the treatment of macular degeneration. Another approach has been to infuse Verteporfin which is then activated by a laser. This is called phototherapy.

Caring for the Skin

It has long been known that over the years, ultraviolet rays from the sun can damage the skin. The damage may be confined to drying and wrinkling of the skin. However, with people living longer in developed societies, precancerous and cancerous skin lesions have gained more prominence.

The conventional wisdom of limiting time spent in the sun, wearing glasses to protect the eyes from damage and cataract formation, wearing clothing that covers, rather than bares, a lot of skin surface, and wearing hats with large brims is still true.

It is important to use sunscreen on skin areas that are exposed to the sun. Some sunscreens, however, protect mainly against ultraviolet B (UVB) rays, without giving protection against ultraviolet A (UVA). Sunscreens should have a protection factor of at least fifteen, and a UVA protection rating of 3-4.

If a new 'mole' or spot appears on the skin, or if an existing area starts to change, it is important to have it evaluated by a dermatologist.

Ideally, a regular examination of the total body surface of skin can be done by a qualified dermatologist, who will identify, examine and evaluate all the spots on the body under a 'blue' light.

Skin Cancer

The commonest form of skin cancer is basal cell carcinoma. Fortunately, although malignant, this tends to be a slow growing and somewhat limited tumor in its potential to spread. Very often, an excision biopsy, by which the tumor is removed with a safe margin of healthy tissue, is adequate for both definitive diagnosis under the microscope in the pathology laboratory and for treatment.

MOHS surgery refers to the specific, layer by layer, removal of tissue until healthy tissue is proven microscopically to be reached, so that no malignant tissue is left behind.

Another form of skin cancer is squamous cell carcinoma. This type of cancer may spread locally and may go to other body sites as well.

Malignant melanoma is a virulent form of skin cancer that has a propensity to spread to lymph nodes and via the blood stream. There may be a genetic predisposition. Too much exposure to the sun as a child, leading to sunburn, especially in fair skinned people, can be a factor.

Early diagnosis is important, so that the tumor may be removed surgically and completely, with a margin of healthy tissue, before lymph node spread can occur. Lymphadenectomy (removal of lymph nodes) is often done. Chemotherapy may be used as well. Intron A (Interferon Alpha 2β) may be of value. The drug can cause a wide range of life-threatening, even fatal, disorders. It should not be used in pregnancy.

Hair

The removal of unsightly hair is often undertaken. One of the most common ways to get rid of this problem is by waxing. Essentially, hot paraffin is placed on the area and then stripped away along with the hair. Depilatory creams can also be used, but some find them irritating. Hair, of course, can judiciously be removed from the legs, and, if necessary, from the pubic area carefully with a razor. Speak to your dermatologist about advanced methods of more permanent hair removal, including destroying the hair follicles themselves, by laser or other means.

Large numbers of people remove unwanted hair on a regular basis. Most of these people are hormonally normal. However, a minority of women have excess body hair because of excess androgenic ("male") hormones, or more rarely because of other hormonal problems or medication use. This includes self medication with nonprescription products containing DHEA (Dihydroepiandrostenedione) and Androstenedione. Even more rarely, there may be a tumor or other disorder in an ovary or in an adrenal gland.

When excess body hair is present in a male pattern, along with acne, baldness of the scalp (alopecia), and infrequent menstruation, there may be androgen excess and insulin resistance. A woman with excess hair should be evaluated by a physician for proper diagnosis before treatment is decided on.

The majority of women who have unwanted hair do not have demonstrable androgen excess, nor do they have male hair distribution (hirsutism). Electrolysis and laser hair removal work, if properly used.

Vaniqa (Eflornithine) is a cream, sold by prescription, that inhibits the growth of facial hair. The cream inhibits the enzyme necessary for hair follicle growth. It should not be used in pregnancy.

Baldness of the scalp in women (alopecia) should be properly investigated, and treated, by a physician. If there is androgen excess, the cause is treated. Specific drugs that suppress androgen secretion are used if needed. Some oral contraceptive pills do suppress ovarian androgens. If insulin resistance is present, it is specifically treated (see chapter on Diabetes). Aldactone (Spironolactone) is an aldosterone antagonist that may be used. Side effects include potentially dangerous effects of elevated potassium (hyperkalemia). The drug may be hazardous in pregnancy.

Rogaine (Minoxidil), which was originally developed as an anti-hypertensive drug, is used extensively to grow back areas of thinning hair on the scalp. It stimulates hair growth. Side effects can include adverse effects in people with heart disease. It should not be used in pregnancy, or while nursing. In fact, no drug should be used by a nursing mother without prior consultation with a qualified physician.

Propecia (Finasteride), which stimulates hair growth, is used in men with male pattern hair loss. It has not been shown to be effective in women and cannot be used in pregnancy.

Cosmetics

The use of cosmetics is an art. It can be practically impossible, unless a person is professionally trained in the theater or visual arts, to see oneself as one is perceived by others. That is why sophisticated people tend to get professional advice on hair care, cosmetics and their total look.

The basic underlying premise is to be as healthy and as fit as possible. Good muscle tone and healthy skin are the foundations of a lustrous and sleek appearance. There are dermatologists today who largely confine their practices to cosmetics, including the appearance of the skin and the hair. A consultation in this area may be a good place to start.

A laser can be used in experienced, qualified, licensed hands to get rid of fine wrinkles. Laser can also be used for permanent body hair removal, by destroying the hair follicles themselves

Dermabrasion is often used to get rid of the superficial layers of the skin, so that new healthy and radiant skin grows in its place. This should be done only by a qualified professional, as going too deep with a such process can lead to actual loss of skin, and permanent scarring. Chemical peels are also used to get rid of superficial skin layers.

Acne can be treated relatively easily today by topical drying agents. Minor surgical procedures can actually remove the areas of eruption. Retin-A (Tretinoin) can be used, but with great caution in any woman who still has the possibility of becoming pregnant, as it is can be quite harmful to a developing fetus, and cannot be used in pregnancy.

The dermatologist will also give advice on makeup, especially hypoallergenic makeup, which is non-irritating.

A cosmetologist should be someone who is well recognized for subtle, quality work. People whose major interest is in selling a lot of products should best be avoided. It is important to be wary of so-called rejuvenating creams and makeup preparations. Despite the investment, these will usually do nothing beyond ordinary skin cover. At worst, they can contain unknown amounts of druglike substances, often including estrogen or progesterone which are female sex hormones. It is important that any female sex hormone taken be properly regulated by a doctor. There is a risk of complications, including breast and uterine cancer. Estrogen can be absorbed through the skin and mucous membranes. Skin creams and oils with hydrocortisone and similar corticosteroids should similarly be used under the supervision of a dermatologist, or other qualified doctor. It is important that all hormonal preparations be avoided in pregnancy.

The overall goal in using makeup is to look healthy and alluring, not to look made up.

Facials are a good thing, and can be very relaxing, as well as helpful to overall appearance. It is important to be knowledgeable about the substances that are being used. Various substances that are used in facials and body massages can cause allergic reactions in some people or are caustic to the skin surface. It is important to know allergy history.

Body massage itself can be soothing and therapeutic. If there is a specific medical condition, the masseuse or masseur should know about it. If necessary, they should consult a physical therapist or sports medicine physician. There are several types of body massage. Two of the more common types are Swedish massage and Shiatsu. The preference can be pretty individual, and what is most comfortable and relaxing should be chosen.

Manicures and pedicures are commonly available. This is the good news and the bad news.

Viral and bacterial infections in the angles of nails are easily spread by instruments used from person to person without adequate sterilization. The most common virus is the wart virus which causes unsightly infections on the side of the nail which can be enormously difficult to get rid of. Also, on occasion, such infected areas can actually turn cancerous. Ideally, for manicures and pedicures, one should have their own set of instruments, or disposable instruments should be used. The fact is, relatively few people do this. It is not realistic to expect the manicurist to do adequate sterilization of instruments in between the manicures. The most effective sterilization techniques are far beyond the capability of most salons, even if they were inclined to use them.

Most people achieve adequate hair care simply by finding a hair stylist who is capable and who follows their wishes. However, in their more mature years some women are faced with thinning hair. Genetics, age and specific health problems can be the cause of this problem. Chemotherapy and radiation can cause temporary or permanent hair loss. It is important in this situation to consult with an experienced dermatologist, who is used to dealing with these conditions. Appearance can be enhanced by one of those excellent hairstylists who knows how to be creative around problem areas. In many cases of chemotherapy, the hair will simply grow back to its formerly lush state. However, where there has been radiation to the scalp, very often total regeneration will not occur. Hair transplantation can be the answer in certain selected cases. There are covering substances available through dermatologists that can camouflage areas where the scalp can show through. Examples of such covering substances are Toppik and Couvre.

Hair should not look artificial and done. It ideally should look lustrous, alluring and soft. It should not have an unnatural color. Blue hair should be left to the adolescents, who are obviously doing it for fun and for shock value.

The ultimate self-indulgence is the spa. In major urban centers in America, there are multitudinous very good day spas, where one can go, relax, and have a number of treatments including facials, massages, manicures, pedicures, herbal wraps, steam baths, saunas, and other pampering. There are also quite famous spas in America and around the world available for anywhere from a long weekend to a week or longer. There are health benefits. Relaxation, eating properly, exercise and feeling better are all good for health.

All the other supposed health benefits should be greeted with a degree of skepticism. Quasitreatments such as unproven alternative cancer therapy, that may take a person's focus away from important life saving measures, should be regarded warily.

The trimmer, the healthier and more fit someone is, the better they will look, and the less they will have to resort to cover up. They will be far more likely to be naturally attractive.

GLOSSARY
MEDICAL TERMS AND THEIR MEANING

ABSCOPAL EFFECT: Radiation given to a targeted tumor causes untreated tumors elsewhere in the body to shrink.
https://www.ncbi.nlm.nih.gov/pmc/articles/PMC6775241/

ACCOUNTABLE CARE ORGANIZATION (ACO): Medical provider organization that incentivizes cost and quality control, for example by reducing inpatient utilization and specialist referrals. Includes **Medicare Shared Savings Program (MSSP),** which sets a target cost of care for patients.

ACE INHIBITOR: Drug that inhibits the angiotensin-converting enzyme, stopping the formation of Angiotensin II which constricts blood vessels. Blood pressure is lowered, because blood vessels are opened up, and blood can flow more freely.
http://www.medicinenet.com/ace_inhibitors/article.htm
https://www.webmd.com/heart-disease/guide/medicine-ace-inhibitors#1
https://www.bmj.com/content/363/bmj.k4209

ACETYLCHOLINE: A neurotransmitter.
http://www.ncbi.nlm.nih.gov/books/NBK11143/

ACNE: Chronic skin condition characterized by seborrhea (oily secretion) and blocked follicles (comedomes) including blackheads and whiteheads that may become infected.
https://online.epocrates.com/diseases/10111/Acne-vulgaris/Key-Highlights

ACRYLAMIDE: Chemical that can form during high heat food preparation of high starch foods from the amino acid asparagine in combination with some sugars. Possible carcinogen in high doses.
https://www.cancer.gov/about-cancer/causes-prevention/risk/diet/acrylamide-fact-sheet

ADDICTION: Physiologic compulsive need for a substance, use of that substance, inability to abstain, development of tolerance to it, and distinctive withdrawal symptoms and signs. See "**Opioid**".
https://www.cdc.gov/drugoverdose/index.html

ADHESION: Abnormal union of surfaces, or fibrous tissue bands between structures.
https://www.ncbi.nlm.nih.gov/pmc/articles/PMC5295619/

ADOPTIVE CELL TRANSFER (ACT): Use of **Tumor-Infiltrating Lymphocytes (TILs)** to overcome immunosuppressive signals and eradicate cancer cells.
https://www.cancer.gov/about-cancer/treatment/types/immunotherapy

ADVANCE DIRECTIVE: Legal document that ensures one's wishes are followed in the event a person cannot make their own decisions. See: The Care of the Older Person: How do I protect my patient?: Randy S. Perskin. RMC Publishing, LLC 2018, 2019
www.careoftheolderperson.com
https://ag.ny.gov/sites/default/files/advancedirectives.pdf

AGING: Gradual loss of physiological functions accompanied by increasing risk of mortality and decreasing fertility. See: The Care of the Older Person: Introduction: Jose Morais. RMC Publishing, LLC 2018, 2019 www.careoftheolderperson.com
http://journal.frontiersin.org/article/10.3389/fgene.2016.00119/full
https://www.nature.com/articles/s41551-017-0093?WT.mc_id=EMI_NBME_1707_JULYISSUE_PORTFOLIO&spMailingID=54556746&spUserID=MTc3MDI4ODk5NQS2&spJobID=1203835636&spReportId=MTIwMzgzNTYzNgS2
https://jamanetwork.com/journals/jama/article-abstract/2703112?utm_source=silverchair&utm_medium=email&utm_campaign=article_alert-jama&utm_content=olf&utm_term=091718
https://www.frontiersin.org/articles/10.3389/fimmu.2019.01614/full?utm_source=F-AAE&utm_medium=EMLF&utm_campaign=MRK_1046250_35_Immuno_20190718_arts_A

AGONIST: Exogenous substance that goes to a cell receptor and produces a response.
https://en.wikipedia.org/wiki/Agonist

AIDS: **A**utoimmune **D**eficiency **S**yndrome: Sexually transmitted infection caused by **H**uman **I**mmunodeficiency **V**iruses HIV-1 and HIV-2 which compromise the immune system.
https://www.aids.gov/
http://www.thelancet.com/journals/lancet/article/PIIS0140-6736(14)60164-1/fulltext
https://jamanetwork.com/journals/jama/article-abstract/2703112?utm_source=silverchair&utm_medium=email&utm_campaign=article_alert-jama&utm_content=olf&utm_term=091718

https://jamanetwork.com/journals/jama/article-abstract/2678246?
utmsource=silverchair&utmmedium=email&utmcampaign=article
alert-jama&utmcontent=

AKATHISIA: A movement disorder with restlessness that may be a drug side effect. See: The Care of the Older Person: Psycho oncology: Living with the Fear of Death: Norman Straker. RMC Publishing, LLC 2018, 2019 www.careoftheolderperson.com
https://www.ncbi.nlm.nih.gov/pmc/articles/PMC1123446/

ALBUMIN: Water soluble single chain protein synthesized in liver. Present in egg white and blood serum.
http://albumin.org/properties-of-human-serum-albumin-and-albumin-atomic-coordinates/

ALDOSTERONE: Mineralocorticoid hormone from adrenal cortex. Increases blood pressure. Implication in alopecia.
https://en.wikipedia.org/wiki/Aldosterone

ALKALINE PHOSPHATASE: Immune protein enzymes that catalyze the hydrolysis of phosphate groups, freeing inorganic phosphate.
http://journal.frontiersin.org/article/10.3389/fimmu.2017.00897/full?utm_source=F-AAE&utm_medium=EMLF&utm_campaign=MRK_352999_35_Immuno_20170808_arts_A

ALLELE: One of the two forms of a gene, derived from either the mother or the father. Genes are carried on chromosomes. Chromosomes are paired, with one chromosome in each pair coming from the father, and one coming from the mother.
http://mcat-review.org/genetics.php

ALLOGRAFT: Transplant from human donor to genetically nonidentical human recipient.

http://ndt.oxfordjournals.org/content/early/2013/04/25/ndt.gft087.full.pdf

ALOPECIA: Baldness
https://www.ncbi.nlm.nih.gov/pmc/articles/PMC3149477/

ALZHEIMER'S DISEASE: AD. Common form of dementia. One characteristic is amyloid plaque deposition in the brain. See: The Care of the Older Person: Update On Alzheimer's Disease Diagnosis and Management: Serge Gauthier: Doctor, My Wife Is Getting Forgetful: Serge Gauthier: Why Does My Patient Have Gait And Balance Disorders ?: Olivier Beauchet; Incontinence In Older Adults: Samer Shamout, Lysanne Campeau, RMC Publishing, LLC 2018, 2019 www.careoftheolderperson.com
http://www.thelancet.com/journals/laneur/article/PIIS1474-4422(16)00062-4/abstract
http://www.ncbi.nlm.nih.gov/pubmed/24028956
http://www.nature.com/nature/journal/v537/n7618/full/537036a.html?WT.feed_name=subjects_neuroscience
http://www.jwatch.org/na42506/2016/10/06/new-biologic-treatment-dramatically-shrinks-plaques
https://www.ncbi.nlm.nih.gov/pubmed/27025652
http://www.nature.com/neuro/multimedia/alzheimers/index.html?WT.mc_id=BAN_NN_1612_Alzheimers
www.nature.com/neuro/multimedia/alzheimers/index.html?WT.mc_id=TOC_NN_1216_Alzheimers&spMailingID=54002625&spUserID=MTc2NTUxNjM5NAS2&spJobID=1160
https://pubs.acs.org/doi/10.1021/acschemneuro.8b00160
https://www.nature.com/articles/s41593-018-0101-9?utm_source=Springer_Nature_website&utm_medium=Website_links&utm_content=AngWan-SN-OD-Neuroscience-Global&utm_campaign=SNOR_USG_SFN18

https://www.alzheimersanddementia.com/article/S1552-5260(18)30068-2/fulltext?rss=yes
https://www.ncbi.nlm.nih.gov/pmc/articles/PMC6194148/
https://alzres.biomedcentral.com/articles/10.1186/s13195-018-0441-4
https://www.nature.com/articles/s41591-018-0311-4?WT.ec_id=NM-201901&sap-outbound-id=D7CBD8E437538AF66B20183215057C627E43F6DB
https://jamanetwork.com/journals/jamaneurology/fullarticle/2722842?guestAccessKey=94b79aa8-7c1d-45f8-9e0b-545a2484647a&utm_source=silverchair&utm_campaign=jama_network&utm_content=weekly_highlights&cmp=1&utm_medium=email
https://www.nature.com/articles/d41586-019-00879-3?WT.ec_id=NATURE-20190321&utm_source=nature_etoc&utm_medium=email&utm_campaign=20190321&sap-outbound-id=01A2C014D0D47D9CED5
https://academic.oup.com/brain/advance-article/doi/10.1093/brain/awz099/5481202

AMINO ACIDS: The building blocks of protein. Some amino acids can be synthesized in the human body. Essential amino acids must be supplied in the diet, as they cannot be synthesized in the human body.
http://www.biology.arizona.edu/biochemistry/problem_sets/aa/aa.html

AMNIOTIC FLUID: The fluid surrounding the developing fetus, contained in the amniotic sac. The thin amniotic membrane is closely applied to the inner walls of the uterus.
http://iaimjournal.com/wp-content/uploads/2014/11/9-Amniotic-fluid-derived-stem-cells.pdf

AMYLOID: Beta amyloid. Protein fragments that can clump in amorphous plaques in degenerative disease.

https://www.nia.nih.gov/alzheimers/publication/part-2-what-happens-brain-ad/hallmarks-ad
http://www.nature.com/nature/journal/v537/n7618/full/nature19323.html

AMYOTROPHIC LATERAL SCLEROSIS: Motor Neuron Disease. Characterized by degeneration of both upper and lower motor neurons leading to muscle weakness and paralysis.
https://www.nature.com/articles/550S105a
https://www.ncbi.nlm.nih.gov/pubmed/17023659
https://jamanetwork.com/journals/jama/fullarticle/2724169?guestAccessKey=cefbe6c9-c210-49d6-aca6-9ebca2eaaf86&utm_source=silverchair&utm_medium=email&utm_campaign=article_alert-jama&utm

ANASTOMOSIS: Relinking of a tubular structure so that the lumen is patent.
http://plasticsurgery.stanford.edu/education/microsurgery/intraoperative.html

ANDROGEN: The "male" sex hormones. Present in women in different amounts than in males. In men, the testicles are the main source of androgens. In women, androgens are mainly derived from the adrenal glands that sit atop the kidneys, and from the ovaries.
https://www.britannica.com/science/androgen
https://www.frontiersin.org/articles/10.3389/fimmu.2018.00794/full?utmsource=F-AAE&utmmedium=EMLF&utmcampaign=MRK63294735Immuno20180508artsA

ANDROGEN RECEPTOR ANTAGONISTS: Drugs that competitively inhibit testosterone from binding to prostate cancer cells.
http://www.nejm.org/doi/full/10.1056/NEJMra1701695?query=main_nav_lg

http://www.nejm.org/doi/full/10.1056/NEJMoa1715546?query=main_nav_lg

ANDROSTENEDIONE: A form of androgen.
https://pubchem.ncbi.nlm.nih.gov/compound/androstenedione#section=Top

ANEMIA: Deficiency of red blood cells or hemoglobin.
https://www.jwatch.org/na45561/2017/11/29/anemia-elderly-review?query=etoc_jwgenmed&jwd=000012066693&jspc=OBG

ANEURYSM: Weakening in a blood vessel wall, leading to a bulge.
http://stroke.ahajournals.org/content/44/12/3613
https://journals.lww.com/cardiologyinreview/Abstract/2016/03000/Abdominal_Aortic_Aneurysms_and_Risk_Factors_for.5.aspx
https://www.jwatch.org/na47426/2018/09/11/natural-history-small-ascending-aortic-aneurysms?query=etoc_jwcard&jwd=000012066693&jspc=OBG

ANGINA (PECTORIS): Chest pain caused by inadequate oxygenation (ischemia) of, and circulation to heart muscle, secondary to arterio-sclerotic disease in the coronary arteries which supply the heart.
https://emedicine.medscape.com/article/150215-overview

ANGIOGENESIS: New blood vessel formation.
http://www.nature.com/nrd/journal/v3/n5/full/nrd1381.html

ANGIOGRAPHY: Radiologic visualization of blood vessels after injecting them with radiopaque dye.
https://emedicine.medscape.com/article/1603072-overview

ANGIOPLASTY: The opening of a narrowed blood vessel by balloon inflation, along with stent placement to preserve patency.
http://www.ncbi.nlm.nih.gov/pubmedhealth/PMH0021296/

ANGIOTENSIN: A vasoconstricting hormone. Stimulates aldosterone release from the adrenal cortex.
http://www.ncbi.nlm.nih.gov/pubmed/8583476

ANGIOTENSIN RECEPTOR BLOCKER: **ARB**. Drug that blocks the angiotensin receptor.
http://www.ncbi.nlm.nih.gov/pmc/artichttps://www.bmj.com/content/363/bmj.k4209les/PMC4395832/

ANHEDONIA: Loss of the capacity to experience pleasure. See: The Care of the Older Person: Psycho oncology: Living with the Fear of Death: Norman Straker. RMC Publishing LLC 2018, 2019.
www.careoftheolderperson.com
https://www.medicinenet.com/script/main/art.asp?articlekey=17900

ANOREXIA: Eating disorder with self starvation and marked weight loss. The Care of the Older Person: Could My Patient Be Malnourished ?: Jose Morais. RMC Publishing, LLC 2018, 2019.
www.careoftheolderperson.com
https://jeatdisord.biomedcentral.com/articles/10.1186/s40337-015-0040-8

ANTHRAX: Serious bacterial infection caused by Bacillus Anthracis. Can be acquired cutaneously, and via the respiratory and gastrointestinal tracts.
https://www.cdc.gov/anthrax/specificgroups/health-care-providers/index.html

ANTIBIOTIC: A drug that kills or inactivates bacteria. Often works by binding and disrupting bacterial ribosomes (see "Ribosome")
http://www.nature.com/nrmicro/journal/v13/n1/full/nrmicro3380.html
http://www.nature.com/ja/journal/v67/n1/full/ja201349a.html
https://en.wikipedia.org/wiki/List_of_antibiotics

http://mdlinx.pdr.net/pharma-news/news-article.cfm/6885214/antibiotic-resistant-bacteria-star-shaped-peptide

ANTIBODY: A substance that reacts with a foreign invader (antigen) inactivating it.
https://www.ncbi.nlm.nih.gov/pmc/articles/PMC4284445/
http://www.nature.com/milestones/mileantibodies/timeline/index.html

ANTIBODY-DRUG CONJUGATES: Antibodies linked to a toxic substance, such as radioactive material, bacterial product, or chemical.
https://www.ncbi.nlm.nih.gov/pubmed/27299281
https://www.ncbi.nlm.nih.gov/pubmed/26589413
https://www.ncbi.nlm.nih.gov/pubmed/24423619

ANTIGEN: Foreign invader of the body.
http://www.annualreviews.org/doi/abs/10.1146/annurev-immunol-032712-095910

ANTIMETABOLITE: Substance that interferes with cell metabolism by inhibiting or replacing a normal metabolite. Used as chemotherapeutic agents in cancer.
http://www.ncbi.nlm.nih.gov/pubmed/23361267
http://www.slideshare.net/OribaDanLangoya/antimetabolites-in-cancer-chemotherapy-23606975

ANTIMULLERIAN HORMONE: Produced by ovarian granulosa cells. Prevents the depletion of follicles in the ovary.
http://www.ncbi.nlm.nih.gov/pubmed/22646322

ANTIOXIDANT: Substance that prevents the chemical combination of oxygen with various other substances, such as fats.

http://dspace.uni.lodz.pl:8080/xmlui/bitstream/handle/11089/17754/bartosz2.pdf?sequence=1&isAllowed=y

ANTISENSE TECHNOLOGY: Turning off genes by introducing pieces of the genetic code.
http://smart-therapeutics.com/Technology/RNAi-Antisense-Technologyb

ANXIETY: Feeling of unease that can rise to the level of panic attacks.
http://www.ajgponline.org/article/S1064-7481(16)30147-6/abstract

AORTA: The main artery from the heart to other parts of the body.
http://teachmeanatomy.info/abdomen/vasculature/arteries/aorta/

APHERESIS: Removing blood from the body for the purpose of eliminating a specific component, then reintroducing the blood into the body.
https://health.ucsd.edu/specialties/apheresis/Documents/2011%20Conventional-apheresis-therapies.pdf

APOLIPOPROTEIN E (ApoE): Protein involved in fat metabolism. A variant is a disease risk factor.
http://www.ncbi.nlm.nih.gov/pubmed/11882522
http://www.ncbi.nlm.nih.gov/pubmed/16432152

APOPTOSIS: Programmed cell death
http://www.ncbi.nlm.nih.gov/pmc/articles/PMC2117903/
https://www.ncbi.nlm.nih.gov/books/NBK26873/
http://journal.frontiersin.org/article/10.3389/fimmu.2017.00961/full?utm_source=F-AAE&utm_medium=EMLF&utm_campaign=MRK_368025_35_Immuno_20170822_arts_A
https://www.frontiersin.org/articles/10.3389/fimmu.2018.00241/full?utm_source=F-AAE&utm_medium=EMLF&utm_campaign=MRK_571163_35_I

https://www.frontiersin.org/articles/10.3389/fimmu.2018.02379/full?utm_source=F-AAE&utm_medium=EMLF&utm_campaign=MRK_812127_35_Immuno_20181030_arts_A

APPENDICITIS: Inflammation of the appendix. Can be treated by minimally invasive surgery. Incidence has possibly been lowered with antibiotic use.
http://www.bmj.com/content/357/bmj.j1703.full

APTAMER: Single stranded DNA or RNA molecule that can bind to preselected targets.
http://www.basepairbio.com/research-and-publications/what-is-an-aptamer-2/

AROMATASE INHIBITORS: The enzyme aromatase catalyzes conversion of testosterone to estradiol. Aromatase inhibitors are drugs that prevent this type of estradiol formation.
http://www.nature.com/nrc/journal/v15/n5/abs/nrc3920.html
http://erc.endocrinology-journals.org/content/20/4/R183.full

ARRHYTHMIA: (Cardiac) Abnormal beating of the heart. Includes tachycardia (abnormally fast heartbeat), bradycardia (abnormally slow heartbeat) and irregular heartbeats.
http://www.clevelandclinicmeded.com/medicalpubs/diseasemanagement/cardiology/cardiac-arrhythmias/

ART: Advanced **A**ssisted **R**eproductive **T**echnology. Techniques that enhance the ability to conceive children, including ovum and sperm retrieval, and ICSI.
http://www.cdc.gov/reproductivehealth/infertility/
http://www.hfea.gov.uk/ICSI.html

ARTERIOSCLEROSIS: Literal meaning is hardening of the arteries. In **atherosclerosis**, a common type, calcified fat deposits build up in the lining of arteries, narrowing and obstructing them.
http://www.ncbi.nlm.nih.gov/pubmed/11001066
http://bmcmedicine.biomedcentral.com/articles/10.1186/1741-7015-11-117

ARTERY: A blood vessel that usually carries oxygenated blood from the heart to other areas of the body. Exceptions are the pulmonary artery, which carries blood from the heart to the lungs for oxygenation, and the umbilical arteries in the fetus, which carry blood from the fetus to the placenta for oxygenation.
https://training.seer.cancer.gov/anatomy/cardiovascular/blood/classification.html

ARTHRITIS: A group of conditions of varying etiology characterized by inflammation in the joints.
http://www.rheumatology.org/Practice-Quality/Clinical-Support/Criteria/ACR-Endorsed-Criteria

ARTHROSCOPY: Direct visualization into the joints by minimally invasive technique.
http://www.arthroscopytechniques.org/
http://www.bmj.com/content/357/bmj.j1982

ARTIFICIAL HEART: Mechanical device that replaces the heart. **Mechanical Cardiac Support** refers to devices that assist the failing heart.
https://www.nature.com/articles/d41586-018-07197-0?WT.mc_id=EMX_NJOBS_1103_NATUREJOBSNEWSLETTER_A&WT.ec_id=EXTERNAL&spMailingID=57708268&spUserID=NjYxMzYyNDIyMjIS1&spJobID=1520347411&spReportId=MTUyMDM0NzQxMQS2

http://www.jhltonline.org/article/S1053-2498(14)00976-0/abstract

ARTIFICIAL INTELLIGENCE: Computer systems able to perform tasks normally attributable to human intelligence. These include visual perception, speech recognition, decision-making and language translation. Ideally, the computer systems would think and act humanly and rationally. Utilizes **Machine Learning** in which data is fed to a computer and statistical techniques are used to help the computer get better at a task without specifically programming it for that. **Deep Learning** is a type of machine learning that runs data inputs through multiple layers of biologically inspired neural network architecture. See **DEEP LEARNING, MACHINE LEARNING**
https://www.lexico.com/definition/artificial_intelligence
https://builtin.com/artificial-intelligence

ASBESTOS: A mined mineral formerly used for insulation and fireproofing. Fibers can be released into the air which can be responsible for asbestosis, a serious lung disease.
http://www.ncbi.nlm.nih.gov/pubmed/25444537

ASTROCYTES: Cells in the brain between neurons.
https://www.nature.com/articles/d41586-018-07197-0?WT.

ATHEROSCLEROSIS: See "Arteriosclerosis"
http://www.atherosclerosis-journal.com/

ATP: **A**denosine **Trip**hosphate: A nucleotide involved in intracellular energy transfer.
https://pubchem.ncbi.nlm.nih.gov/compound/Adenosine_triphosphate

ATROPHY: Wasting of body tissue. **SARCOPENIA** is the loss of skeletal muscle mass and function. **CACHEXIA,** which incorporates sarcopenia, is a complex metabolic wasting syndrome

associated with underlying disease, characterized by unwanted weight loss, muscle atrophy, fatigue, weakness, and loss of appetite.
https://www.ncbi.nlm.nih.gov/pubmed/22773188
https://www.ncbi.nlm.nih.gov/pmc/articles/PMC3940510/
https://www.ncbi.nlm.nih.gov/pubmed/20886766
https://www.ncbi.nlm.nih.gov/pmc/articles/PMC4269139/
https://www.ncbi.nlm.nih.gov/pmc/articles/PMC3117995/

AURA: A perceptual disturbance.
http://www.medicinenet.com/script/main/art.asp?articlekey=2395

AUTOANTIBODY: Immune protein (mainly IgM) produced by the immune system that is directed against (targets) an individual's own proteins, tissues, or organs
https://www.ncbi.nlm.nih.gov/pmc/articles/PMC2703183/
http://journal.frontiersin.org/article/10.3389/fimmu.2017.00603/full?utm_source=F-AAE&utm_medium=EMLF&utm_campaign=MRK_294450_35_Immuno_20170608_arts_A

AUTOIMMUNE DISEASES: Diseases in which the immune response is inappropriately triggered and attacks the individual's own tissues and organs. Includes systemic lupus erythematosus, rheumatoid arthritis, multiple sclerosis and Sjogren's syndrome.
http://www.nature.com/nm/journal/v21/n7/full/nm.3897.html
http://journal.frontiersin.org/article/10.3389/fimmu.2016.00587/full?utm_source=newsletter&utm_medium=email&utm_campaign=Immunology-w52-2016
http://www.clevelandclinicmeded.com/medicalpubs/diseasemanagement/rheumatology/laboratory-evaluation-rheumatic-diseases/
https://www.ncbi.nlm.nih.gov/pmc/articles/PMC4122257/

AUTOPHAGY: Intracellular degradation delivering cytoplasmic constituents to the lysosome. May have implications in anti-aging and starvation adaptation.
http://genesdev.cshlp.org/content/21/22/2861.long
http://journal.frontiersin.org/article/10.3389/fimmu.2016.00657/full?utm_source=newsletter&utm_medium=email&utm_campaign=Immunology-w1-2017

BABY SHAKING SYNDROME: Abusive head trauma. Brain tissue injury, as well as hemorrhage and edema, may result.
https://emedicine.medscape.com/article/1176849-overview

BACTERIUM: (Pleural: Bacteria) An old name for a microscopic organism that can be present in, or invade, humans. A pathogenic bacterium , or microorganism is one that causes disease.
http://www.bode-science-center.com/center/relevant-pathogens-from-a-z.html

BARIATRIC (METABOLIC) SURGERY: Weight loss surgery for selected Type 2 Diabetics and obese patients. Includes gastric binding, stomach stapling, gastric bypass, and stomach shortening sleeve gastrectomy.
https://asmbs.org/patients/bariatric-surgery-procedures

BASAL GANGLIA: Region at the base of the brain with clusters of neurons including the caudate nucleus, putamen, and globus pallidus.
http://webspace.ship.edu/cgboer/basalganglia.html
https://nba.uth.tmc.edu/neuroscience/m/s3/chapter04.html

BASE PAIR: Two (out of four) **nucleic acid bases** on a rung of the spiral ladder of **DNA**. The four nucleic acids involved are adenine

(**A**), cytosine (**C**), guanine (**G**), and thymine (**T**). They code the sequences of amino acids that, in turn, make up the proteins.
http://www.dictionary.com/browse/base-pair

BETA BLOCKER: A drug that lowers blood pressure by taking up the receptor sites that control blood pressure.
http://www.medicinenet.com/beta_blockers/article.htm

BETA CAROTENE: An antioxidant. Precursor of Vitamin A.
http://www.medicalnewstoday.com/articles/252758.php

BILE ACID SEQUESTRANT: Drug that binds bile acids in the intestine, so that they are excreted.
http://www.medicinenet.com/bile_acid_sequestrants/article.htm

BIOENGINEERING: Rearranging DNA. Manufacturing recombinant DNA.
http://www.mdpi.com/journal/bioengineering

BIOFEEDBACK: Training to acquire voluntary control of a body function, such as heart rate.
http://www.ncbi.nlm.nih.gov/pubmedhealth/PMH0070200/

BIORHYTHM: Cyclic pattern of activity; recurring biologic process. See **Circadian Rhythm**

BIOSIMILAR: Product that is highly similar to an approved biologic product
http://www.fda.gov/Drugs/DevelopmentApprovalProcess/HowDrugsareDevelopedandApproved/ApprovalApplications/TherapeuticBiologicApplications/Biosimilars/default.htm
http://jamanetwork.com/journals/jama/fullarticle/2590051
http://jamanetwork.com/journals/jama/article-abstract/2590049

BISPHOSPHONATES: Class of drugs that prevent loss of bone mass by inhibiting bone resorption by blocking osteoclasts. http://www.bmj.com/content/351/bmj.h3783

BLEPHAROPLASTY: Cosmetic eyelid surgery. https://www.ncbi.nlm.nih.gov/pmc/articles/PMC2840922/

BLOCKCHAIN TECHNOLOGY in HEALTHCARE: Interoperable platform that memorializes every event or step ("Block") in a data stream, or chain. Implications in personalized medicine, research, and appropriate healthcare data sharing with enhanced security. http://bulletin.facs.org/2017/12/blockchain-technology-in-health-care-a-primer-for-surgeons/#.WlezLK6nHX4

BODY MASS INDEX: BMI. A calculation of body fat. Weight (kilograms) divided by height (meters squared). The Care of the Older Person: Could My Patient Be Malnourished?: Jose Morais . RMC Publishing, LLC 2018, 2019 www.careoftheolderperson.com

BONE DENSITY: Measurement of Calcium and other minerals in bone.
http://www.ncbi.nlm.nih.gov/pmc/articles/PMC2685234/

BONE DENSITY SCAN: Low exposure Xray to measure bone density. https://www.bones.nih.gov/health-info/bone/bone-health/bone-mass-measurement-what-numbers-mean

BONE SCAN: NUCLEAR: Imaging bone after radiotracer uptake to identify tumors, usually metastatic.
https://www.ncbi.nlm.nih.gov/pmc/articles/PMC4553252/

BOTOX: **Bo**tulinum **tox**in type A. Inhibits acetylcholine release. http://www.ncbi.nlm.nih.gov/pmc/articles/PMC2856357/

BRCA GENES: **Br**east **Ca**ncer Genes 1 and 2. Inherited mutations that predispose to breast and ovarian cancer. BRCA1 may increase risk of endometrial cancer as well.
http://oncology.jamanetwork.com/article.aspx?articleid=2531470
https://www.sgo.org/wp-content/uploads/2016/10/2016-SGO-Genetics-Toolkit3.pdf https://jamanetwork.com/journals/jama/fullarticle/2748515?guestAccessKey=99eb27c0-0cd5-45e6-870f-b8251b23d4be&utm_source=silverchair&utm_medium=email&utm_campaign=article_alert&utm_content=etoc&utm_term=082019

BREAST CANCER: Malignant tumor in breast tissue.
http://www.jwatch.org/na44519/2017/07/06/asco-2017-report-breast-cancer?query=topic_breastcan&jwd=000012066693&jspc=OBG
https://www.acog.org/-/media/Practice-Bulletins/Committee-on-Practice-Bulletins----Gynecology/Public/pb179.pdf?dmc=1&ts=20170710T0228314803
https://tools.bcsc-scc.org/BC5yearRisk/intro.htm
https://insights.ovid.com/crossref?an=00006250-201709000-00035
https://www.partnershipagainstcancer.ca/wp-content/uploads/2019/05/Breast-Cancer-Surgery-Standards-EN-April-2019.pdf

BRONCHITIS: Inflammation of the bronchial passages.
https://www.ncbi.nlm.nih.gov/pubmed/23204254

BULEMIA: Eating disorder. Food consumption followed by self-induced vomiting.
https://www.ncbi.nlm.nih.gov/pmc/articles/PMC2927890/

BUNDLE BRANCH BLOCK: Delay in the pathway of electrical impulses to the left or right ventricle of the heart, resulting in a delay of contraction of that ventricle.
http://www.acc.org/latest-in-cardiology/journal-scans/2016/08/05/11/45/effect-of-the-antihypertensive-and-lipid-lowering-treatment?w_nav=LC

CANCER: Malignant tumor (growth). The hallmark of cancer is its ability to invade normal tissue. Cancer can often metastasize, spreading to distant areas in the body. It is likely to recur even though it has been removed or destroyed at its initial (primary) site. The Care of the Older Person: Cancer in Older Adults: Doreen Wan-Chow-Wah, Cancer Screening in the Older Adult: Catalina Hernandez-Torres, Tina Hsu. RMC Publishing, LLC 2018, 2019
www.careoftheolderperson.com
http://www.cell.com/cell/fulltext/S0092-8674(18)3032-7
http://www.cell.com/pb-assets/consortium/pancanceratlas/pancan/index.html
https://www.cancer.gov/about-cancer/treatment/types/targeted-therapies/targeted-therapies-fact-sheet
https://cancerstaging.org/About/news/Pages/-Cancer-Staging-Manual,-Eighth-Edition,-Just-Released-by-American-Joint-Committee-on-Cancer-(AJCC).aspx
http://www.jcso-ejournal.com/jcso/november_2016?pg=34#pg34
http://journal.frontiersin.org/article/10.3389/fimmu.2017.00374/full?utm_source=F-AAE&utm_medium=EMLF&utm_campaign=MRK_243180_20170411_arts
https://www.nature.com/articles/s41551-017-0067?WT.mc_id=EMI_NBME_1704_APRILISSUE_PORTFOLIO&spMailingID=53957850&spUserID=MTc3MDI4ODk5NQ
http://stm.sciencemag.org/content/9/400/eaan2966

http://science.sciencemag.org/content/early/2018/01/17/science.aar3247
https://www.empr.com/home/news/
fda-approves-tumor-agnostic-oral-cancer-therapy-vitrakvi/
https://www.nature.com/articles/d41586-018-07602-8?utm_source=
briefing-
https://www.nature.com/articles/d41586-018-07602-
8?utm_source=briefing-dy&utm_medium=email&utm_
campaign=briefing&utm_content=20181206dy&utm_
medium=email&utm_campaign=briefing&utm_content=20181206
https://www.frontiersin.org/articles/10.3389/fimmu.2019.00467/
full?utm_source=F-AAE&utm_medium=EMLF&utm_
campaign=MRK_943967_35_Immuno_20190326_arts_A
https://www.frontiersin.org/articles/10.3389/fimmu.2019.00467/
full?utm_source=F-AAE&utm_medium=EMLF&utm_
campaign=MRK_943967_35_Immuno_20190326_arts_A

CANCER MARKER: Substances produced by tumor cells or by other cells in response to a tumor. See: Tumor Specific Antigen (TSA).
https://www.nature.com/articles/s41551-017-0065?WT.mc_id=
EMI_NBME_1704_APRILISSUE_
PORTFOLIO&spMailingID=53957850&spUserID=MTc3MDI4ODk5NQS

CANNABIS: Plant from which cannabinoids are obtained. Tetrahydrocannabinol (THC) is the principal psychoactive compound.
https://medicalmarijuana.procon.org/view.resource.
php?resourceID=000141
https://www.ncbi.nlm.nih.gov/pubmed/16463612
https://www.frontiersin.org/articles/10.3389/fimmu.2018.02009/
full?utm_source=F-AAE&utm_medium=EMLF&utm_
campaign=MRK_779779_35_Immuno_20180927_arts_A
https://www.empr.com/drugs-in-the-pipeline/cannabidiol-
cbd-ischemia-reperfusion-injury-organ-transplantation-

revive-therapeutics-orphan-drug/article/813111/?utm_source=newsletter&utm_medium=email&utm_campaign=mpr-dailydose-cp-20181109&cpn=obg
https://pubchem.ncbi.nlm.nih.gov/compound/cannabidiol#section=Substances-by-Category
https://jamanetwork.com/journals/jamanetworkopen/fullarticle/2716990?utm_source=silverchair&utm_medium=email&utm_campaign=article_alert-jamanetworkopen&utm_content=olf&utm_term=113018
https://www.empr.com/features/medical-marijuana-clinical-practice-geriatric-pain-insomnia-elderly/article/815102/?utm_source=newsletter&utm_medium=email&utm_campaign=mpr-dailydose-cp-201812

CANNABIS WITHDRAWAL SYNDROME: Can include irritability, hostility, nervousness, anxiety, sleeplessness, restlessness, appetite loss, depression, shakiness, tremors, sweating, fever, headaches.
https://www.mailman.columbia.edu/public-health-now/news/more-one-ten-heavy-cannabis-users-experience-withdrawal-after-quitting-cannabis

CARBOHYDRATE: Simple and complex sugars that are the energy source for the body. Excess carbohydrate can be converted to fat for storage.
http://www.fao.org/docrep/w8079e/w8079e0h.htm

CARCINOGEN: Substance or radiation that predisposes to cancer.
http://mdlinx.pdr.net/internal-medicine/news-article.cfm/6931990/?utm_source=in-house&utm_medium=message&utm_campaign=mh-im-nov16
https://en.wikipedia.org/wiki/Carcinogen

CARPAL TUNNEL SYNDROME: CTS: Restriction of the median nerve by the transverse carpal ligament at the wrist resulting in compression neuropathy.
https://www.ncbi.nlm.nih.gov/pmc/articles/PMC3314870/

CAR-T: Chimeric **A**ntigen **R**eceptor **T**-Cell therapy: T-cells genetically modified to enhance tumor destruction.
https://www.cancer.gov/about-cancer/treatment/research/car-t-cells
http://www.nejm.org/doi/full/10.1056/nejmoa1407222#t=article
https://jhoonline.biomedcentral.com/articles/10.1186/s13045-017-0423-1
www.empr.com/news/first-gene-therapy-antigen-receptor-t-cell-acute-lymphoblastic-leukemia/article/685222/?DCMP=EMC-MPR_DailyDose_cp_20170830&cpn=obgyn_all
https://jamanetwork.com/journals/jama/fullarticle/2664338?utm_source=silverchair&utm_medium=email&utm_campaign=article_alert-jama&utm_content=olf&utm_term
The Promise and Challenges of CAR-T Gene Therapy | Genetics and Genomics | JAMA | The JAMA Network

CAT SCAN: Computerized Axial Tomography. An advanced, computerized imaging technique that very quickly takes serial Xrays through the body in thin "slices", so that very small abnormalities can be found. With a helical (spiral) three dimensional CAT scan the Xray tube revolves around the patient. A four dimensional CAT scan takes multiple images during phases of the breathing cycle, particularly useful in cases of lung tumors that have to be precisely localized and that move with respiration. The fourth dimension is Time.
https://radiopaedia.org/articles/computed-tomography
http://www.jwatch.org/na43480/2017/03/16/radiation-exposure-and-cancer-risk-low-dose-ct-lung-cancer?query=etoc_jwgenmed&jwd=000012066693&jspc=OBG

CATALYST: A substance that facilitates a chemical reaction without being changed by that reaction.

CATARACT: Clouding, loss of transparency, of the lens of the eye. http://www.webmd.com/eye-health/cataracts/extracapsular-surgery-for-cataracts

CAUTERY: **(Electrocautery**) Surgical destruction of tissue by direct current heating. **Electrosurgery** utilizes radio frequency (RF) alternating current to heat tissue.
https://en.wikipedia.org/wiki/Electrosurgery

CELL: The basic living microscopic structure in the human body. Each cell is surrounded by a cell membrane. Cells generally have a center, the nucleus, which is itself surrounded by a membrane. The nucleus contains the chromosomes, on which rest the genes.
https://en.wikipedia.org/wiki/Cell_(biology)

CEREBROVASCULAR ACCIDENT: See "**Stroke**"

CERVICAL CANCER: Cancer of the uterine cervix. Most often caused by specific Types of sexually transmitted Human Papilloma Virus (**HPV**), which can also cause **carcinoma of the penis**. Largely preventable by **vaccines**.
https://www.ncbi.nlm.nih.gov/pubmed/12120445
https://www.cancer.gov/about-cancer/causes-prevention/risk/infectious-agents/hpv-vaccine-fact-sheet
https://emedicine.medscape.com/article/2006486-overview

CERVIX: The mouth, or neck, of the uterus, projecting through the vaginal vault. Its opening is the cervical os.
http://www.obgyn.net/gynecological-oncology/identifying-squamous-cancer-colposcopy

CHECKPOINT: T-lymphocyte locus that can shut off T-cell and suppress the immune response. (See T-lymphocyte)
http://www.cgen.com/focus-areas/immuno-oncology/immune-checkpoints
http://journal.frontiersin.org/article/10.3389/fimmu.2017.00692/full?utm_source=F-AAE&utm_medium=EMLF&utm_campaign=MRK_307979_35_Immuno_20170622_arts_A

CHECKPOINT INHIBITOR:(Immune Checkpoint Inhibitor, ICI) Drug that blocks a checkpoint, allowing T-lymphocyte to respond to malignant cell. Ref: Pardoll, Drew: Nature Reviews Cancer 12, 252-264 (April 2012)
http://blog.dana-farber.org/insight/2015/09/what-is-a-checkpoint-inhibitor/
http://ascopubs.org/doi/full/10.1200/JCO.2017.74.6065
http://jamanetwork.com/journals/jama/fullarticle/2653953?amp;utm source=JAMAPublishAheadofPrint&utm_campaign=08-09-2017
http://ard.bmj.com/content/76/10/1747

CHIMERA: A single organism composed of cells from different zygotes. A **chimeric gene** combines portions of different coding sequences to produce a new gene.
https://en.wikipedia.org/wiki/Chimeric_gene

CHIP: Clonal **H**ematopoiesis of **I**ndeterminate **P**otential: Acquired mutations in hematopoietic stem cells that accumulate in bone marrow, associated with an increased risk of heart attack and stroke.
https://www.ncbi.nlm.nih.gov/pmc/articles/PMC4961884/
http://www.nejm.org/doi/full/10.1056/NEJMoa1701719

CHOLESTEROL: Normally occurring lipoproteins in the body. If cholesterol levels, and levels of low density lipoprotein (LDL) are too high, atherosclerosis can result.
http://emedicine.medscape.com/article/121187-overview https://www.ahajournals.org/doi/pdf/10.1161/CIR.0000000000000625
https://www.ahajournals.org/doi/10.1161/CIR.0000000000000625

CHOLESTEROL INHIBITOR: Drug that inhibits the intestine from absorbing cholesterol.
http://www.health.harvard.edu/blog/pcsk9-inhibitors-a-major-advance-in-cholesterol-lowering-drug-therapy-201503157801

CHORIONIC VILLI: Microscopic projections from the placenta in which fetal blood circulates.
https://en.wikipedia.org/wiki/Chorionic_villus_sampling

CHROMATIN: The protein (**histone**)/DNA complex in the cell nucleus that forms the chromosome.
https://en.wikipedia.org/wiki/Chromatin
http://www.nature.com/news/plot-a-course-through-the-genome-1.22553?WT.ec_id=NATURE-20170907&spMailingID=54864391&spUserID=MjA1NjIyNjc4OAS2&spJobID=1244089361&spReportId=MTI0NDA4OTM2MQS2

CHROMOSOME: An elongated, stringlike structure in the nucleus of the cell that carries the genes. There are forty six chromosomes in each cell, arranged in twenty three pairs. One of each pair is originally derived from the mother, and one from the father.
https://www.genome.gov/26524120/chromosomes-fact-sheet/

CILIA: Tiny hairlike projections on cells.

CIRCADIAN RHYTHM: Biologic process that exhibits endogenous circadian (24 hour, diurnal) cycle. Can be influenced by external factors.
https://www.ncbi.nlm.nih.gov/pmc/articles/PMC4353305/
https://en.wikipedia.org/wiki/Circadian_rhythm

CIRRHOSIS: Chronic degeneration of liver cells accompanied by fibrous scarring of the liver.
https://www.niddk.nih.gov/health-information/health-topics/liver-disease/cirrhosis/Pages/facts.aspx

CLAUDICATION: Pain in the legs, or arms, after exercising, usually a symptom of peripheral arterial disease. See: **peripheral artery disease**.
https://www.mayoclinic.org/diseases-conditions/claudication/symptoms-causes/syc-20370952

CLITORIS: The erectile organ above the urethral orifice at the entrance to the vagina.
https://www.ncbi.nlm.nih.gov/pubmed/23169570

CLONE: An exact genetic copy. An identical twin is a clone because the fertilized egg splits in two. A fraternal twin is not a clone because two different eggs, fertilized by two different sperm develop in the uterus at the same time.
https://www.genome.gov/25020028/cloning-fact-sheet/
http://www.cell.com/cell/fulltext/S0092-8674(18)30057-6

COCHLEAR IMPLANT: Medical device that replaces the function of the inner ear, sends signals to the brain via the auditory nerve.
https://www.nidcd.nih.gov/health/cochlear-implants

CODON (TRIPLET): Sequence of three consecutive nucleotides. Part of the genetic code. There are sixty-four codons. Sixty-one code for specific amino acids. The other three codons are stop signals.

See: **Nucleotide** https://www.genome.gov/genetics-glossary/Codon?id=36

COGNITION: Conscious mental activities of thinking, learning, understanding and remembering.
https://www.sciencedaily.com/releases/2016/09/160909095045.htm
http://psychcentral.com/lib/in-depth-cognitive-behavioral-therapy/
https://www.mdlinx.com/family-medicine/medical-news-article/2016/12/13/coffee-chlorogenic-acid-vascular-phenolics-flow-mediated-dilatation-fmd-/6965864/?category=last-month&page_id=1
http://journal.frontiersin.org/article/10.3389/fimmu.2017.01101/full?utm_source=F-AAE&utm_medium=EMLF&utm_campaign=MRK_398354_35_Immuno_20170921_arts_A

COGNITIVE IMPAIRMENT: Mild Cognitive Impairment (**MCI**) is a dysfunction of conscious mental activities with minimal impairment of the instrumental activities of daily life (IADL). In Amnestic MCI memory dysfunction predominates. There can be progression to **Dementia.** The Care of the Older Person: "Doctor, my wife is getting forgetful": Serge Gauthier ; Management of older patients in the Emergency Department: Cyrille Launay ; Assessment of decision-making capacity: Catherine Ferrier. RMC Publishing, LLC 2018, 2019 www.careoftheolderperson.com
http://n.neurology.org/content/90/3/126
http://n.neurology.org/content/90/13/e1158
https://academic.oup.com/brain/article/141/3/877/4818093

COLON, COLORECTAL CANCER: Cancer of the large intestine and rectum. Detectable at precancerous and early stage by colonoscopy and biopsy. Cancer markers can be used in screening.
https://www.ncbi.nlm.nih.gov/pubmed/26151224

https://emedicine.medscape.com/article/1948929-overview
https://cancerstaging.org/references-tools/quickreferences/Documents/ColonMedium.pdf
https://www.cancer.org/cancer/colon-rectal-cancer/detection-diagnosis-staging/how-diagnosed.html
https://gi.org/guideline/colorectal-cancer-screening-recommendations-for-physicians-and-patients-from-the-u-s-multi-society-task-force-on-colorectal-cancer/
https://annals.org/aim/article-abstract/2726664/performance-characteristics-fecal-immunochemical-tests-colorectal-cancer-advanced-adenomatous-polyps
https://www.asco.org/practice-guidelines/quality-guidelines/guidelines/resource-stratified#/3494
https://www.asco.org/practice-guidelines/quality-guidelines/guidelines/resource-stratified#/34946

COLONOSCOPY: Direct inspection of the entire large intestine with a flexible fiberoptic instrument called a colonoscope.
http://www.asge.org/assets/0/71328/9cf71f1d-ef18-4a34-9259-31f487a6213c.pdf

COLOR FLOW DOPPLER: Ultrasound with color coding of blood flow velocity and direction. Doppler effect refers to the measurable difference in sound as it moves away.
https://123sonography.com/content/1821-principles-color-doppler

COMA: Deep, unarousable unconsciousness
https://www.medicinenet.com/script/main/art.asp?articlekey=2803
https://www.ncbi.nlm.nih.gov/pubmed/19001840

CONCUSSION: Traumatic injury to the brain.
https://www.cdc.gov/headsup/basics/concussion_whatis.html
https://www.cdc.gov/traumaticbraininjury/severe.html

https://www.fda.gov/NewsEvents/Newsroom/PressAnnouncements/ucm596531.htm

CONSCIOUSNESS: Awareness.
https://bmcneurosci.biomedcentral.com/articles/10.1186/1471-2202-5-42
https://plato.stanford.edu/entries/consciousness-neuroscience/

CORD BLOOD: Fetal blood in the umbilical cord. Can be banked in order to retrieve stem cells.
http://www.acog.org/Resources-And-Publications/Committee-Opinions/Committee-on-Genetics/Umbilical-Cord-Blood-Banking

COX-1 INHIBITOR: Drugs including aspirin, ibuprofen, and Naprosyn are both COX-1 and COX-2 inhibitors, inhibiting cyclooxygenase-I as well as cyclooxygenase 2.
http://www.ncbi.nlm.nih.gov/pubmed/11566042

COX-2 INHIBITOR: Non-steroidal anti-inflammatory drugs (NSAID's). These drugs target cyclooxygenase-2 (COX-2) enzyme that encourages prostaglandin production, leading to inflammation and pain.
http://journal.frontiersin.org/article/10.3389/fimmu.2016.00375/full?utm_source=newsletter&utm_medium=email&utm_campaign=Immunology-w40-2016

C-REACTIVE PROTEIN: CRP. Plasma protein with increased concentration in the presence of inflammatory disorders. The Care of the Older Person: Could My Patient be Malnourished?: Jose Morais RMC Publishing, LLC 2018, 2019 www.careoftheolderperson.com
https://www.frontiersin.org/articles/10.3389/fimmu.2018.02745/full?utm_source=F-AAE&utm_medium=EMLF&utm_campaign=MRK_838932_35_Immuno_20181129_arts_A.

CRISP R: **C**lustered **R**egularly **I**nterspaced **S**hort **P**alindromic **R**epeats: DNA sequences found in genomes of bacteria. Segments of prokaryocytic DNA containing repetitions of base sequences, followed by segments of spacer DNA. Used in **genome editing**. Useful in detecting viral infection.
https://www.empr.com/news/vitrakvi-larotrectinib-advanced-solid-tumors-ntrk-gene-fusion-approval/article/816725/?utm_source=newsletter&utm_medium=email&utm_campaign=mpr-dailydose-cp-20181129&cpn=obgyn_all,obgyn_md,cambia_august201&hm
https://www.nature.com/articles/d41586-019-00601-3?WT.ec_id=NATURE-20190228&utm_source=nature_etoc&utm_medium=email&utm_campaign=20190228&sap-outbound-id=F3F53CF91C70386022609FDF29CEFA2072F7C0D6

CRISPR-Cas9: Complex of RNA and protein (nucleases): Recognizes sequence of bases in target gene. Cas9 (an enzyme) unwinds double helix. CRISPR RNA sequence binds to target. Cas9 cuts both strands of target DNA. In a modification, DNA sequences are not cut: the Cas9 enzyme carries a molecular switch that turns on target genes.
http://www.ncbi.nlm.nih.gov/pmc/articles/PMC4786927/
http://link.springer.com/article/10.1186/s12977-016-0270-0?view=classic
https://www.nature.com/articles/d41586-019-01824-0?WT.ec_id=NATURE-201906&sap-outbound-id=D57BDD0F2FB94BAE156838EBF274B4C29D863CA1&mkt-key=005056B0331B1ED782E8AD53A869855D
http://www.bloomberg.com/features/2016-how-crispr-will-change-the-world/
http://jamanetwork.com/journals/jama/article-abstract/2600454

https://en.wikipedia.org/wiki/CRISPR
http://journal.frontiersin.org/article/10.3389/fimmu.2016.00375/full?utm_source=newsletter&utm_medium=email&utm_campaign=Immunology-w40-2016
https://www.technologyreview.com/s/608350/first-human-embryos-edited-in-us/
http://jamanetwork.com/journals/jama/fullarticle/2646800?utm_medium=alert&utm_source=JAMAPublishAheadofPrint&utm_campaign=10-08-2017
https://www.nature.com/news/crispr-hacks-enable-pinpoint-repairs-to-genome-1.22884?WT.ec_id=NATURE-20171026&spMailingID=55217903&spUserID=MjA1
https://www.ncbi.nlm.nih.gov/pubmed/27052831
http://www.cell.com/cell/fulltext/S0092-8674(17)31247-3
https://www.extremetech.com/extreme/281232-chinese-scientist-reportedly-creates-genetically-engineered-babies-immune-to-hiv
https://www.technologyreview.com/s/612458/exclusive-chinese-scientists-are-creating-crispr-babies/amp/

CRYOSURGERY: Surgical destruction of tissue by freezing.
http://emedicine.medscape.com/article/1125851-overview

CUL DE SAC: Rectouterine peritoneal pouch between the posterior wall of the uterus and the rectum.
https://en.wikipedia.org/wiki/Recto-uterine_pouch

CYBERNETICS: Control and communication with living tissue, as with a chip implanted in a muscle.
http://www.asc-cybernetics.org/foundations/definitions.htm

CYST: A fluid-filled growth (tumor). May be benign or malignant.
https://www.ncbi.nlm.nih.gov/pubmed/21845969
http://www.pathologyoutlines.com/topic/ovarytumorwhoclassif.html

CYSTOCELE: Bulge of the urinary bladder into the anterior wall of the vagina.
https://www.niddk.nih.gov/health-information/health-topics/urologic-disease/cystocele/Pages/facts.aspx

CYSTOSCOPE: Operating telescope used to visualize the interior of the urinary bladder and the ureteral orifices. P. 237, 238. See : The Care of the Older Person: Incontinence in Older Adults : Samer Shamout, Lysanne Campeau. RMC Publishing, LLC 2018, 2019
www.careoftheolderperson.com
https://www.ncbi.nlm.nih.gov/pmc/articles/PMC4457046/
https://en.wikipedia.org/wiki/Cystoscopy

CYTOKINE: Factor released by a cell that has an effect on other cells. Implications in aging.
http://www.ncbi.nlm.nih.gov/pmc/articles/PMC2785020/
http://journal.frontiersin.org/article/10.3389/fimmu.2017.00930/full?utm_source=F-AAE&utm_medium=EMLF&utm_campaign=MRK_352999_35_Immuno_20170808_arts_A
https://www.frontiersin.org/articles/10.3389/fimmu.2018.00422/full?utm_source=F-AAE&utm_medium=EMLF&utm_campaign=MRK_571163_35_I
https://www.frontiersin.org/articles/10.3389/fimmu.2018.00586/full?utm_source=F-AAE&utm_medium=EMLF&utm_campaign=MRK_608868_35_I
https://www.frontiersin.org/articles/10.3389/fimmu.2019.00480/full?utm_source=F-AAE&utm_medium=EMLF&utm_campaign=MRK_943967_35_Immuno_20190326_arts_A

CYTOPLASM: The contents of a cell outside the nucleus.
https://en.wikipedia.org/wiki/Cytoplasm

D-DIMER: Fibrin degradation product of blood clot degraded by fibrinolysis that can be detected in blood after a pulmonary embolus (blood clot in the lung). Reference values are adjusted for age. https://www.google.com/search?q=d-dimer+definition+medical&rlz=1C1EJFA_enUS783US783&oq=d-dimer+definition+&aqs=chrome.1.69i57j0l5.64272j0j4&sourceid=chrome&ie=UTF-8

DEEP LEARNING: Deep neural network model. Machine learning technique analyzing large amounts of data, enabling prediction of outcomes (prognosis) when new data is presented. May be used to predict cardiovascular disease risk by observation of the eye retina, and to help clarify psychiatric diagnosis.
https://arxiv.org/abs/1708.09843
https://en.wikipedia.org/wiki/Deep_learning https://www.nature.com/articles/s41746-018-0029-1 https://jamanetwork.com/journals/jamapsychiatry/article-abstract/2664960https://jamanetwork.com/journals/jamapsychiatry/article-abstract/2664960

DELIRIUM: Confusional state with altered attention and awareness. See: The Care of the Older Person: How to Diagnose and Manage Delirium: Haibin Yin. RMC Publishing, LLC 2018, 2019
www.careoftheolderperson.com
https://www.ncbi.nlm.nih.gov/pubmed/25300023
https://www.uptodate.com/contents/diagnosis-of-delirium-and-confusional-states

DELIVERY: The birth of the baby as it exits the birth canal.

DEMENTIA: Loss of cognitive functioning. Frontotemporal Dementia refers to a heterogenous group of conditions. See: The Care of the Older Person: Dementia: "Doctor, My Wife is Getting

Forgetful": Serge Gauthier; How do I protect my patient? Randy S. Perskin. RMC Publishing, LLC 2018, 2019 www.careoftheolderperson.com
http://www.ncbi.nlm.nih.gov/pmc/articles/PMC2211335/
http://www.bmj.com/content/347/bmj.f4827
https://www.jwatch.org/na45523/2017/12/05/healthy-life-healthy-brain-lifestyle-factors-and-dementia?query=etoc_jwneuro&jwd=000012066693&jspc=OBG
http://n.neurology.org/content/90/3/126
http://geropsychiatriceducation.vch.ca/docs/edu-downloads/depression/cornell_scale_depression.pdfhttps://jnnp.bmj.com/content/early/2018/08/26/jnnp-2018-318650
https://www.bmj.com/content/361/bmj.k1315
https://www.jwatch.org/na48784/2019/04/16/revisiting-plasma-total-tau-levels-dementia-biomarker?query=etoc_jwneuro&jwd=000012066693&jspc=OBG

DEMOGRAPHY: The study of groups of people and their environment.
http://www.pewresearch.org/fact-tank/2016/03/31/10-demographic-trends-that-are-shaping-the-u-s-and-the-world/

DEPRESSION: Depressive disorder marked by prolonged sadness, mood alteration, often with feelings of loss, anger and frustration. See: The Care of the Older Person: An Overview of Late-Life Depression: Artin Mahdanian, Silvia Monti De Flores. RMC Publishing, LLC 2018, 2019 www.careoftheolderperson.com
http://www.ncbi.nlm.nih.gov/pmc/articles/PMC2922383/
http://geropsychiatriceducation.vch.ca/docs/edu-downloads/depression/cornell_scale_depression.pdf https://ajp.psychiatryonline.org/doi/10.1176/appi.ajp.2018.17060595

DERMABRASION: Surgical procedure to remove skin imperfections by abrading the skin surface.
https://ajp.psychiatryonline.org/doi/10.1176/appi.ajp.2018.17060595
http://emedicine.medscape.com/article/1297069-treatment

DETRUSOR MUSCLE: Muscular coat of the urinary bladder. See: The Care of the Older Person : Incontinence In Older Adults : Samer Shamout, Lysanne Campeau. RMC Publishing, LLC 2018, 2019
www.careoftheolderperson.com
http://emedicine.medscape.com/article/1949017-overview

DHEA: **Dehydroepiandrosterone**. Androgenic steroid hormone secreted largely by adrenal cortex.
https://en.wikipedia.org/wiki/Dehydroepiandrosterone

DIABETES MELLITUS: Chronic disease characterized by abnormally high blood glucose levels. See: The Care of the Older Person: How to manage type 2 diabetes in frail elderly patients : Young-Sang Kim, Jose Morais; Could My Patient Be Malnourished? : Jose Morais ; Frailty : Sathya Karunananthan, Howard Bergman ; Polypharmacy And Deprescribing In The Elderly : Louise Mallet. RMC Publishing, LLC 2018, 2019 www.careoftheolderperson.com
http://www.merckmanuals.com/professional/endocrine-and-metabolic-disorders/diabetes-mellitus-and-disorders-of-carbohydrate-metabolism/diabetes-mellitus-dm
http://www.onlinejacc.org/content/early/2018/11/23/j.jacc.2018.09.020

DIASTASIS RECTI: Widening of the linea alba ("white line") with separation of the rectus abdominis ("ABS") muscles
https://www.ncbi.nlm.nih.gov/pmc/articles/PMC5715079/
https://radiopaedia.org/articles/linea-alba
https://www.ncbi.nlm.nih.gov/pmc/articles/PMC3649122/

DIET: Food intake. See: The Care of the Older Person: Could My Patient Be Malnourished?: Jose Morais. RMC Publishing, LLC 2018, 2019 www.careoftheolderperson.com
http://www.pubfacts.com/detail/27465379/Relation-between-mealtime-distribution-of-protein-intake-and-lean-mass-loss-in-free-living-older-adu
http://jamanetwork.com/journals/jama/fullarticle/2636710
https://www.nature.com/articles/s41398-018-0293-5

DISEASE: Aberrant state of morphology or pathophysiology Boudreau, JD, Cassell, EJ, Fuks, A: Physicianship and the Rebirth of Medical Education. Oxford University Press 2018

DIURETIC: Drug that causes increased passage of fluid by the kidneys. See: The Care of the Older Person: Polypharmacy And Deprescribing In The Elderly: Louise Mallet; Incontinence In Older Adults: Samer Shamout , Louise Campeau. RMC Publishing, LLC 2018, 2019 www.careoftheolderperson.com
http://emedicine.medscape.com/article/2145340-overview

DNA: Deoxyribonucleic acid. DNA makes up the chromosomes that carry the genes. DNA is arranged in a distinctive double helix, three dimensional pattern. It resembles a tight spiral staircase, with rungs (steps) each of which holds two (out of four) nucleic acid bases, called **base pairs**.
https://www.genome.gov/25520880/deoxyribonucleic-acid-dna-fact-sheet/

DNA MICROARRAY: DNA Biochip. Collection of microscopic DNA spots on a surface. Used to measure gene expression patterns.
https://www.genome.gov/10000533/dna-microarray-technology/

DNA MISMATCH REPAIR: During DNA replication, erroneous insertion, deletion and misincorporation of bases can occur in the

daughter DNA strand. Such errors can also occur during DNA recombination. DNA Mismatch Repair involves the recognition and correction of these abnormalities.
https://en.wikipedia.org/wiki/DNA_mismatch_repair
https://jamanetwork.com/journals/jamasurgery/article-abstract/2647248?utm_medium=alert&utm_source=JAMA+SurgLatestIssue&utm_campaign=15-11-2017
https://www.nature.com/scitable/topicpage/dna-is-constantly-changing-through-the-process-6524876

DNA PROBE: A highly specific test to detect the DNA of an individual, or a virus. It is used to detect the human papilloma virus (HPV) that is the usual causative organism of cancer of the cervix. The test is used in the criminal investigation of rape, and in identification. An individual male can be identified by the distinctive DNA in his sperm.
http://www.nature.com/subjects/dna-probesv

DOPAMINE: A neurotransmitter.
http://www.dictionary.com/browse/dopamine

DUODENUM: First part of the small intestine after the stomach.
http://emedicine.medscape.com/article/1948951-overview

DYSKINESIA: Abnormality of voluntary movement.
https://en.wikipedia.org/wiki/Dyskinesia

DYSMENORRHEA: Pain with menses.
https://academic.oup.com/epirev/article/36/1/104/566554

DYSPAREUNIA: Painful intercourse. See: The Care of the Older Person: After the Menopause: Ronald M. Caplan RMC Publishing, LLC 2018, 2019
https://www.ncbi.nlm.nih.gov/pmc/articles/PMC2671314/

DYSPLASIA: An abnormal, benign, microscopic cell change that can be a precursor of cancer.
http://www.cancer.gov/publications/dictionaries/cancer-terms?cdrid=45675

ECTOPIC PREGNANCY: Pregnancy outside of the normal location in the uterus. Usually in a fallopian tube.
https://academic.oup.com/humupd/article/20/2/250/663951

EDEMA: Swelling by accumulation of fluid in tissues. See: The Care of the Older Person: Could My Patient Be Malnourished?: Jose Morais. RMC Publishing, LLC 2018, 2019
www.careoftheolderperson.com
http://www.ncbi.nlm.nih.gov/books/NBK53445/

ELDER ABUSE: The intentional or neglectful causing of harm to an aging person See: The Care of the Older Person: Elder Abuse: Mark J. Yaffe. RMC Publishing, LLC 2018, 2019
www.careoftheolderperson.com
https://online.epocrates.com/diseases/69735/Elder-abuse/Differential-Diagnosis
https://jamanetwork.com/journals/jama/fullarticle/2708121?utm_source=silverchair&utm_medium=email&utm_campaign=article_alert-jama&utm_cont

ELECTROCARDIOGRAM: Noninvasive test that measures the electrical activity of the heart.
https://www.ncbi.nlm.nih.gov/pmc/articles/PMC1614214/

EMBOLIZATION: Therapeutic introduction of a substance into a blood vessel to occlude it. **Transcatheter Arterial Chemoembolization** (**TACE**) combines the introduction of

therapeutic substances into a tumor in conjunction with occlusion of the blood vessels of the tumor.
http://www.hopkinsmedicine.org/liver_tumor_center/treatments/intraarterial_therapies/tace.html

EMBOLUS: Detached thrombus (blood clot) that travels through blood vessels to another site.
http://emedicine.medscape.com/article/300901-overview
http://emedicine.medscape.com/article/1916852-overview

EMBRYO: The developing baby in the uterus during the fourth to eighth weeks of development, to the end of the second month, by which time all major features of the body are recognizable. All the main organ systems in the body have been laid down by the end of the second month.
https://embryology.med.unsw.edu.au/embryology/index.php/Ultrasound
https://www.nature.com/articles/d41586-018-07317-w
https://www.nature.com/articles/d41586-018-07317-w

EMOTION: Affective state of consciousness. Feeling.
https://www.ncbi.nlm.nih.gov/pmc/articles/PMC3950961/

ENDOCRINE GLANDS: Glands that secrete (produce) hormones, including the pituitary gland at the base of the brain, the thyroid gland, the adrenal glands , the ovaries, and the testes.
https://en.wikipedia.org/wiki/Endocrine_gland

ENDOCYTOSIS: Active transport of molecules into the cell in an energy using process
https://www.ncbi.nlm.nih.gov/books/NBK9831/

ENDOMETRIAL BIOPSY: Surgical sampling of the uterine lining.
https://academic.oup.com/humupd/article/23/2/232/2632344

ENDOMETRIAL CANCER: Cancer of the lining of the uterus.
https://www.ncbi.nlm.nih.gov/pmc/articles/PMC5288678/

ENDOMETRIAL HYPERPLASIA: Benign overgrowth condition of the lining of the uterus with crowding of glands. **ATYPICAL (ADENOMATOUS) HYPERPLASIA** of the endometrium is considered to be premalignant.
https://pdfs.semanticscholar.org/3b81/8cfedf864fca863c378a8028f91e0280b299.pdf

ENDOMETRIOSIS: Abnormal deposition of endometrium outside the uterus.
http://www.gponline.com/clinical-review-endometriosis/womens-health/endometriosis-fibroids/article/1150448

ENDOMETRIUM: The lining of the uterus.

ENDORPHINS: Hormones that affect receptors in the brain. May reduce pain by binding to opioid receptors.
http://www.ncbi.nlm.nih.gov/pmc/articles/PMC3104618/

ENDOTHELIN I: A vasoconstrictor.
http://www.ncbi.nlm.nih.gov/pmc/articles/PMC3005421/

ENTEROCELE: True hernia of small bowel covered by peritoneum bulging into the vaginal vault.

ENZYME: An organic catalyst. Enzymes facilitate chemical reactions within the human body.
https://www.mcat.me/review/bb/enzyme-structure-and-function/

EPF: **Early Pregnancy Factor**. Pregnancy-specific protein that is present in pregnant woman's serum 48 hours after fertilization.
http://www.ncbi.nlm.nih.gov/pubmed/9196793

EPIDEMIC: Increase in the number of cases of a disease in a population.
https://www.cdc.gov/ophss/csels/dsepd/ss1978/lesson1/section11.html
https://www.hhs.gov/opioids/about-the-epidemic/index.html

EPIDIDYMIS: Duct behind the testis that carries sperm to the vas deferens.
http://emedicine.medscape.com/article/1949259-overview

EPIGENETIC CLOCK: Essentially refers to DNA Methylation Age. DNA **methylation**: adding a methyl group (CH3) to one of the bases of DNA: is an epigenetic mechanism involved in gene regulation.
https://www.whatisepigenetics.com/dna-methylation/
http://clinicalepigeneticsjournal.biomedcentral.com/articles/10.1186/s13148-019-0656-7 https://www.ncbi.nlm.nih.gov/pmc/articles/PMC6826138/

EPIGENETICS: Study of the processes that regulate the turning on and off of genes. http://epi.grants.cancer.gov/i/epigen-lg.jpg

EPIGENOME: Description of all the chemical modifications to DNA and DNA-associated proteins in the cell which alter gene expression. Epigenetic changes can drive aging. Much of the epigenome is reset when the genome is passed to offspring.
https://www.genome.gov/27532724/
http://www.nature.com/news/an-epigenetics-gold-rush-new-controls-for-gene-expression-1.21513?WT.ec_id=NATURE-20170223&spMailingID=53480287&spUserID=MjA1NjIyNjc4OA

EPIGENOMICS: Analysis of epigenetic changes.
http://anatomyandphysiologyi.com/epithelial-tissue/

EPITHELIUM: A microscopic cellular covering of surfaces, including skin and mucous membranes.
http://anatomyandphysiologyi.com/epithelial-tissue/

EPITOPE: Antigenic determinant. The part of the antigen molecule that is recognized by the antibody, and to which the antibody attaches.
https://www.britannica.com/science/epitope

ERECTILE DYSFUNCTION: ED. Difficulty with achieving or maintaining penile erection. See: The Care of the Older Person: After the Menopause: Ronald M. Caplan RMC Publishing, LLC 2018, 2019
http://www.bmj.com/content/348/bmj.g129

ERYTHROPOIETIN: Stimulates the formation of red blood cells. Produced by recombinant DNA technology.
https://en.wikipedia.org/wiki/Erythropoietin

ESTRADIOL: A form of estrogen produced in the ovaries.
https://pubchem.ncbi.nlm.nih.gov/compound/estradiol

ESTROGEN: Female sex hormones, mainly made in the ovary.
https://en.wikipedia.org/wiki/Estrogen
http://journal.frontiersin.org/article/10.3389/fimmu.2017.00108/full?utm_source=newsletter&utm_medium=email&utm_campaign=Immunology-w7-2017

ESTROGEN REPLACEMENT THERAPY: ERT. Treatment of menopausal symptoms, usually in conjunction with progesterone. See: The Care of the Older Person: After the Menopause: Ronald M. Caplan RMC Publishing, LLC 2018, 2019
http://emedicine.medscape.com/article/276104-overview

EUKARYOTE: Any organism whose cells contain a nucleus which contains DNA within chromosomes.
http://www.dictionary.com/browse/eukaryote

EXERCISE (AEROBIC): Generally refers to sustained physical activity designed to promote oxygen utilization. The Care of the Older Person: Why Does My Patient Have Gait and Balance Disorders?: Olivier Beauchet. Physical Activity as a Countermeasure to Frailty: Guy Hajj Boutros, Antony Karelis: RMC Publishing, LLC 2018, 2019
www.careoftheolderperson.com
http://cardiology.jamanetwork.com/article.aspx?articleid=2530563
https://www.frontiersin.org/articles/10.3389/fimmu.2018.02187/full?utm_source=F-AAE&utm_medium=EMLF&utm_campaig
https://jamanetwork.com/journals/jama/fullarticle/2712935?guestAccessKey=c09863bb-66ff-4c16-88c3-06ab0357f57d&utm_source=silverchair&utm_medium=email&utm_campaign=article_alert-jama&utm
https://jamanetwork.com/journals/jamainternalmedicine/fullarticle/2714300?guestAccessKey=55c4f5ef-9957-470d-9691-071330b0644d&utm_source=silverchair&utm_campaign=jama_network&utm_content=weekly_highlights&cmp=1&utm_medium=email
https://jamanetwork.com/journals/jama/fullarticle/2712935?guestAccessKey=2364bbfc-d62a-4d49-9fdb-9d0114d00fc8&utm_source=silverchair&utm_medium=email&utm_campaign=article_alert-jama&utm_content=etoc&utm_term=112018https://n.neurology.org/content/92/9/e905 https://jamanetwork.com/journals/jamanetworkopen/fullarticle/2724776?utm_source=silverchair&utm_medium=email&utm_campaign=article_alert-jamanetworkopen&utm_content=etoc&utm_term=030119

EXOSOME: Extracellular vesical involved in cell communication and immune function. Role in cancer cells.
https://www.frontiersin.org/articles/10.3389/fgene.2018.00092/full

EXTRAPYRAMIDAL SYSTEM: Part of the motor system network incorporating the Basal Ganglia, involved with involuntary actions performed at a subconscious level. Distinguished from the tracts of the motor cortex that travel through the pyramids of the Medulla.
https://www.sciencedirect.com/topics/neuroscience/extrapyramidal-system

FABRY'S DISEASE: Alpha-galactosidase-A deficiency: enzyme utilized in lipid metabolism. Rare X-linked lysosomal storage disease.
http://www.ninds.nih.gov/disorders/fabrys/fabrys.htm

FALLOPIAN TUBE: The fine tubular structure arising from each side of the uterus near the fundus, ending in fingerlike projections called fimbria that are close to each ovary, essentially forming the "pickup" mechanism for the egg released at ovulation.

FERTILITY: The ability to conceive children.
http://emedicine.medscape.com/article/274143-overview

FERTILIZATION: The fusion of the ovum (oocyte, egg) and the spermatozoon (sperm).
https://en.wikipedia.org/wiki/Human_fertilization

FETUS: The baby developing in the uterus is known as the fetus from the beginning of the third month until the baby is born. The fetal period is the longest period of intrauterine life.
http://www.nature.com/news/secrets-of-life-in-a-spoonful-of-blood-1.21430?WT.ec_id=NATURE-20170209&spMailingID=53380605&spUserID=MjA1NjIyNjc4OAS2&spJobID=1101425398&spRepo

rtId=MTEwMTQyNTM5OAS2 https://www.nature.com/articles/d41586-018-07317-w

FHIT GENE: Fragile **hi**stidine **t**riad. Aberrant transcripts from this gene are found in some cancers, notably esophageal, stomach and colon cancer.
http://www.ncbi.nlm.nih.gov/gene/2272

FIBEROPTICS: Light images sent through fine fibers of glass or plastic. http://www.laserfocusworld.com/articles/2011/01/medical-applications-of-fiber-optics-optical-fiber-sees-growth-as-medical-sensors.html

FIBRIN: In blood clotting, thrombin causes fibrinogen to polymerize, forming fibrin. Polymerized fibrin and platelets form a hemostatic plug , or clot.
https://www.britannica.com/science/fibrin

FIBROID: A benign solid tumor of the uterus.

FIBROMA: A benign solid tumor that can occur in the breast or ovary.

FISTULA: An abnormal passage from one body cavity to another, or out to the body surface.

FOLLICLE (OVARIAN): The fluid-filled structure surrounding the developing egg (ovum)in the ovary.
http://www.embryology.ch/anglais/cgametogen/oogenese02.html

FRAILTY SYNDROME: Weakness, slowness, minimal physical activity, exhaustion and low energy, weight loss. See: The Care of the Older Person: Frailty: Sathya Karunananthan, Howard Bergman. RMC Publishing,LLC 2018, 2019 www.careoftheolderperson.com https://jamanetwork.com/journals/jamasurgery/article-abstract/2656841

http://www.ncbi.nlm.nih.gov/pubmed/17634320
http://annals.org/aim/article-abstract/2668215/effect-physical-activity-frailty-secondary-analysis-randomized-controlled-trial
https://documentcloud.adobe.com/link/track?uri=urn%3Aaaid%3Ascds%3AUS%3Af24df018-1e90-454d-af5f-7a345b6d5190
https://jamanetwork.com/journals/jamanetworkopen/fullarticle/2733174?utm_source=silverchair&utm_medium=email&utm_campaign=article_alert-jama
https://jamanetwork.com/journals/jamanetworkopen/fullarticle/2740784?utm_source=silverchair&utm_medium=email&utm_campaign=article_alert-jamanetworkopen&utm_content=wklyforyou&utm_term=08022019

FREE RADICAL: Short lived uncharged molecule
https://documentcloud.adobe.com/link/track?uri=u
https://jamanetwork.com/journals/jamanetworkopen/fullarticle/2733174?utm_source=silverchair&utm_medium=email&utm_campaign=article_alert-
jaman%3Aaaid%3Ascds%3AUS%3Af24df018-1e90-454d-af5f-7a345b6d5190
http://www.ncbi.nlm.nih.gov/pmc/articles/PMC3249911/

FSH: Follicle stimulating hormone.
http://www.ncbi.nlm.nih.gov/pubmed/9741710

GABA: **G**amma-**a**mino**b**utyric **a**cid. A neurotransmitter.
http://www.webmd.com/vitamins-supplements/ingredientmono-464-gaba%20gamma-aminobutyric%20acid.aspx?activeingredientid=464&

GALACTOGRAPHY: Mammography with injection of contrast to image milk ducts.

GAMETE: A germ (sex) cell: the female ovum, or the male spermatozoon. https://www.khanacademy.org/science/biology/cellular-molecular-biology/meiosis/a/phases-of-meiosis

GENE: The determinant of human characteristics and behavior from a cellular level on upwards. Each gene is a section on a DNA molecule and usually resides at a specific point (locus) on a chromosome. Each gene has a counterpart on the other chromosome that makes up the pair. The genes elaborate proteins. http://www.ncbi.nlm.nih.gov/genbank/

GENE EDITING (Genome Editing): A form of **Genetic Engineering.** Insertion, deletion or replacement of DNA at a specific site on the genome using engineered nucleases ("molecular scissors") See **CRISP R**
https://www.technologyreview.com/s/608350/first-human-embryos-edited-in-us/
https://www.horizondiscovery.com/gene-editing
http://jamanetwork.com/journals/jama/fullarticle/2646800?utm_medium=alert&utm_source=JAMAPublishAheadofPrint&utm_campaign=10-08-2017
https://www.technologyreview.com/s/612458/exclusive-chinese-scientists-are-creating-crispr-babies/amp/?__twitter_impression=true

GENE EXPRESSION PROFILING: Measurement of activity (expression) of thousands of genes, giving a picture of cellular functioning. In breast cancer for example, identifies distinct molecular entities associated with differential prognoses and response to cytotoxic drugs.
http://www.ncbi.nlm.nih.gov/pubmed/11823860
https://www.mdedge.com/hematology-oncology/clinical-edge/summary/

breast-cancer/optimizing-gene-expression-profiling-early?utm_source=ClinEdge_OP_cedge_110816&utm_medium=email&utm_content=Gene%20Profiling%20in%20Early%20BC%20|%20CTC%20Clusters%20and%20MBC%20|%20Impact%20of%20Chemo%20Events%20|%20

GENE SILENCING: Regulation of gene expression. siRNA: small interfering RNA potentially can inhibit genes in genetic disease (See RNAi)
http://www.ncbi.nlm.nih.gov/probe/docs/applsilencing/
https://jamanetwork.com/journals/jama/fullarticle/2712406?guestAccessKey=22414c3e-162a-4ff0-8b50-5477ff58735b&utm_source=silverchair&utm_campaign=jama_network&utm_content=weekly_highlights&cmp=1&utm_medium=email
https://www.ncbi.nlm.nih.gov/pmc/articles/PMC5542916/

GENE THERAPY: Treating a disorder by inserting a gene into cells.
http://www.ama-assn.org/ama/pub/physician-resources/medical-science/genetics-molecular-medicine/current-topics/gene-therapy.page?
https://www.frontiersin.org/articles/10.3389/fimmu.2018.00554/full?utm_source=F-AAE&utm_medium=EMLF&utm_campaign=MRK_589856_35_Immuno_20180403_arts_A

GENETIC ENGINEERING: Manipulating the genome.
http://www.fda.gov/AnimalVeterinary/DevelopmentApprovalProcess/GeneticEngineering/
https://www.frontiersin.org/articles/10.3389/fimmu.2018.00153/full?utm_source=F-AAE&utm_medium=EMLF&utm_campaign=MRK_536191_35

GENOME: The complete DNA sequence. The human genome project deciphered the complete DNA sequence of humans.
http://www.ncbi.nlm.nih.gov/projects/genome/guide/human/

NEXT GENERATION SEQUENCING: Technologies that sample multiple DNA sequences in parallel.
https://www.cancer.gov/publications/dictionaries/genetics-dictionary/def/next-generation-sequencing

GENOTYPE: The individual genes of each person. The expression of the person's genetic code. **SNP genotyping** refers to variations in Single Nucleotide Polymorphisms between individuals.
https://www.niehs.nih.gov/news/assets/docs_p_z/snp_genotyping_508.pdf
http://www.nature.com/tpj/journal/v3/n2/full/6500167a.html
https://www.britannica.com/science/genotype

GERD: Gastroesophageal Reflux Disease.
https://gi.org/guideline/diagnosis-and-managemen-of-gastroesophageal-reflux-disease/

GERIATRICS: Medical specialty that focuses on health care, diseases, and issues of elderly people, and the aging process. See: The Care of the Older Person: Introduction: Jose Morais. RMC Publishing, LLC 2018, 2019 www.careoftheolderperson.com
http://www.merckmanuals.com/professional/geriatrics/provision-of-care-to-the-elderly/overview-of-geriatric-care
http://bulletin.facs.org/2016/12/improving-quality-in-geriatric-surgery-a-blueprint-from-the-american-college-of-surgeons/

GERONTOLOGY: The multidisciplinary study of aging and its issues in all its aspects
http://biomedgerontology.oxfordjournals.org/content/59/1/M24.full

GEROPROTECTOR: Drug that targets the fundamental mechanisms of aging
https://www.nature.com/articles/d41586-018-01668-0?utm_source=briefing-dy&utm_medium=email&utm_campaign=20180215

GLAND: Organ that synthesizes and secretes a substance required by the body.
http://www.histology.leeds.ac.uk/glandular/exocr_endocr_properties.php

GLAUCOMA: Condition that causes optic nerve damage and vision loss, often by an increase in intraocular pressure.
https://www.ncbi.nlm.nih.gov/pubmed/24825645vg

GLOBULINS: Include **alpha globulins**, beta **globulin**, and **gamma globulin, including (Ig)A, (Ig)G: immunoglobulin G, (Ig)M, (Ig)E and (Ig)D** synthesized by B lymphocytes, important in the immune response. Identified by **serum protein electrophoresis**, which separates the proteins.
https://www.aafp.org/afp/2005/0101/p105.html
https://www.ncbi.nlm.nih.gov/pmc/articles/PMC2715434/
https://www.reference.com/science/gamma-globulin-2944770f90b33e6c?aq=Gamma+Globulins&qo=cdpArticles

GLOBUS PALLIDUS: A subcortical structure in the brain. Part of the basal ganglia.
http://webspace.ship.edu/cgboer/basalganglia.html

GLOMERULONEPHRITIS: Lesions of kidney glomeruli (capillary networks that filter blood) resulting from deposition or formation of immune complexes. In the acute phase, hematuria (blood in the

urine), proteinuria (protein in the urine), and red blood cell casts in the urine are seen.
http://emedicine.medscape.com/article/239278-overview#a4
http://www.sci.utah.edu/~macleod/bioen/be6000/prevnotes/L18-kidney.pdf

GLP-1R: Glucagon-like peptide 1 receptor agonist. Used in treatment of Type 2 (adult onset) Diabetes.
http://www.diabetesincontrol.com/newly-updated-glp-1-agonist-medications-chart/

GLYCOENGINEERING: Altering a cell surface so that infused tumor-specific immunocytes can enter the tumor parenchyma (functional tissue).
https://www.frontiersin.org/articles/10.3389/fimmu.2018.03084/full?utm_source=FAAE&utm_medium=EMLF&utm_campaign=MRK_889258_35_Immuno_20190122_arts_A

GOITER: Enlargement of the thyroid gland.
http://www.uptodate.com/contents/clinical-presentation-and-evaluation-of-goiter-in-adults

GNRH: Gonadotropin releasing hormone from the hypothalamus.
http://emedicine.medscape.com/article/255152-overview

GRAFT: Healthy tissue taken from one part of the body to replace diseased or damaged tissue in another part.

GRANULOSA CELL: A cell in the lining of an ovarian follicle. Granulosa cells manufacture estrogen, and to a lesser extent androgens and progestins. Conversion of androgens to estrogen takes place in granulosa cells.
https://embryology.med.unsw.edu.au/embryology/index.php/Granulosa_cell

GREENHOUSE GASES: Include carbon dioxide, sulfur dioxide, nitrous oxide, methane.
https://www.epa.gov/ghgemissions/overview-greenhouse-gases

GROWTH HORMONE: Somatotropin. Secreted by the pituitary gland.
http://www.ncbi.nlm.nih.gov/pubmed/20020365

HCG: **Human chorionic gonadotropin**. Produced by the placenta.
http://www.fda.gov/Drugs/ResourcesForYou/Consumers/BuyingUsingMedicineSafely/MedicationHealthFraud/ucm281834.htm

HEART FAILURE: Congestive heart failure. Heart muscle contraction not sufficiently strong to properly circulate blood. Fluid accumulates.
http://heartfailure.onlinejacc.org/article.aspx?articleid=1568320

HEMORRHAGE: Excessive bleeding.

HER-2 GENE: Human Epidermal Growth Factor Receptor-2. Linked to breast cancer.
http://www.cancer.gov/research/progress/discovery/HER2

HEREDITY: Parent to child transmission of traits, by inheritance of genes.
https://ghr.nlm.nih.gov/primer/inheritance/inheritancepatterns

HERNIA: Intraabdominal contents enclosed by peritoneum bulging into a weakened wall.

HIGH DENSITY LIPOPROTEIN: **HDL**. Complex of lipids and proteins that transports cholesterol in the blood to the liver.
http://www.ncbi.nlm.nih.gov/pmc/articles/PMC3787738/
https://www.jwatch.org/na45882/2018/01/17/continuing-enigma-hdl?query=topic_lipid&jwd=000012066693&jspc=OBG

HIPPOCAMPUS: Area of the brain involved with spatial memory which is important in navigation, and episodic memory (remembering autobiographical events). Located in the medial temporal lobe of the brain. Includes a gray matter ridge on the floor of each lateral ventricle.
https://en.wikipedia.org/wiki/Hippocampus
https://www.nature.com/nature/journal/vaop/ncurrent/full/nature22067.html
https://en.wikipedia.org/wiki/Episodic_memory

HIRSUTISM: Excess hair growth.
http://emedicine.medscape.com/article/121038-overview

HISTOCOMPATIBILITY: Antigenic similarities between tissue donor and recipient so that a transplant is not rejected.
https://www.hindawi.com/journals/jtrans/2012/842141/

HISTONE: Protein in chromosomes that binds to DNA, giving shape to the chromosome. Role in controlling gene activity.
https://www.cancer.gov/publications/dictionaries/cancer-terms/def/histone

HMO: Health maintenance organization. Essentially a health insurance plan.

HOLOGRAPHY: The scattered light from an object is captured, then illuminated by a beam. Multiple two dimensional pictures are assembled into a three dimensional display.
http://holocenter.org/what-is-holography

HOMOCYSTEINE: Amino acid derived from the dietary amino acid methionine. Homologue of the amino acid cysteine.
http://www.ncbi.nlm.nih.gov/pmc/articles/PMC4146172/

HOMOGRAFT: Transplanted tissue from another human individual.
http://bja.oxfordjournals.org/content/108/suppl_1/i29.full

HORMONE: A substance formed in an endocrine gland and carried by the blood stream to other organs which it affects. Such organs are called end organs. For example, follicle stimulating hormone and luteinizing hormone from the pituitary gland act on the ovary, controlling ovarian secretion of estrogen and progesterone. Estrogen and progesterone act on the endometrium lining the uterus.
http://biology.freeoda.com/chemical_composition_of_the_hormones.htm
http://www.news-medical.net/health/Hormone-Interactions-with-Receptors.aspx

HORMONE REPLACEMENT THERAPY: HRT. Treatment of menopausal symptoms with estrogen and progesterone.
http://press.endocrine.org/doi/abs/10.1210/jc.2015-2236

HOT FLASHES: Sudden onset of a feeling of heat and flushing of short duration.
http://theoncologist.alphamedpress.org/content/16/11/1658.long

HUMAN CONNECTOME PROJECT: Mapping the human brain connectivity
http://www.humanconnectomeproject.org/

HYALURONIC ACID: An anionic nonsulfated glycosaminoglycan. Component of skin.
http://www.ncbi.nlm.nih.gov/pmc/articles/PMC3583886/

HYDROFLUOCARBONS: HFC. Several organic compounds. Decreasingly used as refrigerants.
https://www.britannica.com/science/hydrofluorocarbon

HYPERGLYCEMIA: Abnormally increased blood glucose levels.
https://ccforum.biomedcentral.com/articles/10.1186/cc12514
http://joe.endocrinology-journals.org/content/204/1/1.full.pdf

HYPERPLASIA: Overgrowth of tissue. Increase in cellular reproduction rate.
http://journals.lww.com/jaapa/Fulltext/2016/08000/Benign_prostatic_hyperplasia__A_clinical_review.2.aspx
http://emedicine.medscape.com/article/269919-overview

HYPERTENSION: High blood pressure. Recently defined as 130 mm Hg systolic (pressure during heart muscle contraction), and 80 mm HG diastolic (pressure during relaxation).
http://jaha.ahajournals.org/content/4/12/e002315.full
http://www.jwatch.org/na43262/2017/03/02/pharmacologic-treatment-hypertension-older-adults?query=etoc_jwgenmed&jwd=000012066693&jspc=OBG
http://hyper.ahajournals.org/content/early/2017/11/10/HYP.0000000000000065
https://jamanetwork.com/journals/jama/fullarticle/2664350?utm_source=silverchair&utm_medium=email&utm_campaign=article_alert-jama&utm_content=olf&u
https://jamanetwork.com/journals/jama/fullarticle/2664350?&utm_source=191323&utm_medium=BulletinHealthCare&utm_term=120217&utm_content=Mornin

HYPOTENSION, ORTHOSTATIC: Low blood pressure on standing.
http://www.ncbi.nlm.nih.gov/pubmed/27225359?access_num=27225359&link_type=MED&dopt=Abstract

HYPOTHALAMUS: Part of the brain below the thalamus. Forms the major portion of the ventral region of the diencephalon. Forms part of the wall of the third ventricle.
http://press.endocrine.org/doi/abs/10.1210/jc.2015-2236

HYSTERECTOMY: Surgical removal of the uterus.

HYSTEROSALPINGOGRAM: Injection of radiopaque dye into the uterus via the cervix to radiologically visualize the uterine cavity, the fallopian tubes, and their patency.

HYSTEROSCOPY: A minimally invasive surgical technique in which a fiberoptic telescope (hysteroscope) is introduced through the cervical os into the uterine cavity. The endometrial lining of the uterus and the interior openings of the fallopian tubes can be seen.

ICSI: **I**ntra**c**ytoplasmic **s**perm **i**njection.
http://americanpregnancy.org/infertility/intracytoplasmic-sperm-injection/

IMMUNE SYSTEM: The system that allows the body to ward off invasion by foreign substances, including infectious agents. Cells including T-lymphocytes that go to infected sites are elaborated in bone marrow and other areas. Antibodies (immunoglobulins) that target specific invaders (antigens) circulate in the bloodstream. Infected areas drain through lymphatic channels to the lymph nodes, where invading organisms are processed.
http://emedicine.medscape.com/article/1948753-overview

IMMUNOCYTE: Leukocyte that induces immune response by antibody production in reaction to an antigen.
http://www.feinsteininstitute.org/programs-researchers/immunology/immunocytes-cytokine-biology/

IMMUNOGLOBULIN: Ig. Proteins that function as antibodies and bind to antigens.
http://www.ebioscience.com/knowledge-center/antigen/immunoglobulin.htm

IMMUNOME (CELLULAR): Immune cell subset phenotype and activation/functional status. Used to predict whether a patient will respond to immunotherapy.
https://www.frontiersin.org/articles/10.3389/fimmu.2019.01767/full?utm_source=F-AAE&utm_medium=EMLF&utm_campaign=MRK_1064098_35_Immuno_20190808_arts_A

IMMUNOSENESCENCE: Age associated immune change, notably with a reduction in peripheral blood naïve cells , and a relative increase of memory cells, along with the inflammatory changes that accompany aging, so-called "inflamm-aging"
https://www.frontiersin.org/articles/10.3389/fimmu.2019.02247/full?utm_source=F-AAE&utm_medium=EMLF&utm_campaign=MRK_1111535_35_Immuno_20191001_arts_A

IMMUNOSUPPRESSION: Suppression of the immune response.
http://emedicine.medscape.com/article/432316-overview

IMMUNOTHERAPY: Prevention or treatment of disease with substances that stimulate the immune response. Blocking the shut-off of the immune response. Anticancer vaccines. https://www.mdanderson.org/treatment-options/immunotherapy.html
http://journal.frontiersin.org/article/10.3389/fimmu.2016.00621/full?utm_source=newsletter&utm_medium=email&utm_campaign=Immunology-w1-2017
http://journal.frontiersin.org/article/10.3389/fimmu.2016.00621/full?utm_source=newsletter&utm_medium=email&utm_campaign=Immunology-w1-2017

http://www.mdedge.com/jcso/article/135689/gastroenterology/meeting-potential-immunotherapy-new-targets-provide-rational/pdf?channel=213
http://journal.frontiersin.org/article/10.3389/fimmu.2017.00555/full?utm_source=F-AAE&utm_medium=EMLF&utm_campaign=MRK_275249_35_Immuno_20170518_arts_A
https://www.frontiersin.org/articles/10.3389/fimmu.2018.00384/full?utm_source=F-AAE&utm_medium=EMLF&utm_campaign=MRK_571163_35_

IMPLANTATION: The sperm fertilizes (fuses with) the egg (ovum) in the fallopian tube. The fertilized egg then migrates from the fallopian tube into the uterus at a specific time , when the endometrium is most receptive, and attaches to and burrows into the uterine lining.

IMPRINTING: (Genomic Imprinting) The process by which only the copy of a gene from one parent gets switched on in an offspring.
https://www.genome.gov/27532724/
https://ghr.nlm.nih.gov/primer/inheritance/updimprinting

INDUCED PLURIPOTENT STEM CELLS: IPS. Cells from an adult human that have been reprogrammed into an embryonic-like state.
http://stemcells.nih.gov/info/basics/pages/basics10.aspx
http://www.nature.com/news/japanese-man-is-first-to-receive-reprogrammed-stem-cells-from-another-person-1.21730?WT.ec_id=NEWS-20170330&spMailingID=53740049&sp
https://www.nature.com/articles/d41586-019-00656-2?utm_source=Nature+Briefing&utm_campaign=fb45cec6f6-briefing-dy-20190225&utm_medium=email&utm_term=0_c9dfd39373-fb45cec6f6-42544483

INFARCT: Cutoff of blood supply causing tissue death, resulting in a scarred area.
http://www.omicsonline.org/biomarkers-in-acute-myocardial-infarction-2155-9880.1000222.pdf

INFECTION: Invasion of foreign organisms, such as bacteria or viruses, into the body.
http://www.ph.ucla.edu/epi/faculty/detels/epi220/detels_agents.pdf

INFLAMMATION: The body's response to infection or injury, including redness, swelling, and heat. The specific responses are geared to killing the infectious agent and repairing the damaged tissue.
http://journal.frontiersin.org/article/10.3389/fimmu.2017.00017/full?utm_source=newsletter&utm_medium=email&utm_campaign=Immunology-w4-2017

INFLUENZA: Contagious respiratory illness caused by influenza virus.
http://journals.lww.com/epidem/Abstract/2015/11000/Review_Article___The_Fraction_of_Influenza_Virus.13.aspx
http://www.cdc.gov/mmwr/volumes/65/rr/rr6505a1.htm

INFORMATION TECHNOLOGY: IT. Computerized paperless data keeping, analysis, and transmission.
https://www.intel.com/content/www/us/en/healthcare-it/collaborative-care.html?cid=sem43700013297809532&intel_term=technology+for+healthcare&gclid=Cj0KEQjw6am-BRCTk4WZhLfd4-oBEiQA3ydA3lK6NZjCN51AIK72GMKucyGNX297Xgy6h66th96XBwcaAhYO8P8HAQ&gclsrc=aw.ds

INHIBINS: Peptides made in granulosa cells of ovarian follicles that inhibit secretion of follicle stimulating hormone (FSH).
http://www.medicinenet.com/script/main/art.asp?articlekey=22571
http://press.endocrine.org/doi/abs/10.1210/endo-124-1-552

INSOMNIA: Sleeplessness.

INSULIN: Polypeptide hormone, produced by the beta cells of the islets of Langerhans in the pancreas, that regulates blood glucose http://onlinelibrary.wiley.com/doi/10.1002/bip.20734/full

INSULIN RESISTANCE: Lowered level of response to insulin. http://emedicine.medscape.com/article/122501-overview

INTEGRIN: A receptor glycoprotein on a cell surface involved in the adhesion of the cell to other cells such as T-cells. https://www.ncbi.nlm.nih.gov/books/NBK26867/

INTELLIGENCE: Ability to acquire and apply knowledge and skills. https://www.lexico.com/en/definition/intelligence

INTERFERON: A protein that can inhibit virus replication. https://www.drugs.com/drug-class/interferons.html http://journal.frontiersin.org/article/10.3389/fimmu.2017.00062/full?utm_source=newsletter&utm_medium=email&utm_campaign=Immunology-w7-2017

INTERSTITIAL CYSTITIS: Painful Bladder Syndrome (BPS). http://emedicine.medscape.com/article/2055505-overview

INTERSTITIAL SPACE: Small, narrow, fluid containing space between tissues
https://www.ncbi.nlm.nih.gov/pmc/articles/PMC3139075/
https://www.thefreedictionary.com/interstitial+space

INTERSTITIUM: Fluid filled interstitial space draining to lymph nodes, supported by a network of collagen bundles. Visualized by laser endomicroscopy in relation to the extrahepatic bile duct, and other tissues that are subject to intermittent compression, including the submucosa of the gastrointestinal tract, and the urinary bladder. https://www.nature.com/articles/s41598-018-23062-6

INTRAUTERINE ENVIRONMENT: The environment in which the growing fetus lives.

INTRAUTERINE GROWTH RETARDATION: IUGR. Fetal growth restriction.
http://www.uptodate.com/contents/fetal-growth-restriction-evaluation-and-management

ISCHEMIA: Inadequate blood supply to an organ, resulting in inadequate oxygenation.

KAPOSI'S SARCOMA: Malignancy with cutaneous lesions caused by HHV8: human herpesvirus 8. Tends to occur in immunosuppressed individuals, notably those with AIDS (Autoimmune Deficiency Syndrome).
http://emedicine.medscape.com/article/279734-overview

KERATOPLASTY: Conductive keratoplasty. CK. Eye surgery utilizing radio frequency energy to change the shape of the cornea.

KILLER CELL: Natural killer (**NK**) cells are derived from hematopoietic stem cells in bone marrow. They kill cancer cells by secreting **perforins** (cytolytic proteins) and **granzymes** (proteases : enzymes that catalyze degradation of protein)
https://www.ncbi.nlm.nih.gov/pmc/articles/PMC4346487/
https://en.wikipedia.org/wiki/Granzyme
http://medical-dictionary.thefreedictionary.com/perforin
http://www.dictionary.com/browse/protease
http://journal.frontiersin.org/article/10.3389/fimmu.2016.00492/full

http://journal.frontiersin.org/article/10.3389/fimmu.2017.00293/full?utm_source=newsletter&utm_medium=email&utm_campaign=Immunology-w12-2017
http://journal.frontiersin.org/article/10.3389/fimmu.2017.00683/full?utm_source=F-AAE&utm_medium=EMLF&utm_campaign=MRK_307979_35_Immuno_20170622_arts_A
http://journal.frontiersin.org/article/10.3389/fimmu.2017.00760/full?utm_source=F-AAE&utm_medium=EMLF&utm_campaign=MRK_320984_35_Immuno_20170706_arts_A
http://journal.frontiersin.org/article/10.3389/fimmu.2017.00930/full?utm_source=F-AAE&utm_medium=EMLF&utm_campaign=MRK_352999_35_Immuno_20170808_arts_A
http://journal.frontiersin.org/article/10.3389/fimmu.2017.00774/full?utm_source=F-AAE&utm_medium=EMLF&utm_campaign=MRK_333189_35_Immuno_20170720_arts_A
http://journal.frontiersin.org/article/10.3389/fimmu.2017.01061/full?utm_source=F-AAE&utm_medium=EMLF&utm_campaign=MRK_398354_35_Immuno_20170921_arts_A

KINASE: Enzyme important in the carbohydrate metabolism and energy output of cells. **Protein-Tyrosine Kinases (PTK's)** regulate signaling in the cell. If PTK signaling is disrupted, malignant transformation of the cell can result.
http://www.ncbi.nlm.nih.gov/pubmed/10966463
http://www.sciencedirect.com/science/article/pii/S1043661813001771
https://www.empr.com/news/vitrakvi-larotrectinib-advanced-solid-tumors-ntrk-gene-fusion-approval/article/816725/?utm_source=newsletter&utm_medium=email&utm_campaign=mpr-dailydose-cp-20181129&cpn=obgyn_all%2cobgyn_md%2ccambia_august2018&hmS

LABOR: Period from the onset of regular uterine contractions with dilatation and effacement of the cervix and descent of the fetus through the birth canal culminating in delivery of the baby.

LACTIC ACIDOSIS: Increased plasma lactate. See: The Care of the Older Person: How To Diagnose And Treat Delirium: Haiban Yin. RMC Publishing, LLC 2018, 2019 www.careoftheolderperson.com http://emedicine.medscape.com/article/167027-overview

LACTOSE INTOLERANCE: Inability to digest lactose, a disaccharide in milk made up of glucose and galactose. http://emedicine.medscape.com/article/187249-overview

LAPAROSCOPY: a minimally invasive surgical technique in which a fiberoptic telescope (laparoscope) is introduced into the abdominal cavity through a small incision near the lower margin of the umbilicus.

LASER: **L**ight **A**mplification by **S**timulated **E**mission of **R**adiation. A narrow, often powerful, beam of light which does not spread and is monochromatic. This is a directed light beam, not nuclear radiation. http://www.azooptics.com/Article.aspx?ArticleID=44 https://www.nature.com/articles/s41551-016-0008?WT.mc_id=EMI_NBME_1701_LAUNCHISSUE_PORTFOLIO&spMailingID=53217285&spUserID=MTc3MDI4ODk5NQS2&spJobID=1083253126&spReportId=MTA4MzI1MzEyNgS2

LEPTIN: Hormone produced by adipocytes involved in fat storage regulation. Acts on hypothalamus to suppress appetite. http://www.sciencedirect.com/science/article/pii/S0083672905710128

LEUKEMIA: Malignant form of white blood cells in the blood stream, commonly arising from the bone marrow. http://www.ncbi.nlm.nih.gov/pmc/articles/PMC3396664/

LIBIDO: Sexual drive. See: The Care of the Older Person: After the Menopause: Ronald M. Caplan RMC Publishing, LLC 2018, 2019
https://en.wikipedia.org/wiki/Flibanserin
http://www.medscape.com/viewarticle/871481?nlid=110609_2581&src=WNL_mdplsnews_161111_mscpedit_obgy&uac=66536PR&spon=16&impID=1232827&faf=1
https://www.fda.gov/news-events/press-announcements/fda-approves-new-treatment-hypoactive-sexual-desire-disorder-premenopausal-women
http://www.addyi.com

LIFE EXPECTANCY: The age to which a person or a selected population group might live. See: The Care of the Older Person: Introduction: Jose Morais. RMC Publishing, LLC 2018, 2019
www.careoftheolderperson.com
https://www.zionmarketresearch.com/report/home-healthcare-market
http://science.sciencemag.org/content/360/6396/1459
http://onlinelibrary.wiley.com/doi/10.1002/sres.2420/full
http://www.cdc.gov/nchs/data/hus/2011/022.pdf
http://www.statcan.gc.ca/tables-tableaux/sum-som/l01/cst01/health26-eng.htm
http://www.cdc.gov/nchs/data/databriefs/db267.pdf
http://mdlinx.pdr.net/internal-medicine/news-article.cfm/6986115/?utm_source=in-house&utm_medium=message&utm_campaign=mh-im-dec16
http://journals.plos.org/plosbiology/article?id=10.1371/journal.pbio.2002458#pbio.2002458.ref039 http://science.sciencemag.org/content/360/6396/1459
https://www.cdc.gov/nchs/data/hus/2017/027.pdf

https://www.jwatch.org/fw114817/2018/11/30/us-life-expectancy-down-overdose-and-suicide-rates?query=pfwTOC&jwd=000012066693&jspc=OBG

LIPOSUCTION: Surgical removal of fat by suction.

LIQUID BIOPSY: Blood testing for circulating tumor DNA (ctDNA). Identifies cancer mutations useful as biomarkers, many associated with targeted drug.
http://www.ncbi.nlm.nih.gov/pmc/articles/PMC4356857/
http://www.nature.com/nrclinonc/posters/liquidbiopsies/nrclinonc_liquidbiopsies_poster_web.pdf
http://www.nature.com/news/liquid-biopsies-success-highlights-power-of-combining-basic-and-clinical-research-1.21883?WT.ec_id=NATURE-20170427&spMailingID=53937339&
https://www.nature.com/articles/s41551-017-0065?WT.mc_id=EMI_NBME_1704_APRILISSUE_PORTFOLIO&spMailingID=53957850&spUserID=MTc3MDI4ODk5NQS

LOW DENSITY LIPOPROTEIN: LDL. Complex of lipids and proteins that transports cholesterol in the blood. Significant factor in the formation of arteriosclerotic plaques.
http://www.ncbi.nlm.nih.gov/pubmed/10073963

LUNG CANCER: Malignant tumor in the lung. Major cause of cancer deaths. Predominant type is Non- Small Cell Lung Cancer (**NSCLC**), strongly linked to tobacco smoking.
https://cancerstaging.org/references-tools/quickreferences/Documents/LungMedium.pdf
https://www.ncbi.nlm.nih.gov/pmc/articles/PMC3864624/
https://www.ncbi.nlm.nih.gov/pmc/articles/PMC4367711/
https://www.ncbi.nlm.nih.gov/pmc/articles/PMC5107578/

http://www.jtcvsonline.org/article/S0022-5223(17)31171-6/fulltext#sec1.6

LUTEINIZING HORMONE: LH. Secreted by the anterior pituitary, surges prior to ovulation. Acts on the ovary.
http://emedicine.medscape.com/article/2089268-overview

LYME DISEASE: Tick-borne illness caused by Borrelia burgdorferi. Other tick-borne illnesses include babesiosis, anaplasmosis, ehrlichosis, and Rocky Mountain Spotted Fever.
http://www.ncbi.nlm.nih.gov/pmc/articles/PMC3542482/

LYMPH NODE: Small and bean shaped, lymph nodes are present throughout the body. They are composed of lymphoid tissue, and are connected by lymph channels. The lymphatic system is important in the immune response, in fighting infection. Cancerous cells can enter the lymphatic system and drain to lymph nodes, enlarging them. Cancer surgery often involves the removal of affected lymph nodes, or lymph nodes that are likely to be affected by a cancer.
https://www.boundless.com/physiology/textbooks/boundless-anatomy-and-physiology-textbook/lymphatic-system-20/lymph-cells-and-tissues-193/lymph-nodes-963-3100/

LYMPHOCYTE: A form of white blood cell. B cells and T cells are two main types.
http://www.ncbi.nlm.nih.gov/pubmedhealth/PMHT0022042/

LYMPHOMA: A solid malignant tumor often composed of cells that resemble lymphocytes. Can arise at various sites within the body and invade the bloodstream.
http://www.bloodjournal.org/content/125/1/22

LYNCH SYNDROME: Autosomal dominant inherited predisposition for colon and endometrial cancers
https://www.ncbi.nlm.nih.gov/pmc/articles/PMC2933058/
https://www.sgo.org/wp-content/uploads/2016/10/2016-SGO-Genetics-Toolkit3.pdf

LYSOSOMES: Organelles in the cell containing enzymes that degrade biologic polymers including proteins, carbohydrates and lipids.
https://www.ncbi.nlm.nih.gov/books/NBK9953/

MACHINE LEARNING: How computers learn from data. Intersection of statistics and computing algorithms.
https://www.ncbi.nlm.nih.gov/pmc/articles/PMC5831252/
https://www.sciencedirect.com/science/article/pii/S093336571730009X
https://www.techemergence.com/machine-learning-in-pharma-medicine/
https://www.healthcareitnews.com/projects/ai-and-machinelearning?mkt_tok=eyJpIjoiWVRJNE5qTmpPRE01WmpabSIsInQiOiJCckta VzljSVRpVVpWQ3FYa2lEazc1WHlQSGc5bUV3YXlwTFVtbEdv M2RjSVY

MACROPHAGE: A large phagocytic white blood cell.
http://www.cell.com/immunity/fulltext/S1074-7613(14)00235-0

MACULAR DEGENERATION: Deterioration of the macula, the area surrounding the fovea near the center of the retina in the eye.
https://www.ncbi.nlm.nih.gov/pmc/articles/PMC3732788/
https://www.nature.com/articles/nbt.4114.epdf?referrer_access_token=8BtrAvy5kx0RIQxVHmwBfNRgN0jAjWeI9jnR3ZoTv0PJSqIFs 8CVMGLKXeHOLTvVGIDHNZm

MALNUTRITION: Improper intake and processing of foodstuffs. See: The Care of the Older Person: Could My Patient Be

Malnourished? Jose A. Morais, RMC Publishing, LLC 2018, 2019
www.careoftheolderperson.com
https://www.ncbi.nlm.nih.gov/pubmed/16782522

MAMMOGRAPHY: Xray breast imaging.
http://emedicine.medscape.com/article/346529-overview
http://www.jwatch.org/na42993/2016/12/13/when-stop-surveillance-mammography-older-breast-cancer?query=etoc_jwwomen&jwd=000012066693&jspc=OBG

MAO INHIBITORS: Monoamine oxidase inhibitors, sometimes still used in the treatment of depression. Monoamine oxidase enzymes catalase oxidation and inactivation of monoamine neurotransmitters, including dopamine, noradrenaline, adrenaline and serotonin.
http://www.webmd.com/depression/symptoms-depressed-anxiety-12/antidepressants

MEDIASTINUM: Space in the thorax between the pleural sacs, notably containing the heart and its great vessels.
https://www.youtube.com/watch?v=2POIlBe2xR4
MEDULLA (OBLONGATA): Part of the brain in the brainstem that controls involuntary activities necessary for life. https://www.neuroscientificallychallenged.com/blog/know-your-brain-medulla-oblongata

MEIOSIS: Cell division resulting in cells (gametes) with a single set of chromosomes, half the number of chromosomes present in the parent cell.
https://www.khanacademy.org/science/biology/cellular-molecular-biology/meiosis/a/phases-of-meiosis

MELANOMA: Tumor of melanin-forming cells.
http://www.medicaljournals.se/acta/content/?doi=10.2340/00015555-2035&html=1
https://www.cell.com/cell/fulltext/S0092-8674(17)30952-2

MENOPAUSE: Cessation of menses. See: The Care of the Older Person: After the Menopause: Ronald M. Caplan RMC Publishing, LLC 2018, 2019
https://www.ncbi.nlm.nih.gov/pmc/articles/PMC3285482/

MENSTRUATION: Blood and shedding endometrium from the uterus beginning approximately fourteen days after ovulation in a non-pregnant cycle.
https://www.ncbi.nlm.nih.gov/pubmed/16160098

METABOLIC ACIDOSIS: Increase in plasma acidity. Excess production of acid with inadequate buffer, bicarbonate, to neutralize it. Insufficient renal excretion of acid.
http://www.nature.com/nrneph/journal/v6/n5/abs/nrneph.2010.33.html

METABOLIC SYNDROME: Central (abdominal)obesity, hypertension, and insulin resistance. High levels of triglycerides, low levels of HDL.
http://www.ncbi.nlm.nih.gov/pmc/articles/PMC3966331/

METABOLISM: Molecular chemical reactions within living tissue.
http://www.biology-pages.info/C/CellularRespiration.html

METAPLASIA: A benign cell change. In a common type, glandular epithelium is transformed into squamous epithelium.
https://en.wikipedia.org/wiki/Squamous_metaplasia

METASTASIS: Cancer cells at a distance from the primary tumor.
https://www.nature.com/articles/d41586-018-05445-x?utm_source=briefing-dy&utm_medium=email&utm_campaign=briefing&utm_content=20180618
https://www.cancer.gov/publications/dictionaries/cancer-terms/def/metastasis

METFORMIN: Oral anti-hyperglycemic agent used in Type 2 Diabetes. Decreases hepatic glucose production. Implications in other disease states, weight loss and possibly lifespan
https://www.ncbi.nlm.nih.gov/pmc/articles/PMC3398862/

MICROBIOME: Bacteria that inhabit the gut.
http://jamanetwork.com/journals/jama/fullarticle/2594788

MICROGLIA: Immune, phagocytic, central nervous system (brain and spinal cord) cells implicated in Alzheimer's.
https://www.frontiersin.org/articles/10.3389/fimmu.2019.00790/full?utm_source=F-AAE&utm_medium=EMLF&utm_campaign=MRK_973135_35_Immuno_20190425_arts_A

MICROSURGERY: Surgery performed with visualization through a microscope, often involving anastomoses of small blood vessels.

MIGRAINE: Vascular headaches involving the blood vessels of the brain.
http://www.ncbi.nlm.nih.gov/pmc/articles/PMC3663475/
https://www.jwatch.org/fw113584/2017/11/30/migraine-prevention-two-calcitonin-gene-related-peptide?query=pfwTOC&jwd=000012066693&jspc=OBG
http://www.pdr.net/drug-summary/Imitrex-Tablets-sumatriptan-succinate-201
https://www.ncbi.nlm.nih.gov/pubmed/29800211

https://www.thelancet.com/journals/lancet/article/PIIS0140-6736(18)32534-0/fulltext
https://www.empr.com/ajovy/drug/34876/
https://www.ptcommunity.com/journal/article/full/2018/10/616/emerging-therapies-patients-difficult-treat-migraine?utm_source=PT_NL_2018-10-16_nsp_v9&utm_campaign=PT+NL+18-10-16&utm_medium=email https://www.empr.com/news/ajovy-migraine-prevention-fremanezumab-vfrm-preventative-migraine/article/796090/?utm_source=newsletter&utm_medium=email&utm_campaign=mpr-promo-20181105&chttps://jamanetwork.com/journals/jamaneurology/fullarticle/2681442
https://jamanetwork.com/journals/jamaneurology/fullarticle/2681442
https://onlinelibrary.wiley.com/doi/10.1111/head.13456

MITOCHONDRIA: Intracellular organelle in which respiration and energy production occur.

https://jamanetwork.com/journals/jamaneurology/fullarticle/2681442
http://citeseerx.ist.psu.edu/viewdoc/download?doi=10.1.1.572.8830&rep=rep1&type=pdf
http://www.cell.com/cell-metabolism/fulltext/S1550-4131(16)30502-2
http://mdlinx.pdr.net/neurology/news-article.cfm/6907659?utm_source=in-house&utm_medium=message&utm_campaign=medhead
https://link.springer.com/article/10.1007/s10815-017-1006-3/fulltext.html?wt_mc=alerts.TOCjournals
https://www.deepdyve.com/lp/springer-journal/quantitative-and-qualitative-changes-of-mitochondria-in-human-Gh20vR9aBa?key=bioportfolio

MITOSIS: Cell division resulting in daughter cells identical to the parent cell.
https://www.khanacademy.org/science/biology/cellular-molecular-biology/meiosis/a/phases-of-meiosis

MOBILITY: Ability to move freely and easily. See The Care of the Older Person: Why Does My Patient Have Gait and Balance Disorders?: Olivier Beauchet RMC Publishing, LLC 2018, 2019
https://www.mayoclinic.org/diseases-conditions/movement-disorders/symptoms-causes/syc-20363893
https://en.oxforddictionaries.com/definition/mobility

MOHS SURGERY: Surgery in which thin layers of cancer containing skin are stepwise removed and examined microscopically, until only cancer free tissue remains.
http://emedicine.medscape.com/article/2212475-overview

MOLECULAR PROFILING (of cancer patients): The use of Next Generation Sequencing (NGS) gives rise to Personalized therapy with selective genome and immune-targeted drugs (see Precision Medicine, NGS)
https://www.nature.com/articles/s41591-019-0407-5

MONOCLONAL ANTIBODY: An antibody that will go to a specific receptor site. "Monoclonal" refers to the fact that the antibody protein is derived from one clone of cells, all of which are identical.
http://www.ncbi.nlm.nih.gov/pmc/articles/PMC4491443/

MONTREAL COGNITIVE ASSESSMENT: MoCA: Test to detect mild cognitive impairment and Alzheimer's disease. The Care of the Older Person: Chapter: "Doctor, my wife is getting forgetful": Serge Gauthier RMC Publishing, LLC 2018, 2019
www.careoftheolderperson.com

http://dementia.ie/images/uploads/site-images/MoCA-Test-English_7_1.pdf
http://www.mocatest.org/
https://www.sciencedirect.com/topics/neuroscience/montreal-cognitive-assessment

MRI: **Magnetic Resonance Imaging**. An advanced imaging technique that uses a powerful magnet to alter polarity.
https://onlinelibrary.wiley.com/doi/full/10.1002/jmri.23642

MSG: Monosodium glutamate.
http://www.mayoclinic.org/healthy-lifestyle/nutrition-and-healthy-eating/expert-answers/monosodium-glutamate/faq-20058196

MOTORIC COGNITIVE RISK SYNDROME (MCR): Predementia syndrome combining cognitive complaint and slow gait.
http://biomedgerontology.oxfordjournals.org/content/71/8/1081

MULTIPLE MYELOMA: Plasma cell (a type of white blood cell derived from B cell) malignancy. Anemia and osteolytic (bone reabsorbing) skeletal lesions usually present. A monoclonal (M) protein can usually be detected in the blood serum and urine.
https://www.mdedge.com/oncologypractice/article/154492/multiple-myeloma/crb-410-update-multiple-myeloma-response-rates?oc_slh=1de3dcf7eb6395af6b796baf8538c
https://www.ncbi.nlm.nih.gov/pmc/articles/PMC5223450/
https://www.cancer.gov/publications/dictionaries/cancer-terms?cdrid=46230
https://www.cancer.gov/publications/dictionaries/cancer-terms?cdrid=45810

MUTATION: Abnormal recombinations of the chromosomes. Permanent alteration in DNA sequence. Alteration in a genome, that may or may not be harmful to the individual.
http://www.nature.com/scitable/definition/recombination-226
http://www.ncbi.nlm.nih.gov/pubmed/23266571
https://academic.oup.com/annonc/article/29/1/30/4616649

MYELIN: Insulating sheath around nerve fibers.
http://www.news-medical.net/health/Myelin-Function.aspx

MYELODYSPLASTIC SYNDROME (MDS): Bone marrow cancer with insufficient presence of normal blood cells, and presence of abnormal blood cells.
https://www.cancer.gov/publications/dictionaries/cancer-terms/def/myelodysplastic-syndrome

MYELOPEROXIDASE: MPO. Enzyme in neutrophils linked to cardiovascular disease.
http://www.ncbi.nlm.nih.gov/gene/4353
http://www.ncbi.nlm.nih.gov/pubmed/26567811/

MYOCARDIAL INFARCTION: Irreversible injury to heart muscle.
http://www.clevelandclinicmeded.com/medicalpubs/diseasemanagement/cardiology/acute-myocardial-infarction/
https://arxiv.org/abs/1708.09843

MYOCARDIUM: Heart muscle.
https://www.boundless.com/physiology/textbooks/boundless-anatomy-and-physiology-textbook/cardiovascular-system-the-heart-18/the-heart-172/myocardial-thickness-and-function-867-10251/

MYOCYTE: Heart muscle cell.
https://www.sciencedaily.com/releases/2016/04/160421145756.htm

MYOMECTOMY: Surgical removal of fibroids from the uterus.

NANOTECHNOLOGY: Engineering of tiny machines, often for the monitoring, prevention, and treatment of disease.
http://tedx.tumblr.com/post/35204848311/fight-cancer-with-nanotechnology-sylvain-martel
https://iopscience.iop.org/journal/0957-4484;jsessionid=3420F74BB331365A7161E71B24C8121C.c4.iopscience.cld.iop.org
https://www.frontiersin.org/articles/10.3389/fimmu.2017.00069/full?utm_source=newsletter&utm_medium=email&utm_campaign=Immunology-w6-2017
https://www.nature.com/articles/s41551-017-0029?WT.mc_id=LDN_NBME_1801_FIRSTANNIVERSARY_PORTFOLIO

NARRATIVE MEDICINE: Narrative competence: Listening to and understanding related stories , and appropriately responding.
http://www.ncbi.nlm.nih.gov/pmc/articles/PMC3034473/

NEPHROPATHY: Kidney disease or damage.
http://www.ncbi.nlm.nih.gov/pmc/articles/PMC3084647/
https://en.wikipedia.org/wiki/Kidney_disease

NEPHROSIS: Generally refers to degenerative disease of the renal (kidney) tubules
http://medical-dictionary.thefreedictionary.com/nephrosis

NEPHROTIC SYNDROME: Excretion of significant amounts of protein in the urine, along with decreased serum albumin (a protein), and edema (swelling due to fluid accumulation)
http://emedicine.medscape.com/article/244631-overview

NEURAL TUBE DEFECT: Birth defect of brain, spine, or spinal cord. http://www.ncbi.nlm.nih.gov/pmc/articles/PMC4023229/

NEURODEGENERATION: Progressive loss of brain function associated with aging. https://www.ncbi.nlm.nih.gov/pubmed/30258237

NEURODEGENERATIVE DISEASES: Diseases which cause progressive loss of cognitive and/or motor function.
https://www.ncbi.nlm.nih.gov/pubmed/23305823
https://www.ncbi.nlm.nih.gov/pubmed/30258237

NEUROGENESIS: Formation of neurons
https://www.nature.com/articles/nature25975https://www.nature.com/articles/s41591-019-0375-9?utm_source=nm_etoc&utm_medium=email&utm_campaign=toc_41591_25_4&utm_content=20190405&WT.ec_id=NM-201904&sap-outbound-id=A2CA93DADBF79C1C13E7D04CDCA72468DD68FEE3

NEUROIMMUNE COMMUNICATION: Interaction between the nervous and immune systems, influencing each other.
http://www.nature.com/ni/journal/v18/n2/full/ni.3676.html
http://www.nature.com/neuro/journal/v20/n2/full/nn.4496.html

NEUROMORPHIC ENGINEERING: Designing hardware and physical models of neural and sensory systems.
https://www.frontiersin.org/journals/neuroscience/sections/neuromorphic-engineering
http://compneuro.uwaterloo.ca/research/nef/overview-of-the-nef.html

NEURON: Specialized nervous system cell that can be stimulated and conducts impulses.
http://www.ncbi.nlm.nih.gov/books/NBK21535/
https://www.nature.com/articles/s41593-018-0205-2.

epdf?shared_access_token=60bklwIRkphHPPY3R_u069RgN0jAjWel9jnR3ZoTv0M_ZnMCyHI8KbNyV63mNxsudkNYBmXFIhQDgOHiquMVMmq6S_Ta_jrenQf

NEUTROPHIL: A white blood cell containing granules that are enzyme containing sacs.
http://jem.rupress.org/content/210/7/1283.full

NEXT GENERATION SEQUENCING (NGS): Rapid (high throughput) DNA sequencing. Used for molecular profiling of tumor samples in order to individualize treatment.
https://www.ncbi.nlm.nih.gov/pmc/articles/PMC5808190/
https://www.ncbi.nlm.nih.gov/pmc/articles/PMC4494749/

NICOTINAMIDE RIBOSIDE: NR: A form of Vitamin B3 (nicotinic acid, Niacin). Converts to **NAD**, Nicotinamide Adenine Dinucleotide, a coenzyme in cells that is involved in energy metabolism
http://www.ctl.cornell.edu/events/ctvf12/Sauve.pdf
http://jpet.aspetjournals.org/content/324/3/883.full

NITRITES: Ester or salt of nitrous acid. Vasodilator.
http://circ.ahajournals.org/content/117/16/2151

NUCLEAR POWER: Energy produced by atomic reaction.
http://www.nei.org/Knowledge-Center/How-Nuclear-Reactors-Work

NUCLEAR WASTE: Radioactive byproducts usually from operation of a nuclear reactor.
http://www.nrc.gov/reading-rm/doc-collections/fact-sheets/radwaste.html

http://www.nrc.gov/reading-rm/doc-collections/fact-sheets/radwaste.html

NUCLEASE: Enzyme that catalyzes the cleavage of phosphodiester bonds between nucleotides.
http://www.nature.com/onc/journal/v21/n58/full/1206135a.html?foxtrotcallback=true
https://www.ncbi.nlm.nih.gov/pubmed/24690881
https://www.ncbi.nlm.nih.gov/pubmed/24690881

NUCLEIC ACID: Substance found in the cytoplasm of cells, as well as in chromosomes, and in viruses. Four specific nucleic acids: **adenine** (A), **cytosine** (C), **guanine** (G), and **thymine** (T) are arranged in pairs on each rung of the ladder of DNA. They code the sequences of amino acids that make up proteins.
http://www.rsc.org/Education/Teachers/Resources/cfb/nucleicacids.htm

NUCLEOSOME: The basic structural unit of chromatin.
https://en.wikipedia.org/wiki/Chromatin
https://www.nature.com/scitable/topicpage/dna-packaging-nucleosomes-and-chromatin-310

NUCLEOTIDE: Building block (subunit) of nucleic acid. Nitrogenous base plus ribose or deoxyribose plus one or more phosphate groups.
https://en.wikipedia.org/wiki/Nucleotide

NUCLEUS: A central structure, surrounded by its own membrane, in the cell. The nucleus contains the chromosomes.
https://micro.magnet.fsu.edu/cells/nucleus/nucleus.html
https://micro.magnet.fsu.edu/cells/nucleus/nucleus.html

NURSING: Breastfeeding.

OBESITY: More than 20% above expected body weight, Body Mass Index (BMI) of 30 or more.
http://www.ncbi.nlm.nih.gov/pubmed/22171945
https://www.ncbi.nlm.nih.gov/pubmed/27386756
http://www.cell.com/cell/fulltext/S0092-8674(16)30213-6
https://www.frontiersin.org/articles/10.3389/fimmu.2017.01745/full?utm_source=F-AAE&utm_medium=EMLF&utm_campaign=MRK_491010_35_I
https://jamanetwork.com/journals/jama/article-abstract/2685153?utm_source=silverchair&utm_campaign=jama_network&utm_content=weekly_highlights&cmp=1&utm_medium=email

ONCOLOGIST: Physician who specializes in the treatment of cancer.
http://www.oncologypractice.com/jcso/specialty-focus/lung/single-article-page/genomic-oncology-moving-beyond-the-tip-of-the-iceberg/0a952f61278bdd07e9d7db4e7c6d1fcb.html

OPHTHALMIC NERVE: Branch of the trigeminal nerve that gives sensory fibers to the ciliary muscle of the eye, lacrimal gland, eyelids, forehead, and mucous membrane of the nose.
http://www.ncbi.nlm.nih.gov/pubmed/11842844

OPIOID: Naturally occurring and synthetic potentially addictive substances that act on specific (opioid) receptors to produce effects including pain relief. Major cause of drug abuse, addiction, and death.
https://www.drugabuse.gov/drugs-abuse/opioids
https://www.drugabuse.gov/drugs-abuse/opioids/opioid-crisis
https://www.fda.gov/Drugs/DrugSafety/InformationbyDrugClass/ucm337066.htm

OSTEOBLAST: Cell that synthesizes bone.
www.nature.com/articles/boneres20169

OSTEOCLAST: Cell that reabsorbs bone. The Care of the Older Person: After the Menopause: Ronald M. Caplan RMC Publishing, LLC 2018, 2019 www.careoftheolderperson.com
http://www.ncbi.nlm.nih.gov/pubmed/1873485
https://www.nature.com/articles/s41413-018-0040-9

OSTEOPENIA: Reduced bone mass. Less severe than osteoporosis.
medicine.medscape.com/article/330598-overview

OSTEOPOROSIS: Reduced bone mass due to depletion of calcium and bone protein.
https://www.karger.com/Article/FullText/431091
http://www.thelancet.com/journals/lancet/article/PIIS0140-6736(17)31613-6/fulltext
https://mydigimag.rrd.com/publication/?i=470718&ver=html5&p=30&utm_source=PT+eTOC+2018-02+prospect+no+spons&utm_campaign=PT1802_Digital_Edition_Alert&utm_medium=email#{"page":"30"
https://www.medscape.com/viewarticle/914567?src=WNL_recnl_190722_MSCPEDIT_obgyn&uac=66536PR&impID=2036955&faf=1

OVARIAN CANCER: Cancer of the ovary.
https://www.ncbi.nlm.nih.gov/pmc/articles/PMC5365187/
https://www.uptodate.com/contents/screening-for-ovarian-cancer

OVARY: The primary female sex organ. Almond shaped, 3 centimeters long. Two ovaries, one on either side of the uterus in the pelvis.
http://emedicine.medscape.com/article/1949171-overview

http://www.fertstert.org/article/S0015-0282(17)31879-4/fulltext?elsca1=etoc&elsca2=email&elsca3=0015-0282_201710_108_4_&elsca4=Obstetrics%20and%20Gyn
https://www.fertstert.org/article/S0015-0282(18)31744-8/fulltext?dgcid=raven_jbs_etoc_email
https://www.frontiersin.org/articles/10.3389/fimmu.2018.02009/full?utm_source=F-AAE&utm_medium=EMLF&utm_campaign=MRK_779779_35_Immuno_20180927_arts_A

OVULATION: During the menstrual cycle, several fluid filled follicles, each containing an ovum, develop. One becomes the dominant follicle. The other follicles regress. At midcycle, the dominant follicle ruptures, releasing the egg, which is then picked up by the fimbria of the fallopian tube.
https://www.ncbi.nlm.nih.gov/books/NBK279054/

OVUM: Pleural: ova. The oocyte. The egg. A single cell present in the female ovary that eventually can be fertilized by a single sperm cell from the male. The ovum before fertilization has only twenty three chromosomes. These pair with the twenty three chromosomes from the spermatozoon to create a genetically new individual with forty six chromosomes.
http://www.theodora.com/anatomy/the_ovum.html

PALLIATIVE CARE: Team support system of enhanced physical, psychosocial, and spiritual quality of life in the face of life-threatening illness. Prevention and relief of suffering and pain. Affirmation of life, and regarding dying as a normal process.
http://www.who.int/cancer/palliative/definition/en/
https://www.surgical.theclinics.com/article/S0039-6109(19)30088-X/pdf
https://www.sciencedirect.com/science/article/pii/S0039610919300891?dgcid=author

PAPANICOLAOU SMEAR: Cells in cervical mucus examined microscopically .
https://www.google.com/search?q=photographs+of+normal+and+ascus+cells&rlz=1C1CHBF_enUS694US694&espv=2&biw=1745&bih=883&tbm=isch&tbo=u&source=univ&sa=X&ved=0ahUKEwittZaMp57PAhUELyYKHeGjBJcQsAQIGw

PARATHYROID HORMONE: PTH. Secreted by parathyroid glands. Regulates blood levels of calcium and phosphorus.
http://www.ncbi.nlm.nih.gov/pubmed/19395963

PARKINSONISM: Parkinson disease. Chronic progressive debilitating neurologic condition arising in the basal ganglia of the brain. Loss of dopaminergic cells. Decreased dopamine production in substantia nigra. The Care of the Older Person: Why Does My Patient Have Gait & Balance Disorders?: Olivier Beauchet. RMC Publishing, LLC 2018, 2019 www.careoftgheolderperson.com
http://www.neurobiologyofaging.org/article/S0197-4580(16)30060-4/abstract
https://www.nature.com/articles/s41531-017-0015-3?WT.mc_id_EMI_PARKD_1708_PMC&WT.ec_id=INTERNAL&spMailingID=54985332&spUserID=MTc3MDI4ODk
https://www.frontiersin.org/articles/10.3389/fneur.2018.00809/full
https://jamanetwork.com/journals/jamanetworkopen/fullarticle/2723412?utm_source=silverchair&utm_medium=email&utm_campaign=article_alert-jamanetworkopen&utm_content=etoc&utm_term=030119

PATHOLOGIST: Physician specializing in the diagnosis of disease by inspecting organs and tumors, both by direct vision and microscopically.

PATIENT-GENERATED HEALH DATA: PGHD: Wearable monitoring devices.
https://pages.mobihealthnews.com/WP-Fitbit-Mediashark-2018-10_LP-Multiplying-the-Value-of-Wearables-and-Patient-Generated-Health-Data2.html?topic=analytics%2C%20mobile%2C%20patientengagement&utm_source=epush&utm_medium=email&utm_campa

PCI: Percutaneous coronary intervention. Coronary angioplasty. Stent introduced by catheter and placed in coronary artery.
http://emedicine.medscape.com/article/161446-overview
http://emedicine.medscape.com/article/161446-technique

PEPTIDE: Two or more amino acids linked together.
https://www2.chemistry.msu.edu/faculty/reusch/virttxtjml/protein2.htm

PERIMENOPAUSE: The time shortly before menopause.

PERIPHERAL ARTERY OCCLUSIVE DISEASE: Narrowing and blockage of smaller arteries. **CLAUDICATION:** Thigh pain with exercise is a symptom.
http://emedicine.medscape.com/article/460178-overview

PERSONALITY TYPE: Psychologic classification of individuals.
http://mbtitoday.org/carl-jung-psychological-type/

PESSARY: Device placed in the vagina for support.

PET SCAN: Positron Emission Tomography. The person being imaged is given sugar, which is tagged by radioactive isotope. Malignant cells tend to metabolize sugar at a higher rate, because they are actively growing and dividing. The increased radioactive

uptake measured at a given site in the body infers that there may be a malignant tumor at that site.
https://journals.lww.com/thoracicimaging/Fulltext/2013/01000/Overview_of_Positron_Emission_Tomography,_Hybrid.4.aspx

PHAGOCYTOSIS: The engulfing of a cell fragment or foreign body by a cell.
http://www.dictionary.com/browse/phagocytosis

PHENOTYPE: The observable properties, characteristics and traits of an organism produced by the interaction of the genotype and the environment.
https://en.wikipedia.org/wiki/Phenotype

PHEROMONE: Chemical substance released by an individual that stimulates the behavior of other individuals.
http://www.scientificamerican.com/article/are-human-pheromones-real/

PHLEBITIS: Inflammation of the walls of a vein.
http://emedicine.medscape.com/article/463256-overview

PHYTOESTROGENS: Naturally occurring estrogen like compounds in plants.
http://www.ncbi.nlm.nih.gov/pmc/articles/PMC3074428/

PITUITARY GLAND: Endocrine gland attached to the base of the brain that secretes hormones that act on other endocrine glands.
http://teachmeanatomy.info/neuro/structures/pituitary-gland/

PLACENTA: Disc-shaped organ that forms in pregnancy, nourishes and supports the developing fetus, and secretes hormones. The surface that is in contact with the mother's uterine wall is composed of many tiny villi. The fetal blood circulates

within these villi, which are bathed on their outside by maternal blood from arteries in the uterine wall. Exchange between mother and fetus of nutrients, waste products of metabolism, oxygen and carbon dioxide continuously occurs through the external lining of each villus. After the baby is delivered, the placenta detaches from the wall of the uterus, and is itself delivered.
https://www.nichd.nih.gov/about/meetings/2014/Documents/BurtonWashington2014.pdf

PLASMA (BLOOD): Fluid part of the blood that carries the blood cells
https://www.ncbi.nlm.nih.gov/pubmedhealth/PMHT0022021/

PLASMID: Circular molecule of DNA found in bacteria.
https://www.nature.com/scitable/definition/plasmid-plasmids-28

PLATELET: Cell fragment in blood involved in blood clotting.
https://www.ouhsc.edu/platelets/platelets/platelets%20intro.html

PMDD: Premenstrual dysphoric disorder. Premenstrual mood and behavioral changes.

PMS: Premenstrual syndrome. Various symptoms just prior to, or with the onset of, a period. May include depression, anxiety, bloating, constipation, diarrhea, breast tenderness, weight gain, and headache.

PNEUMONIA: Lung inflammation with congestion.
https://www.ncbi.nlm.nih.gov/pmc/articles/PMC4072047/
https://www.ncbi.nlm.nih.gov/pmc/articles/PMC4072047/
https://www.ncbi.nlm.nih.gov/pmc/articles/PMC4072047/

POLAR BODY: Small cells resulting from two meiotic divisions of the oocyte. Contain the same DNA as the oocyte.
http://www.ncbi.nlm.nih.gov/pmc/articles/PMC3164815/

POLLUTION: Presence in, or introduction into, the environment of harmful substances.

POLYGENIC RISK SCORE: (Genetic Risk Score) Estimating the risk conferred by a number of DNA variants in genes to result in a disease onset or other outcome.
https://jamanetwork.com/journals/jama/fullarticle/2730627?guestAccessKey=6579bb87-9479-4cfd-a93c-d39102a0fb5f&utm_source=silverchair&utm_medium=email&utm_campaign=article_alert-jama&utm_

POLYP: Benign growth arising from a stalk. Polyps occur in the interior of the uterus and may protrude out the cervical os. Polyps in the large intestine may be malignant. Polyps can grow on the vocal cords, and other areas.

POLYPHARMACY: Simultaneous use of multiple drugs, more than are medically necessary. See: The Care of the Older Person: Polypharmacy and Deprescribing in the Elderly: Louise Mallet RMC Publishing LLC 2018, 2019 www.careoftheolderperson.com
https://www.ncbi.nlm.nih.gov/pmc/articles/PMC3864987/
https://jamanetwork.com/journals/jama/fullarticle/2714515?guestAccessKey=06cab41f-eab9-4441-85a3-53b6c4725e5e&utm_source=silverchair&utm_medium=email&utm_campaign=article_alert-jama&utm

POSTMENOPAUSAL BLEEDING: Vaginal bleeding occurring after the menopause.
https://www.ncbi.nlm.nih.gov/pmc/articles/PMC3951032/

PRECISION MEDICINE: Studying how the genomic variation in an individual or their disease (tumor sample) influences drug response. Identification of the specific mutations in a tumor, so

that targeted therapy can be brought to bear. See Next Generation Sequencing (NGS)
http://stm.sciencemag.org/content/7/300/300ps17.full
https://academic.oup.com/annonc/article/29/1/30/4616649

PREIMPLANTATION GENETIC DIAGNOSIS: PGD. Chromosomal analysis of the polar body (See: Polar body), or of a single embryonic cell.
http://emedicine.medscape.com/article/273415-overview

PRETERM INFANT: Formerly called prematurity. A baby born before thirty eight weeks of intrauterine life.
http://www.adelaide.edu.au/news/news88982.html

PROBIOTICS: Microorganisms, usually bacteria, with health benefits.
http://www.medicinenet.com/script/main/art.asp?articlekey=11901

PROGENITOR CELL: Activated in tissue repair; differentiate to replace damaged tissue. If signal to differentiate not processed, progenitor cells can keep on reproducing, leading to mutations
http://stemcell.childrenshospital.org/about-stem-cells/adult-somatic-stem-cells-101/what-are-progenitor-cells/

PROGESTERONE: A female sex hormone, made in the ovary, prominent in the second half of the menstrual cycle.
https://en.wikipedia.org/wiki/Progesterone

PROGESTIN: A progesterone-like substance.

PROGRAMMED CELL DEATH: See Apoptosis for references

PROKARYOTE: Single celled organism without a distinct nucleus and no specialized organelles (except ribosomes). Includes Bacteria.
http://www.dictionary.com/browse/prokaryote

PROLACTIN: Hormone secreted by the anterior pituitary that stimulates lactation.
http://www.ncbi.nlm.nih.gov/pubmed/11015620

PROLAPSE: Downward displacement of an organ.
http://emedicine.medscape.com/article/276259-overview

PROSTAGLANDINS: Group of fatty acids that stimulate contractility of uterine and other smooth muscle.
http://www.ncbi.nlm.nih.gov/pmc/articles/PMC3081099/

PROSTATE: Gland located below the bladder and surrounding the urethra in males. Prostatic fluid is secreted via ducts that open into the urethra.
http://www.ncbi.nlm.nih.gov/pubmedhealth/PMH0072475/
http://www.ncbi.nlm.nih.gov/pmc/articles/PMC4633657/
http://jamanetwork.com/journals/jama/fullarticle/2618352?utm_medium=alert&utm_source=JAMAPublishAheadofPrint&utm_campaign=11-04-2017

PROSTATE CANCER: Cancer of the prostate gland.
https://www.ncbi.nlm.nih.gov/pubmed/28655021
http://www.nejm.org/doi/full/10.1056/NEJMoa1715546?query=main_nav_lg

PROTEIN: A specific sequence of amino acids. Specific proteins are elaborated by specific genes. Proteins have vital functions within the body. They make up the structure of various organs and are involved in their function. They make up the hormones, and the enzymes which facilitate chemical reactions in the body. They are involved in immune response.
https://en.wikipedia.org/wiki/Proteome

PROTEOMICS: The study of all the proteins in the body, how they function and interact.
http://proteomics.cancer.gov/whatisproteomics

PROTON PUMP INHIBITORS: Drugs that inhibit acid secretion by gastric parietal cells. Used in gastroesophageal reflux disease (**GERD**).
https://www.ncbi.nlm.nih.gov/pmc/articles/PMC5221858/

PTK: Protein-tyrosine kinase. Regulates signaling in the cell.
http://www.ncbi.nlm.nih.gov/pubmed/9393984

PULMONARY EMBOLUS: PE. Blood clot in the lung.
http://emedicine.medscape.com/article/300901-overview

RADIATION: Emission of energy as electromagnetic waves or as moving subatomic particles, especially high energy particles that cause ionization. Ionizing radiation has enough energy to remove electrons from the orbit of an atom, causing the atom to be charged (ionized).
http://www.who.int/ionizing_radiation/about/what_is_ir/en/

RECEPTOR SITE: Distinctively shaped area on a cell surface, designed to receive a specific substance.
http://www.merckmanuals.com/professional/clinical-pharmacology/pharmacodynamics/drug%E2%80%93receptor-interactions
https://www.empr.com/news/vitrakvi-larotrectinib-advanced-solid-tumors-ntrk-gene-fusion-approval/article/816725/?utm_source=newsletter&utm_medium=email&utm_campaign=mpr-dailydose-cp-20181129&cpn=obgyn_all,obgyn_md,cambia_august2018&hmS

RECOMBINANT DNA TECHNOLOGY: Rearranging DNA molecules, manufacturing recombinant DNA. Recombinant DNA

molecule constructed from segments obtained from different DNA molecules.
https://en.wikipedia.org/wiki/Recombinant_DNA

RECOMBINATION: Genetic recombination. Interchange of chromosomal parts or genes. Breaking and rejoining DNA strands, forming new DNA molecules.
https://en.wikipedia.org/wiki/Genetic_recombination
https://www.nature.com/scitable/topicpage/dna-is-constantly-changing-through-the-process-6524876

RECTOCELE: Bulging of the anterior wall of the rectum into the posterior wall of the vagina.
https://www.ncbi.nlm.nih.gov/pmc/articles/PMC2967328/

REGENERATIVE MEDICINE: Creation of new organs, tissues, and body parts from stem cells, which are placed on a dissolvable matrix: tissue engineering, along with self-healing by the body's systems.
http://www.nature.com/articles/npjregenmed20167
https://www.nature.com/articles/s41536-017-0008-1?WT.mc_id=EMI_RegMed_1704&spMailingID=53890539&spUserID=MTc3MDI4ODk5NQS2&spJobID=114328
https://www.nature.com/articles/npjregenmed20167?WT.mc_id=EMI_RegMed_1706&spMailingID=54243481&spUserID=MTc3MDI4ODk5NQS2&spJobID=1181517

REJECTION: HOST VS GRAFT: Immunologic response by organ recipient to allograft, damaging it. Immune cells in the transplanted organ can also attack the host: Graft vs. host response.
http://emedicine.medscape.com/article/430449-overview#a4

RENIN: Proteolytic enzyme elaborated by juxtaglomerular cells of the kidneys that acts on angiotensin.
https://www.britannica.com/science/renin-angiotensin-system

RENIN-ANGIOTENSIN SYSTEM: RAS. A mechanism of acute renal hypertension. Renal artery compression or occlusion causing ischemia of the renal cortex results in renal juxtaglomerular cells converting prorenin into renin. Renin acts on angiotensinogen in the bloodstream from the liver, converting it to angiotensin I, which is converted to angiotensin II by angiotensin-converting enzyme. Angiotensin II acts on aldosterone producing cells in the adrenal cortex, causing aldosterone production, leading to sodium retention and increased plasma volume. This leads to an increase in blood pressure, and increased blood flow, including to the kidneys, resulting in stretching of renal afferent arterioles, giving negative feedback so that renin secretion tends to return towards normal. Renin-angiotensin systems are present in various other tissues, in addition to the kidneys.
http://www.ncbi.nlm.nih.gov/pubmed/17878513

REPROGRAMMING: (Cellular Reprogramming): Using the expression of four genes (**Yamanaka Factors**) to convert any cell into **induced pluripotent stem cells (iPSCs)**
https://www.salk.edu/news-release/
turning-back-time-salk-scientists-reverse-signs-aging/
http://www.cell.com/cell/fulltext/S0092-8674(16)31664-6

RESVERATROL: Polyphenolic compound in red wine that may be partly responsible for the beneficial cardiovascular effects that have been attributed to red wine
http://lpi.oregonstate.edu/mic/dietary-factors/phytochemicals/
resveratrol

RETICULOENDOTHELIAL SYSTEM, also called: **MONONUCLEAR PHAGOCYTE SYSTEM (MPS):** Widespread system in reticular (thin banding fibers) connective tissue that forms antibodies to counteract foreign antigens. https://en.wikipedia.org/wiki/Mononuclear_phagocyte_system

RETINOPATHY: Disease of the retina http://www.ncbi.nlm.nih.gov/pmc/articles/PMC3874488/

RH ISOIMMUNIZATION: Immune response of Rh Negative mother to her Rh positive fetus. First Rh positive child usually not affected. http://emedicine.medscape.com/article/797150-overview

RIBOSOME: The protein manufacturing machine. Complex molecular machine one millionth of an inch in diameter. Tiny organ (organelle) in the cytoplasm of the cell. Made up of proteins and ribosomal RNA (rRNA)- the active component in protein synthesis. At the ribosome, the genetic code is read and translated into proteins. Amino acids are carried to the ribosome by transfer RNA (tRNA) . The genetic code instructions for making a protein are carried to the ribosome by messenger RNA (mRNA) from the DNA in the cell nucleus. At the ribosome, the tRNA recognizes the sequence of the genetic code on the mRNA and lines up the amino acids in the proper order. The ribosome catalyzes the formation of bonds between the amino acids. https://micro.magnet.fsu.edu/cells/ribosomes/ribosomes.html

RNA: Ribonucleic acid. Messenger RNA (mRNA) is essentially a copy of a piece of one strand of DNA. Proteins are not made from the DNA of the gene. A template of RNA is made from the gene DNA. The RNA is then processed. The processing involves splicing of RNA. This spliced RNA, the template upon which the protein

is made (protein synthesis), is called messenger RNA (mRNA). mRNA goes to the ribosome in the cell cytoplasm, where it meets the transfer RNA (tRNA) carrying the amino acids. Under the influence of ribosomal RNA (rRNA), the amino acids are bound together to form the protein (see Ribosome).
http://www.nature.com/scitable/definition/ribonucleic-acid-rna-45
https://jamanetwork.com/journals/jama/fullarticle/2712406?guestAccessKey=22414c3e-162a-4ff0-8b50-5477ff58735b&utm_source=silverchair&utm_campaign=jama_network&utm_content=weekly_highlights&cmp=1&utm_medium=email

RNA INTERFERENCE: RNAi : Pathway that regulates gene expression
https://jamanetwork.com/journals/jama/fullarticle/2712406?guestAccessKey=22414c3e-162a-4ff0-8b50-5477ff58735b&utm_source=silverchair&utm_campaign=jama_network&utm_content=weekly_highlights&cmp=1&utm_medium=email https://www.ncbi.nlm.nih.gov/probe/docs/techrnai/
https://www.nature.com/nrg/multimedia/rnai/animation/index.html
https://www.ncbi.nlm.nih.gov/pmc/articles/PMC5542916/
https://www.nature.com/articles/d41586-018-05867-7?WT.ec_id=NATURE-20180816&utm_source=nature_etoc&utm_medium=email&utm_campaign=20180816&spMailingID=57190125&spUserID=MjA1NjIyNjc4OAS2&spJobID=1462154550&spReportId=MTQ2MjE1

ROBOTICS: A robot is a machine capable of automatically carrying out complex actions, programmable by computer.
https://jamanetwork.com/journals/jama/fullarticle/2712406?guestAccessKey=22414

c3e-162a-4ff0-8b50-5477ff58735b&utm_source=silverchair&utm_campaign=jama_network&utm_content=weekly_highlights&cmp=1&utm_medium=emailt

Robotic surgery is carried out via robotic telemanipulation. The surgeon's movements at a console are translated to surgical instruments previously placed into the patient by minimally invasive technique.
http://allaboutroboticsurgery.com/surgicalrobots.html

SARCOMA: A virulent form of malignant, solid tumor.
http://sarcomahelp.org/reviews/who-classification-sarcomas.html

SARS: **S**evere **a**cute **r**espiratory **s**yndrome.
http://www.cdc.gov/sars/about/fs-sars.html

SCAR: Cicatrix. Connective tissue in which fibroblasts form granulation tissue. Older scars are composed of dense collagenous tissue.

SCURVY: Disease caused by lack of Vitamin C (ascorbic acid).
http://www.medicalnewstoday.com/articles/155758.php

SELF-DESTRUCT GENES: Genes that cause cell death (apoptosis).
http://www.nature.com/mt/journal/v23/n9/full/mt2015139a.html

SENOLYTICS: Drugs that kill **senescent**, non-dividing cells that accumulate in aging organs.
https://www.nature.com/news/to-stay-young-kill-zombie-cells-1.22872?WT.ec_id=NEWS-20171026&spMailingID=55224149&spUserID=MTc2NjY4OTM5NgS2&s
http://www.cell.com/cell/fulltext/S0092-8674(17)30246-5
https://www.ncbi.nlm.nih.gov/pubmed/22048312

https://www.ncbi.nlm.nih.gov/labs/journals/j-am-geriatr-soc/new/2017-09-05/
http://onlinelibrary.wiley.com/wol1/doi/10.1111/jgs.14969/full

SENSITIVITY: (In medical testing) Probability that a test result will be positive when the disease is present.
https://www.medcalc.org/calc/diagnostic_test.php

SEPSIS: Systemic inflammatory response to infection.
http://www.ncbi.nlm.nih.gov/pmc/articles/PMC3684427/
Consensus Definitions for Sepsis and Septic Shock | Critical Care Medicine | JAMA | The JAMA Network

SERM: Specific estrogen receptor modulator. A class of drugs used during the menopause to prevent osteoporosis. Some drugs in this class are protective against the formation of breast cancer.
http://www.ncbi.nlm.nih.gov/pmc/articles/PMC3624793/

SEROTONIN: 5HT. 5-hydroxytryptamine. A monoamine neurotransmitter derived from tryptophan.
https://en.wikipedia.org/wiki/Serotonin

SEROTONIN/NOREPINEPHRINE REUPTAKE INHIBITORS: SNRI'S. Medications used in depression. See: The Care of the Older Person: An Overview of Late-Life Depression: Artin Mahdanian, Silvia Monti De Flores. RMC Publishing, LLC 2018, 2019
www.careoftheolderperson.com
http://pharmacologycorner.com/serotonin-5ht-receptors-agonists-antagonist/#serotonin%20agonists

SHBG: Sex hormone binding globulin. Protein elaborated in the liver that binds and transports testosterone, dihydrotestosterone (DHT), and estradiol as inactive forms in blood.
https://en.wikipedia.org/wiki/Sex_hormone-binding_globulin

SHINGLES: Delayed cutaneous manifestation by **Herpes Zoster** (Varicella: chicken pox) virus. Preventive vaccine available. http://annals.org/aim/fullarticle/2671913/recommended-immunization-schedule-adults-aged-19-years-older-united-states http://bmjopen.bmj.com/content/4/6/e004833

SIALOMUCIN: Mucopolysaccharide containing sialic acid. Component of lung airway secretion. http://www.ncbi.nlm.nih.gov/gene/8763

SICKNESS (ILLNESS): Inability of individuals to pursue their goals and purposes because of impairments in function considered to be in the domain of medicine Boudreau, JD, Cassell, EJ, Fuks, A: Physicianship and the Rebirth of Medical Education. Oxford University Press 2018

SIGNAL TRANSDUCTION (CELL SIGNALING): Transmission of molecular signals from cell surface receptors to the cell interior. https://www.tocris.com/pharmacologicalBrowser.php?ItemId=187888#.V8hjh7ZTFwE

SINGLE CELL BIOLOGY: The study of the individual cell. https://genomebiology.biomedcentral.com/articles/10.1186/s13059-016-0941-0
http://www.nature.com/news/single-cell-biology-1.22241
https://www.frontiersin.org/articles/10.3389/fimmu.2018.02425/full?utm_source=F-AAE&utm_medium=EMLF&utm_campaign=MRK_812127_35_Immuno_20181030_arts_A

SIRTUIN GENES: Genes that exert anti-aging effect in yeast. Increased sirtuin activity may be related to the mechanism by which caloric restriction extends life span. https://www.ncbi.nlm.nih.gov/pubmed/18419308

SOMATIC CELL NUCLEAR TRANSFER: Therapeutic cloning. Nucleus is taken from an adult cell and placed into an ovum whose own nucleus has been removed. These embryonic stem cells are induced to form specialized cells needed by the adult from whom the adult cell nucleus was taken.
http://www.hhmi.org/biointeractive/somatic-cell-nuclear-transfer-animation

SPECIFICITY:(In medical testing) Probability that a test result will be negative when the disease is not present.
https://www.medcalc.org/calc/diagnostic_test.php

SPERMATOZOON: The male germ (sex) cell, derived from the testicle. It has a head, body and tail, and is motile. The spermatozoon swims up the female reproductive tract, eventually fertilizing (fusing with) the egg (ovum) in the fallopian tube.
https://www.boundless.com/physiology/textbooks/boundless-anatomy-and-physiology-textbook/the-reproductive-system-27/physiology-of-the-male-reproductive-system-253/spermatogenesis-1234-9350/

SPINDLE NUCLEAR TRANSFER: Removal of the nuclear spindle from a maternal oocyte and transferring that spindle to a donor oocyte from which the spindle has been removed, in order to obviate a mitochondrial mutation. The donor oocyte containing the maternal nuclear spindle is then fertilized.
https://www.ncbi.nlm.nih.gov/pmc/articles/PMC4005382/
https://www.sciencenews.org/blog/science-ticker/first-%E2%80%98three-parent-baby%E2%80%99-born-nuclear-transfer

SPLICING: The reattaching of the two ends of a stringlike material, after a piece has been removed. In **GENE SPLICING,** DNA is cut and a gene inserted.

http://www.premierbiosoft.com/tech_notes/gene-splicing.html

SSRI: Selective serotonin reuptake inhibitor. Medications used in depression. See: The Care of the Older Person: An Overview of Late-Life Depression; Artin Mahdanian, Silvia Monti De Flores. RMC Publishing, LLC 2018, 2019. www.careoftheolderperson.com
http://www.rxlist.com/the_comprehensive_list_of_antidepressants-page2/drugs-condition.htm#ssris

STATINS: Drugs that reduce circulating LDL (low density lipoprotein) by encouraging the LDL receptor to increase uptake. Decreased production of LDL-C (low density lipoprotein cholesterol) results.
https://www.drugs.com/drug-class/hmg-coa-reductase-inhibitors.html

STEM CELL: An undifferentiated cell that has the potential to become a specialized cell with a specific function, such as a blood cell or a muscle cell.
http://stemcells.nih.gov/info/basics/1.htm
http://fhs.mcmaster.ca/main/news/news_2016/life_saving_blood_stem_cells.html

STEM CELL TRANSPLANT: Injection of stem cells into the body to replace damaged or diseased tissue, blood.
http://www.cancer.gov/about-cancer/treatment/types/stem-cell-transplant
http://journal.frontiersin.org/article/10.3389/fimmu.2016.00470/full

STENT: Self expanding tube placed in a blood vessel to keep that vessel patent. May be drug-eluting.
https://www.sciencedaily.com/releases/2015/03/150316135610.htm

STEREOTACTIC RADIOSURGERY: SRS. Precisely focused radiation to scar and close the blood vessels of an arteriovenous malformation (AVM) in the brain.
http://www.irsa.org/radiosurgery.html

STEREOTAXIS: Method in neurosurgery for locating points within the brain using an external three dimensional frame.

STROKE: Cerebrovascular accident. Damage to the brain by a blood clot in a vessel supplying the brain, or by hemorrhage into the brain.
http://www.neurology.org/content/early/2016/09/16/WNL.0000000000003238.abstract
http://www.empr.com/news/repatha-heart-attack-stroke-prevention-pcsk9-inhibitor/article/711332/?DCMP=EMC-MPR_DailyDose_cp_20171204&cpn=obgyn_all&hmSubId=&hmEmail=hIe6FnTBLUDNqAesd8d7sd9Sz-y1cfMN0&NID=1538223656&c_id=&dl=0&spMailingID=18599771&spUserID=MTgxMDk3OTQyMDM0S0&spJobID=1160335565&spReportId=MTE2MDMzNTU2NQS2
http://www.acc.org/latest-in-cardiology/ten-points-to-remember/2018/01/29/12/45/2018-guidelines-for-the-early-management-of-stroke hs://www.nature.com/articles/s41746-017-0015-z?utm_source=Springer_Nature_website&utm_medium=Website_links&utm_content=AngWan-SN-OD-Neuroscience-Global&utm_campaign=SNOR_USG_SFN18ttp

SUBUNIT: Ribosomal nucleic acid (rRNA) molecules (see "Ribosome")
http://www.microbe.net/simple-guides/fact-sheet-ribosomal-rna-rrna-the-details/

SUDDEN INFANT DEATH SYNDROME: SIDS, Unexplained death during sleep of a seemingly healthy baby.
http://emedicine.medscape.com/article/804412-overview

SUICIDE: Intentional, voluntary taking of own life. Contributory factor influencing average lifespan.
http://healthjournalism.org/blog/2014/04/exploring-risk-factors-rates-of-suicide-in-seniors/

SUPERAGER: Person 80 years or older with episodic memory ability at least as good as average middle-age adult. Significantly thicker brain cortex than same-age peers.
http://jamanetwork.com/journals/jama/article-abstract/2614177

T-LYMPHOCYTE: **T-Cell**. White blood cell that is immunologically competent. Responsible for cell-mediated immunity. Can attack surface antigens on malignant cells, if activated by prior presentation of the antigen.
https://en.wikipedia.org/wiki/T_cell
https://www.frontiersin.org/articles/10.3389/fimmu.2018.00233/full?utm_source=F-AAE&utm_medium=EMLF&utm_campaign=MRK_554072_35_Immuno_20180227_arts_A

TALENS: **T**ranscription **A**ctivator-**L**ike **E**ffector **N**ucleases. Utilized to alter genes. See **Transcription, Nuclease.**
https://www.ncbi.nlm.nih.gov/pmc/articles/PMC3547402/

TARGETED AREA CORRECTION SEQUENCING: Detection of mutations and rearrangements indicative of cancer in cell-free plasma DNA.
https://www.ncbi.nlm.nih.gov/pmc/articles/PMC4755822/
http://journals.plos.org/plosgenetics/article?id=10.1371/journal.pgen.1005816
http://journals.plos.org/plosone/article?id=10.1371/journal.pone.0064271
http://journals.plos.org/plosgenetics/article?id=10.1371/journal.pgen.1005816

TARGETED THERAPY: Drug designed to reverse the effects of a specific mutation
http://www.ncbi.nlm.nih.gov/pubmed/23470539

TELOMERASE: Enzyme that maintains and repairs the telomere.
http://study.com/academy/lesson/what-is-telomerase-definition-function-structure.html

TELOMERE: The end of a chromosome. It is made up of DNA. The telomere gives stability to the end of the chromosome, preventing abnormal recombinations (mutations). The Care of the Older Person: Introduction: Jose Morais. RMC Publishing, LLC, 2018, 2019.
www.careoftheolderperson.com
https://en.wikipedia.org/wiki/Telomere
https://link.springer.com/article/10.1007/s10815-017-0967-6/fulltext.html?wt_mc=alerts.TOCjournals

TEMPLATE: The pattern from which copies are made.
https://engineering.ucsb.edu/~shell/che170/DNA-notes.pdf

TESTIS: The male gonad.
http://emedicine.medscape.com/article/1949259-overview

TESTOSTERONE: The prominent androgen in the male. Male sex hormone. Present in lesser amounts in women.
http://www.livescience.com/38963-testosterone.html

THALLIUM STRESS TEST: Radioisotope uptake monitoring and myocardial perfusion assessment while patient is on a treadmill.
http://pubs.rsna.org/doi/full/10.1148/rg.317115090

THROMBOPHLEBITIS: Inflammation of the wall of a vein in conjunction with thrombosis.

THROMBOSIS: Blood clotting in a blood vessel.

THYMUS GLAND: Lymphoid gland of the immune system located in the neck that produces T-Cells.
http://biology.about.com/od/anatomy/ss/thymus.htm

TIA: Transient ischemic arteriospasm. Constriction of blood vessels in the brain with no permanent damage.

TISSUE ENGINEERING: Combining cells, scaffolds, and biologically active molecules to create new tissue.
https://www.nibib.nih.gov/science-education/science-topics/tissue-engineering-and-regenerative-medicine

TISSUE TYPING: Tissue antigens of prospective organ donor and recipient compared for histocompatibility. HLA (human leukocyte antigen) typing.
http://www.encyclopedia.com/topic/Tissue_Typing.aspx

TOTIPOTENTIALITY: Capability of a cell to differentiate into unlimited number of cell types.
http://medical-dictionary.thefreedictionary.com/totipotential+cell

TOXEMIA: The hypertensive disorders of pregnancy.

TPA: Tissue plasminogen activator. Protein involved in the breakdown of blood clots.
http://pharmacologycorner.com/thrombolytic-agents-mechanism-of-action-indications-contraindications-and-side-effects/
http://atvb.ahajournals.org/content/29/8/1151.full

TRABECULA: Supporting structures of connective tissue.

TRANSCRIPTION: Transfer of genetic code information between nucleic acids. The process by which the genetic code on the DNA gets into the mRNA template (see DNA, RNA).
http://www.vcbio.science.ru.nl/en/virtuallessons/cellcycle/trans/

TRANSCRIPTOME: Gene readouts (transcripts) of all the DNA in a cell by RNA
https://www.genome.gov/13014330/transcriptome-fact-sheet/

TRANSFORMATION ZONE: The outer cervix is lined by squamous cells, much like the vaginal lining. The inner canal of the cervix is lined by tall cylindrical cells. Where these two layers meet, there is an area of microscopic activity where the cylindrical columnar cells are being transformed, or over-ridden, by squamous cells. This is a benign process called **squamous metaplasia**. This area is called the transformation zone. It is in this area of cell activity that cancer of the cervix most commonly arises.

TRANSLATION: The process by which the genetic code of mRNA becomes proteins.
https://bioweb.uwlax.edu/GenWeb/Molecular/Theory/Translation/translation.htm

TRANSLATIONAL MEDICINE: Mechanisms by which new drugs and tests get from the laboratory into the hands of physicians for administration to patients, and the mechanisms for ensuring that patients get necessary services.
https://www.ncbi.nlm.nih.gov/pmc/articles/PMC2829707/
http://www.medscape.com/viewarticle/871305nlid=110427_2581&src=WNL_mdplsnews_161104_mscpedit_obgy&uac=66536PR&spon=16&impID=1228473&faf=1

TRANSPLANTATION: Transfer of organ or tissue from one individual to another.
http://www.ajog.org/article/0002-9378(70)90382-0/abstract?cc=y=
http://www.who.int/transplantation/organ/en/

TRIGEMINAL NERVE: The fifth cranial nerve.
http://emedicine.medscape.com/article/1873373-overview

TRIGLYCERIDE: Ester formed from glycerol and three molecules of fatty acids.
https://en.wikipedia.org/wiki/Triglyceride

TRIPTANS: Serotonin (5HT) receptor agonists. Medications that constrict blood vessels in the brain and are used in the treatment of migraine.
http://archneur.jamanetwork.com/article.aspx?articleid=782346

TROPHOBLAST: Outer ring of cells around the blastocyst cavity that becomes the placenta.
http://discovery.lifemapsc.com/in-vivo-development/trophoblast/trophoblast

TROPONINS: Proteins released when heart muscle is damaged. Can be detected in blood circulation and be used to predict cardiovascular disease (CVD) risk.
https://www.ahajournals.org/doi/pdf/10.1161/CIRCULATIONAHA.118.038772

TUBERCULOSIS: Infectious disease especially affecting the lungs caused by mycobacterium tuberculosis.
http://www.thelancet.com/journals/lanres/article/PIIS2213-2600(15)00063-6/abstract

TUMOR: Abnormal growth. May be benign or malignant.

TUMOR GRADE: Appearance, abnormality of malignant tumor cells.
https://www.cancer.gov/about-cancer/diagnosis-staging/prognosis/tumor-grade-fact-sheet

TUMOR INFILTRATING LYMPHOCYTE (TIL): Immune cell from a patient's blood that has moved into a tumor to attack it. TIL's can be removed from the tumor, activated, then given back to the patient.

https://www.cancer.gov/publications/dictionaries/cancer-terms/def/tumor-infiltrating-lymphocyte

TUMOR SPECIFIC ANTIGEN (TSA): Protein or other molecule produced in tumor cells that sets off an immune response in the host. Used as tumor markers to identify tumor cells in the body. Used in the immunologic treatment of cancer. Also, **Tumor Associated Antigens (TAA)** that are significantly more abundant in cancer cells than in other tissue. CEA Antigen, Prostate-Specific Antigen, CA125, CA19-9
https://www.researchgate.net/publication/9314460_Demonstration_of_Tumor-Specific_Antigens_in_Human_Colonic_Carcinomata_by_Immunological_Tolerance_and_Absorption_Techniques
https://www.researchgate.net/publication/12453745_Self_recognition_in_the_Ig_superfamily_Identification_of_precise_subdomains_in_carcinoembryonic_antigen_required_for_intercellular_adhesion

TUMOR STAGE: Extent of the malignant tumor: its size and spread.
https://www.cancer.gov/about-cancer/diagnosis-staging/staging

TUMOR SUPPRESSOR GENE (Antioncogene): Genes, such as the TP59 gene, that elaborate tumor suppressor proteins that control cell growth. Mutations (DNA changes) in these genes are associated with cancer. Tumor Protein 53 (TP53) that also has a role in germ cell survival, is another example.
https://www.cancer.gov/publications/dictionaries/cancer-terms?cdrid=46657

https://www.nature.com/articles/d41586-017-07291-9?WT.ec_id=NEWSDAILY-20171123&utm_source=briefing&utm_medium=email&utm_campaig
http://www.fertstert.org/article/S0015-0282(17)32096-4/fulltext?elsca1=etoc&elsca2=email&elsca3=0015-0282_201801_109_1_&elsca4=Obstetrics%20and%20Gyn

TURBINATES: Shelves of bone covered by thick mucous membrane that project into the nasal passages.
http://emedicine.medscape.com/article/874771-overview

UBIQUITIN-PROTEASOME SYSTEM : A protein clearance mechanism with implications in aging and age-related diseases
https://link.springer.com/article/10.1007/s10815-016-0842-x?wt_mc=alerts.TOCjournals
http://www.nature.com/ncomms/2014/141208/ncomms6659/fig_tab/ncomms6659_F1.html

ULTRASONOGRAPHY: Imaging by reflecting high energy "sound" waves off objects. The waves have higher frequency than sound that can be heard by humans. Four dimensional sonography refers to images being seen in real time.
https://www.ncbi.nlm.nih.gov/pubmed/20541656
http://medical-dictionary.thefreedictionary.com/ultrasonography

ULTRAVIOLET RAYS: UV. Short wavelength solar rays that are invisible to the human eye.
http://medical-dictionary.thefreedictionary.com/ultraviolet+rays

UMBILICAL CORD: The cord that connects the developing fetus to the placenta. Blood circulates in the cord via two arteries and one vein: the umbilical vein carrying nutrients and oxygen from the placenta to the fetus, and the umbilical arteries carrying waste

products of metabolism and carbon dioxide away from the fetus, back to the placenta.
https://www.ncbi.nlm.nih.gov/books/NBK53254/

UMBILICAL CORD BLOOD: Fetal blood that circulates via the umbilical cord.
http://www.webmd.com/parenting/baby/features/banking-your-babys-cord-blood#1
http://journal.frontiersin.org/article/10.3389/fimmu.2017.00087/full?utm_source=newsletter&utm_medium=email&utm_campaign=Immunology-w6-2017
https://www.nature.com/nature/journal/vaop/ncurrent/full/nature22067.html

URETHRA: The passage from the urinary bladder to the vulva in the female, and to the penile meatus in the male.

URETHROCELE: Bulging of the urethra into the anterior vaginal wall.

URINARY INCONTINENCE: Involuntary loss of urine. Stress incontinence, urgency incontinence and neurogenic incontinence are types. See: The Care of the Older Person: Incontinence In Older Adults: Samer Shamout, Lysanne Campeau. RMC Publishing, LLC, 2018, 2019. www.careoftheolderperson.com
http://jamanetwork.com/journals/jama/article-abstract/2595508

UTERUS: The womb. Its endometrial lining undergoes decidual change to receive the implanting fertilized egg (zygote). During labor, muscular rhythmic contractions of the uterine wall gradually send the fetus through the birth canal.

VACCINE: Usually a killed, or attenuated (variant) virus given by mouth or injection to activate the body's immune system against the actual dangerous virus. If a vaccinated person comes in contact

with the actual virus, the person's activated immune system kills the virus before it can cause harm. Anticancer vaccines that target malignant cells are now being developed and are in use. The Care of the Older Person: Are the Immunizations of my patient Up To Date? Dominique Tessier. RMC Publishing, LLC 2018, 2019
www.careoftheolderperson.com
https://www.jci.org/articles/view/80009
http://journal.frontiersin.org/article/10.3389/fimmu.2017.00800/full?utm_source=F-AAE&utm_medium=EMLF&utm_campaign=MRK_333189_35_Immuno_20170720_arts_A tps://jamanetwork.com/journals/jama/fullarticle/2714651?guestAccessKey=1f4ca6ea-c69b-48ab-909f-713499b43cf8&utm_source=silverchair&utm_medium=email&utm_campaign=article_alert-jama&utm_content=etoc&utm_term=120518
https://jamanetwork.com/journals/jama/fullarticle/2714651?guestAccessKey=1f4ca6ea-c69b-48ab-909f-713499b43cf8&utm_source=silverchair&utm_medium=email&utm_campaign=article_alert-jama&utm_content=etoc&utm_term=1205181

VAGINA: The female genital tract extending inwards from the vulva. Closed at rest with the anterior wall resting on the posterior wall. Its muscular, elastic wall is lined by a mucous membrane that has a normal secretion. The cervix protrudes into the inner end, the vaginal vault.

VALUE-BASED MEDICAL CARE: Quality of care relative to its cost. Quality is assessed in the areas of outcomes, safety and service. Outcomes includes measurement of mortality rates, complications, and resultant functional status of patients. Safety includes attention to infection rates, accidental falls, and

medication errors. Service assesses patient satisfaction, wait times, access to treatment and procedures, and affordability.
https://wire.ama-assn.org/education/value-based-care-elusive-concept-enters-curriculum?&utm_source=BHClistID&utm_medium=BulletinHealthCare&utm_term=120616&utm_content=MorningRounds&utm_campaign=BHCMessageID
http://jamanetwork.com/journals/jama/fullarticle/2594716

VARICOSE VEINS: Veins that bulge out due to damage to their valves.
http://emedicine.medscape.com/article/462579-treatment

VASOPRESSIN: Antidiuretic hormone (**ADH**). Formed in the hypothalamus and released from the posterior pituitary. Acts on renal collecting system, increasing water permeability and decreasing urine formation. Acts on vascular smooth muscle, causing vasoconstriction.
http://www.cvphysiology.com/Blood%20Pressure/BP016

VEGETATIVE SYMPTOMS: Disturbances of functions necessary to maintain life: See: The Care of the Older Person: An Overview of Late-Life Depression: Artin Mahdanian, Silvia Monti De Flores. RMC Publishing, LLC 2018, 2019 www.careoftheolderperson.com
https://en.wikipedia.org/wiki/Vegetative_symptoms

VEGF: Vascular Endothelial Growth Factor. Angiogenic factor that promotes growth in vascular endothelial cells. Has a role in tumor angiogenesis.
http://www.nature.com/nrc/journal/v8/n8/full/nrc2403.html
http://perspectivesinmedicine.cshlp.org/content/2/10/a006577.full

VEIN: A blood vessel that carries blood from the body towards the heart, usually transporting carbon dioxide and waste products of metabolism. Exceptions include the pulmonary vein, which carries oxygenated blood from the lungs to the heart for redistribution throughout the body, and the umbilical vein in the fetus, which carries oxygenated blood from the placenta to the fetal heart for redistribution throughout the fetal body.

VILLUS: A tiny projection from a surface

VIRUS: An infecting agent so small that it cannot be seen under a light microscope. Viruses are made up of DNA or RNA. They can only replicate (divide) by invading into a host cell and causing that cell to manufacture more virus.
http://www.ncbi.nlm.nih.gov/books/NBK21523/

VITAL ORGAN: Organ necessary for life, including the heart, lungs, brain, kidneys and liver.

VITAMIN: A substance that in small amounts is essential to metabolism, that naturally occurs in food. The Care of the Older Person: Could My Patient Be Malnourished?: Jose Morais. RMC Publishing, LLC 2018, 2019 www.careoftheolderperson.com
http://annals.org/article.aspx?articleid=1767855

VULVA: The female external genitalia. Includes: labia majora, labia minora, clitoris, vestibule, urethral orifice, mons pubis.

WEST NILE VIRUS: A mosquito borne flavivirus that can cause encephalitis and meningitis.
http://www.cdc.gov/westnile/symptoms/

XENOBOT: Tiny robot constructed from living (frog} cells with the aid of Artificial Intelligence (AI)
https://www.smithsonianmag.com/innovation/scientists-assemble-frog-stem-cells-first-living-machines-180973947/

YAMANAKA FACTORS: Four genes that are important in cellular reprogramming to pluripotent stem cells.
https://www.ncbi.nlm.nih.gov/pubmed/19030024

ZIKA VIRUS: Mosquito borne. The fetuses of infected pregnant women have an increased incidence of microcephaly. There is an increased incidence of Guillain-Barre Syndrome with flaccid paralysis. Ref: Yale School of Medicine News, 08/26/2016
http://www.bloomberg.com/news/articles/2016-08-19/zika-may-cause-brain-damage-in-adults-too
http://www.contagionlive.com/news/zika-research-reveals-virus-may-negatively-impact-adult-neural-stem-cells?utm_source=Informz&utm_medium=Contagion+Live&utm_campaign=Contagion_Live_Trending_News_9-5-16
http://jamanetwork.com/journals/jama/fullarticle/2593701
https://www.mdlinx.com/obstetrics-gynecology/top-medical-news/article/2017/01/02/3?utm_source=in-house&utm_medium=message&utm_campaign=in-the-news-jan17

ZONA PELLUCIDA: The glycoprotein outer envelope of the ovum.
http://www.ncbi.nlm.nih.gov/pubmed/10497324

ZYGOTE: Fertilization (fusion of ovum and spermatozoon) results in a new cell: the zygote, which has forty six chromosomes including either an X or Y chromosome from the spermatozoon, and an X chromosome from the ovum. The zygote is therefore either XX (female) or XY (male). The zygote develops to a blastocyst stage with an inner cell mass that becomes the embryo, a fluid filled blastocyst cavity, and an outer ring of cells around the blastocyst cavity called the trophoblast, which becomes the placenta.
http://www.biology-online.org/dictionary/Zygote

BIBLIOGRAPHY & SUPPLEMENTAL BIBLIOGRAPHY

See www.rcaplanmd.com

ABOUT THE AUTHOR

Ronald M. Caplan MD, is an Obstetrician Gynecologist and medical author who has spent the greater part of his life studying and treating the medical conditions that impact humanity, and their relation to the evolving society in which we all live.

He did his medical and postgraduate training at McGill University, where his interest in renal disease in pregnancy and homotransplantation culminated in the first delivery of a baby from a mother who had received a deceased donor kidney transplant.

After serving on the Faculty of McGill University, he transferred to New York City, and a long career at the Joan and Sanford I. Weill Medical College of Cornell University, where he became one of the early proponents of minimally invasive surgery, and where he is now Clinical Associate Professor Emeritus of Obstetrics and Gynecology.

He is a Fellow of the American College of Surgeons, the American College of Obstetrics and Gynecology, and the Royal College of Surgeons (Canada).

He previously edited the textbooks Principles of Obstetrics, which was translated into both Spanish and Portuguese, and Advances in Obstetrics and Gynecology, which was translated into Spanish. He is now an editor of The Care of the Older Person, an e-textbook presently in its third edition. He authored another four mass market medical books in multiple editions. Prestigious medical and comprehensive libraries around the world hold copies of his work.

Medical Text Books and e-textbooks edited by Dr. Caplan:

The Care of the Older Person: First, Second and Third Editions: RMC Publishing, LLC 2018, 2019. www.careoftheolderperson.com

Principles of Obstetrics: Williams and Wilkins, Baltimore 1982

Portuguese Edition: 1986 Fundacao Calouste Gulbenkian, Lisboa

Spanish Edition: 1987 Editorial Limusa, S.A. Mexico

Advances in Obstetrics and Gynecology: Williams &Wilkins, Baltimore, 1978

Spanish Edition: 1982 Espax, S.A. Espana

Other books written by Dr. Caplan:

Your Pregnancy: (with Betty Rothbart) Quill William Morrow, 1992

The Doctor's Guide to Pregnancy after Thirty: Ivy Books (Ballantine) 1987, Macmillan 1986

Pregnant is Beautiful: Pocket Books (Simon & Schuster) 1985, Appleton 1981

Long Life: A Survival Strategy: Morgan James Publishing 2008

Made in the USA
Monee, IL
04 November 2026

67387508R00256